FERTILITY PRESERVATION

FERTILITY PRESERVATION

ADVANCES AND CONTROVERSIES

Editors

Mohamed A Bedaiwy MD PhD FACOG
Professor and Division Head
Reproductive Endocrinology and Infertility
Department of Obstetrics and Gynecology
Faculty of Medicine
University of British Columbia
Vancouver, BC, Canada

Botros RMB Rizk MD MA FRCOG FRCS HCLD FACOG FACS
Professor and Head
Reproductive Endocrinology and Infertility
Department of Obstetrics and Gynecology
University of South Alabama
Mobile, Alabama, USA

Foreword

Victor Gomel

JAYPEE

JAYPEE BROTHERS MEDICAL PUBLISHERS (P) LTD

New Delhi • London • Philadelphia • Panama

Jaypee Brothers Medical Publishers (P) Ltd

Headquarters

Jaypee Brothers Medical Publishers (P) Ltd
4838/24, Ansari Road, Daryaganj
New Delhi 110 002, India
Phone: +91-11-43574357
Fax: +91-11-43574314
Email: jaypee@jaypeebrothers.com

Overseas Offices

J.P. Medical Ltd
83, Victoria Street, London
SW1H 0HW (UK)
Phone: +44-2031708910
Fax: +02-03-0086180
Email: info@jpmedpub.com

Jaypee-Highlights Medical Publishers Inc
City of Knowledge, Bld. 237, Clayton
Panama City, Panama
Phone: + 507-301-0496
Fax: + 507-301-0499
Email: cservice@jphmedical.com

Jaypee Medical Inc
The Bourse
111 South Independence Mall East
Suite 835, Philadelphia, PA 19106, USA
Phone: + 267-519-9789
Email: joe.rusko@jaypeebrothers.com

Jaypee Brothers Medical Publishers (P) Ltd
17/1-B Babar Road, Block-B, Shaymali
Mohammadpur, Dhaka-1207
Bangladesh
Mobile: +08801912003485
Email: jaypeedhaka@gmail.com

Jaypee Brothers Medical Publishers (P) Ltd
Bhotahity, Kathmandu
Nepal
Phone: +977-9741283608
Email: kathmandu@jaypeebrothers.com

Website: www.jaypeebrothers.com
Website: www.jaypeedigital.com

Fertility Preservation: Advances and Controversies

First Edition: **2014**

ISBN 978-93-5090-986-7

Printed at Replika Press Pvt. Ltd.

Dedicated to

Our Parents, Families,
Mentors and Patients

CONTRIBUTORS

Alper Mumcu MD
Montreal Reproductive Center
Montreal, Quebec, Canada

Amanda N Kallen MD
Department of Obstetrics, Gynecology and Reproductive Sciences
Yale University School of Medicine
New Haven, CT, USA

Amjad Hossain PhD
Division of Reproductive Endocrinology and Infertility
Department of Obstetrics and Gynecology
University of Texas Medical Branch
Galveston, TX, USA

Ayman Al-Talib MD
Fellow, Reproductive Endocrinology and Infertility
Department of Obstetrics and Gynecology
McGill University
Montreal, Quebec, Canada

Ayse Seyhan MD
Fellow, McGill Reproductive Center
Department of Obstetrics and Gynecology
McGill University
Montreal, Quebec, Canada

Baris ATA MD MSc
Associate Professor
Division of Reproductive Endocrinology and Infertility
Department of Obstetrics and Gynecology
Uludağ University, School of Medicine
Görükle, Bursa, Republic of Turkey

Bonnie Patel MD
Department of Obstetrics and Gynecology
University Hospitals Case Medical Center
Case Western Reserve University
Cleveland, Ohio, USA

Botros RMB Rizk MD MA FRCOG FRCS HCLD FACOG FACS
Professor and Head
Reproductive Endocrinology and Infertility
Department of Obstetrics and Gynecology
University of South Alabama
Mobile, Alabama, USA

Candice P Holliday JD
Research Assistant
Division of Reproductive Endocrinology and Infertility
Department of Obstetrics and Gynecology
University of South Alabama
Mobile, Alabama, USA

Demeestere Isabelle MD PhD
Research Laboratory on Human Reproduction
Université Libre de Bruxelles
Erasme Hospital
Brussels, Belgium

Drisana Henry MS
Case Western Reserve University School of Medicine
Cleveland, Ohio, USA

Edmund S Sabanegh Jr MD
Professor and Chairman
Department of Urology
Cleveland Clinic
Cleveland, Ohio, USA

Edmund Y Ko MD
Assistant Professor
Department of Urology
Loma Linda University
Loma Linda, CA, USA

Elizabeth Ginsburg MD
Associate Professor
Department of Obstetrics, Gynecology and Reproductive Biology
Medical Director
In Vitro Fertilization Program I
Center for Infertility and Reproductive Surgery
Brigham and Women's Hospital and Harvard Medical School
Boston, Massachusetts, USA

Eman Elgindy MD
Professor
Department of Obstetrics and Gynecology
Zagazig University
Zagazig, Egypt

Englert Yvon MD
Research Laboratory on Human Reproduction
Université Libre de Bruxelles, Erasme Hospital
Brussels, Belgium

Faten F Abdelhafez MD
Lecturer
Department of Obstetrics and Gynecology
Assiut University School of Medicine
Assiut, Egypt

Hai Ying Chen MD MSc
Senior Embryologist
Montreal Reproductive Center
Montreal, Quebec, Canada

John Phelps III MD
Division of Reproductive Endocrinology and Infertility
Department of Obstetrics and Gynecology
University of Texas Medical Branch
Galveston, TX, USA

Kristine Zanotti MD
Department of Obstetrics and Gynecology
University Hospitals Case Medical Center
Case Western Reserve University
Cleveland, Ohio, USA

Lamiya Mohiyiddeen MD
Consultant
Department of Reproductive Medicine
St Mary's Hospital
Manchester, UK

Luciano G Nardo MD
Reproductive Medicine and Surgery Unit
GyneHealth
Manchester, UK

Mohamed A Bedaiwy MD PhD FACOG
Professor and Division Head
Reproductive Endocrinology and Infertility
Department of Obstetrics and Gynecology
Faculty of Medicine
University of British Columbia
Vancouver, BC, Canada

Nina Desai PhD
Cleveland Clinic Foundation
Cleveland, Ohio, USA

Pasquale Patrizio MD MBE
Department of Obstetrics, Gynecology and
Reproductive Sciences
Yale University School of Medicine
New Haven, CT, USA

Peter N Schlegel MD
Department of Urology
Weill Cornell Medical College
James Buchanan Brady Foundation
New York-Presbyterian Hospital
New York, USA

Rachel Pope MD
Department of Obstetrics and Gynecology
University Hospitals Case Medical Center
Case Western Reserve University
Cleveland, Ohio, USA

Seang Lin Tan MD MBBS FRCOG FRCSC FACOG
MMed (O&G) MBA
James Edmund Dodds Chair of
Obstetrics and Gynecology Professor
McGill University
Medical Director
Montreal Reproductive Center
Montreal, Quebec, Canada

Shaikat Hossain MSc
Division of Reproductive Endocrinology and Infertility
Department of Obstetrics and Gynecology
University of Texas Medical Branch
Galveston, TX, USA

Sherman J Silber MD
Infertility Center of St Louis
St Luke's Hospital
St Louis, MO, USA

Togas Tulandi MD MHCM
Professor and Academic Vice Chairman
Department of Obstetrics and Gynecology
Milton Leong Chair in Reproductive Medicine
McGill University
Montreal, Quebec, Canada

Wayland Hsiao MD
Assistant Professor
Department of Urology
Emory University
Georgia, Atlanta, USA

Wayne Lin MD MPH
Clinical Fellow
Center for Infertility and Reproductive Surgery, Brigham
Women's Hospital and Harvard Medical School, Boston
Massachusetts, USA

William W Hurd MD MSc MPH
Professor and Director
Division of Reproductive Endocrinology and Infertility
Department of Obstetrics and Gynecology
Duke University School of Medicine
Durham, NC, USA

FOREWORD

Fertility preservation has become an increasingly important issue for women in reproductive age. In turn, it has become an important aspect of reproductive medicine due to the recent advances in cancer treatment and innovations in assisted reproductive technologies.

Women diagnosed with cancers during their reproductive years, often, face the consequences of treatment-induced reproductive and endocrine impairment. Fertility impairment is a consequence of exposure to radical surgery, radiotherapy and chemotherapy. Over the past few decades, there has been a gradual improvement in cancer survival, which is quite significant. Furthermore, the focus has shifted from simply survival driven approach to maximizing the quality of life of cancer survivors. Preserving fertility and maintaining normal ovarian endocrine function are key components of the quality of life of cancer survivors in reproductive age group of women.

Further, in parallel, there has been a gradual and significant delay in childbearing for women in the past four decades, especially in industrialized countries, many of which have such low birth rates resulting in overall population decline. It is evident that fertility declines with increasing age due to decrease in oocyte quality. Many women wish to preserve their fertility until such time as they are ready to have a child. The data for all in vitro fertilization (IVF) clinics in the USA clearly indicates that the majority of the women treated (61.1%) were 35 years of age and more, and only 38.9% were under 35 years. Impairment of men reproductive functions occurs in a similar way consequential to cancer therapy in young age. In addition to fertility impairment, gonadal insufficiency causes many deleterious effects, and significant impairment in the quality of life. These are the most common indications for fertility preservation not related to cancer.

Physicians in various specialties, caring for such patients, will find this book valuable in addressing the different fertility preservation strategies for women and men alike.

The editors are physician scientists with extensive experience in fertility, and internationally known in their field. Dr Mohamed A Bedaiwy is Professor and Division Head of Reproductive Endocrinology and Infertility at the University of British Columbia, Vancouver, BC, Canada; and Dr Botros RMB Rizk is Professor and Head of Reproductive Endocrinology and Infertility at University of South Alabama, Mobile, Alabama, USA. Their goal was to produce a comprehensive, up-to-date book that presented the different medical and surgical strategies for fertility preservation for both women and men. They achieved their goal by recruiting for each chapter, internationally renowned authors for their expertise in the specific field.

The book is clinically oriented with a strong scientific basis; it even has a chapter on basic cryobiology. The book is concise, well-written with frequent use of pictures, tables and algorithms, and contains up-to-date and established references. It represents a current, comprehensive review of an important topic. It will serve as reference to trainees, practicing clinicians and scientists alike.

Victor Gomel MD FRCS
Professor Emeritus
Department of Obstetrics and Gynecology
Faculty of Medicine
University of British Columbia
Vancouver, BC, Canada

PREFACE

Few areas in medicine have witnessed significant progress such as fertility preservation in the last decade. In 2013, it is estimated that over 1,665,000 men and women will be afflicted with cancer. A significant proportion of these cancers will be during the reproductive age. The fertility impairment associated with cancer therapy can result in significant impairment of the quality of life. Recent advances in cancer therapy resulted in significant improvement in cancer-free survival. This was paralleled by increased number of reproductive age women requiring access to fertility preservation. With the recent advances in technology, cryopreservation of spermatozoa, oocytes and embryos become very successful. Moreover, the cryopreservation of testicular tissue and ovarian tissue added to the armamentarium of options that could be offered to these patients. In addition, there is an increasing hope that a pharmacological approach to prevent the chemotherapy-induced gonadal toxicity is within the reach. With this plethora of information comes the need to have a practically acceptable and readable guide to serve as a resource to healthcare providers.

This book is written with the primary goal of providing an up-to-date, concise, yet informative guide about fertility preservation options for both men and women. Throughout the chapters, the biological basis of the different treatment strategies is thoroughly discussed. To enhance the multidisciplinary approach to such a unique problem, the chapters are written by experts in their field. This book is divided into two major sections, sharing a similar approach to discuss the different fertility preservation strategies for both men and women. Also, an evidence-based approach is adopted to present relevant clinical recommendations about each strategy. The currently available laboratory techniques such as sperm cryopreservation, embryo cryopreservation and oocyte cryopreservation are discussed thoroughly as viable alternatives when indicated. Experimental approaches such as ovarian tissue cryopreservation are touched upon in the context of possibly becoming a viable option in the near future. The guidelines of the respected committees in the field are quoted and integrated in the respective chapters. To our readers, we put in your hands a book that we hope will assist you to provide cutting edge and evidence-based treatment to your patients.

Mohamed A Bedaiwy
Botros RMB Rizk

CONTENTS

SECTION 2
Fertility Preservation Strategies in the Male

Section 1

Fertility Preservation Approaches in the Female

1

Fertility Preservation in Female Patients: An Overview

Mohamed A Bedaiwy, Candice P Holliday, Botros RMB Rizk

CHAPTER OUTLINE

INTRODUCTION

Female fertility can be adversely influenced by cancer therapies that affect the ovary and uterus. At the ovarian level, pelvic irradiation and chemotherapy can decrease ovarian reserve and result in ovarian failure. Moreover, pelvic irradiation can adversely affect the uterus, increasing the subsequent risk of obstetrical complications such as intrauterine fetal growth restriction and preterm birth.[1] A number of potential options are currently available, however, to help preserve a woman's future fertility, thanks to a better understanding of the intricate mechanisms governing human reproduction. They are: [a] storage of frozen embryos, [b] storage of frozen ovarian tissue or the whole ovary for future transplantation, [c] storage of frozen ovarian tissue or isolated follicles for in vitro growth and maturation, [d] ovarian transposition before radiotherapy, [e] ovarian protection during chemotherapy with either GnRH analogs or antiapoptotic agents (e.g. sphingosine-1-phospate), [f] uterine transplant after successful cancer treatment where a functional uterus no longer exists and [g] in vitro fertilization (IVF) with embryo cryopreservation prior to cancer therapy.

Of those, only the last one—IVF followed by oocyte cryopreservation or embryo cryopreservation—is considered a clinically proven option for women requiring cancer treatment.[2] The remaining strategies are considered experimental largely due to unproven efficacy or lack of adequate long-term follow-up.

In this review, the consequences of irradiation and chemotherapy on ovarian function and fertility as well as current and future fertility preservation strategies in female cancer patients will be discussed.

EVOLUTION OF HUMAN OOGENESIS

By the end of the first trimester of pregnancy, the human ovaries are almost fully formed. By the seventh week of intrauterine life, primordial germ cells reach their final destination in the gonadal ridge after migrating from the yolk sac endoderm. They differentiate into oogonia and eventually into primary oocytes by mitosis. Before the twelfth week, some primary oocytes enter their first meiotic division, which becomes arrested in the dictyotene stage of prophase I. This process resumes with the first ovulation. Contrary to spermatogenesis, oogenesis in humans does not continue after birth. The maximum number of primary oocytes (6 to 7 million) is attained at 20 weeks of intrauterine life. That number falls dramatically to 400,000 at birth and approximately 200,000 at the time of puberty.[3,4] Oocyte reserve continues to diminish both in quantity and quality throughout the remaining life cycle.

A multitude of endocrine, paracrine, autocrine and intracrine factors govern the fate of each ovarian follicle.[5] During the menstrual cycle, follicles mature in a series of stages (primordial, primary, secondary and tertiary) in a process called folliculogenesis, which is independent of gonadotropin stimulation. The vast majority of follicles undergo atresia after differentiation into tertiary follicles with an antral cavity. During any ovarian cycle, one or two follicles mature to the preovulatory stage as a result of gonadotropin-induced folliculogenesis.[5] Throughout reproductive life, the main source of ovarian estrogens remains the mature Graafian follicle.[6] Many genes, hormones, proteins and factors are responsible for governing the intricate process of folliculogenesis in humans.[7-14] The dynamic nature of folliculogenesis makes it a principal target for the cytotoxic treatment.[15] Intrafollicular communication between the cells controls follicular dynamics; exposure to cancer therapy frequently results in the death of many neighboring cells too.[6,7,12,13]

Traditionally, it has been well-established that the germline cells (primordial follicles) are non-renewable. This concept was challenged by 2 recent reports stating that germline cells may be renewed locally[16] or from bone marrow stem cells.[17] However, these new and exciting findings were not reproduced by other groups and were challenged by the opinion of some other experts in the field.[18-20]

ANTICANCER THERAPY-INDUCED PREMATURE OVARIAN FAILURE (POF)

POF Induced by Chemotherapy

Premature ovarian failure (POF) occurs after exposure to many anticancer drugs. Chemotherapeutic agents can be mainly classified into alkylating agents (e.g. cyclophosphamide, mechlorethamine, etc.), antitumor antibiotics (e.g. bleomycin, adriamycin, etc.), plant alkaloids (e.g. taxanes, vinblastine, etc.), antimetabolites (e.g. 5-fluorouracil, methotrexate, etc.), topoisomerase inhibitors (e.g. etoposide phosphate, etc.) and others (e.g. cisplatin).[21] Fifty percent of women over the age of 25 and 25% of women under the age of 25, will develop POF after being treated with mechloroethamine, vincristine, procarbazine and prednisone.[22] Unfortunately, chemotherapy-induced ovariotoxicity is almost always an irreversible insult. After treatment with ovariotoxic drugs, the ovary exhibits a spectrum of histological changes ranging from decreased numbers of follicles to absent follicles to fibrosis.[23] The variable effects of different anticancer regimens on ovarian functions have been reported by many other investigators.[24,25]

The incidence of chemotherapy-induced POF cannot be precisely estimated because of the multifactorial nature of the insult. However, a number of factors can increase the risk:

- The cumulative dose
- The patient's age at the start of treatment. POF increases with advancing age owing to progressive age-dependent follicular depletion
- The degree of gonadotoxicity. This varies from one chemotherapeutic drug to another.

Cell cycle specificity of the chemotherapeutic agent is the major determinant for the magnitude of ovarian injury; cell cycle–nonspecific chemotherapeutic agents are more ovariotoxic than cell cycle–specific ones. Alkylating agents are the most gonadotoxic of all cell cycle–nonspecific anticancer drugs. Cyclophosphamide, a common treatment for breast cancer, is the most ovariotoxic of its group. Given the fact that breast cancer is the most common malignancy in women, most cases of chemotherapy-induced ovariotoxicity are induced by cyclophosphamide. Patient age and cumulative dose most strongly influence the POF rate in those taking this drug.[23] Less than 50% of women treated with cyclophosphamide, who are younger than 30 years old develop POF. On the other hand, approximately 60% of women between the ages of 30 and 40 years, will develop POF and hypergonadotropic amenorrhea.[23]

Consequently, the risk of POF is not the same in all patients receiving multiagent gonadotoxic chemotherapy. Women with the highest risk for developing POF are those who receive high-doses of alkylating agents with pelvic irradiation. In contrast, young women with Hodgkin's disease treated with multiagent chemotherapy and radiation to a field that does not include the ovaries will often remain fertile, although usually for a shorter period of time than that of age-matched controls.[26] In one case report, a young woman treated with repeated courses of ifosfamide combined with pelvic irradiation for Ewing's sarcoma of the pelvis who developed POF was able to achieve a spontaneous pregnancy.[27]

POF Induced by Radiotherapy

Among young women of reproductive age, radiotherapy is standard treatment for many genital as well as extragenital cancers, including cervical, vaginal and anorectal cancers, some germ cell tumors, Hodgkin's disease and central nervous system (CNS) tumors. Pelvic radiotherapy cannot only damage the ovaries, but also the uterus. The patient's age, total dose of radiation reaching the ovaries and the number of sessions needed to deliver the total dose are the prominent factors that determine both the extent and duration of ovarian damage. This is quite similar to the impact of chemotherapy.

Fractionating the total dose of radiotherapy significantly reduces the extent of ovarian damage.[28] Single-dose radiation is more toxic than fractionated therapy. The approximate threshold for radiation-induced ovarian failure is 300cGy to the ovaries; only 11% to 13% of women developed POF at doses below 300cGy versus 60% to 63% at doses above that threshold.[29] Standard pelvic irradiation to the ovaries will consistently result in POF; this is compounded by co-administered chemotherapy.[30,31]

Ionizing radiation is particularly deleterious to ovarian follicles, resulting in radiation-induced DNA damage, ovarian atrophy and a significant depletion of ovarian follicles.[32] Oocytes exhibit a rapid onset of pyknosis, disruption of the nuclear envelope, chromosome condensation and cytoplasmic vacuolization. Within 4 to 8 weeks after exposure to radiation, serum levels of FSH and LH progressively rise while serum E2 levels fall.[32,33] Radiotherapy results in a dose-dependent reduction in the follicular pool.[33] Fifty percent of the oocyte population is destroyed by a radiation dose < 2 Gy (LDL50 < 2 Gy).[34]

CHEMOTHERAPY/RADIOTHERAPY-INDUCED POF: DIAGNOSIS AND PREDICTION

The diagnostic and prognostic implications of predicting POF in cancer patients cannot be overemphasized. Researchers are currently looking for a biomarker that can reliably predict chemotherapy- or radiotherapy-induced POF with satisfactory sensitivity and specificity. Among those potential markers are anti-Mullerian hormone (AMH), serum FSH, inhibin B and basal antral follicle counts (AFC).

AMH is produced by the granulosa cells of virtually all types of follicles, from the primary to early antral stages. Growing follicles progressively lose their ability to produce AMH, which is why peripheral AMH concentrations decrease during ovarian stimulation. Unlike all other hormonal biomarkers, which are dependent on the stage of follicular development, AMH is independent of FSH, LH and inhibin levels.

Serum FSH levels were elevated in cancer survivors with regular menstrual cycles, whereas AMH levels were lower than those of age-matched controls.[35] Despite the smaller ovarian volume in cancer patients, AFC were similar between cancer survivors and controls.[35] In pre-pubertal girls receiving anticancer chemotherapy, serum levels of inhibin B transiently decreased. Consequently, serum FSH, coupled with serum inhibin B, was proposed as a potential biomarker of the ovariotoxic effects of cancer chemotherapy in pre-pubertal girls.[36]

Basal AFC have been used extensively alone or with other markers to predict POF. An AFC < 5 is predictive of poor ovarian reserve.[37] Measurement of serum AMH levels could be a quantitative and possibly a qualitative biomarker of granulosa cell health and activity.[38] For pre-pubertal girls undergoing sterilizing cancer therapy, AMH may have promising prospects.

WHEN IS FERTILITY PRESERVATION INDICATED IN WOMEN?

Breast cancer is the most common malignancy seen during the reproductive years that requires an immediate fertility-preserving intervention. One of every 7 breast cancer patients is younger than 40 years old.[39, 40] Unfortunately, breast cancer in young women exhibits a high ductal infiltrating effect and most of these women are required to undergo highly gonadotoxic chemotherapy for treatment.[41] Another common malignancy seen in younger women that requires fertility-preserving intervention is cervical cancer. Of the 13,000 new cervical cancer cases diagnosed in the United States each year, 50% are estimated to occur in women younger than 35 years of age.[42] Moreover, owing to the peculiar anatomic location of the cervix, fertility preservation is even more challenging in those cases. Because it is usually difficult to estimate infertility risk, it is essential to perform conservative surgery when fertility preservation is offered.[43]

The indications of fertility preservation in women currently include ovariotoxic radiotherapy/chemotherapy for cancer as well as for the treatment of a multitude of nonmalignant conditions such as systemic lupus erythematosus, acute glomerulonephritis, and Behcet's disease. On the other hand, many other patients with extragenital cancers are candidates for fertility-preserving procedures, including those with hematopoietic cancers such as leukemias and lymphomas, musculoskeletal cancers such as Ewing's sarcoma and osteosarcoma, neuroblastomas and Wilms' tumor. Women receiving chemotherapy while undergoing bone marrow transplantation or umbilical cord stem-cell transplantation are potential candidates as well as patients with non-gynecologic cancers including lymphomas, sarcomas and colorectal carcinoma. Some of the salient indications of fertility preservation in women are summarized in **Table 1**.

STRATEGIES FOR FERTILITY PRESERVATION

A spectrum of potentially promising strategies has been assessed for fertility preservation. Although the currently available armamentarium encompasses an ever expanding list, most of those are more experimental than practical. Moreover, none have been tested in a prospective randomized controlled trial (RCT).

Pharmacologically-Based Protection

The theoretical rationale behind pharmacologically-based protection came from the intriguing observation that the pre-menarchal ovary is less sensitive to the effects of ovariotoxic agents. Consequently, researchers have studied pretreatment with a GnRH agonist, as well as many other medications that suppress the hypothalamic pituitary ovarian axis, in an endeavor to maintain the pre-pubertal ovarian quiescence during chemotherapy.[44,45] Meanwhile, a direct ovarian effect

TABLE 1 Situations necessitating fertility preservation in women

1. Nonmalignant conditions treated with ovariotoxic radiotherapy or chemotherapy:
   - A. Multi-system disorders:
     - Acute glomerulonephritis
     - Behcet's disease
     - Systemic lupus erythematosus (SLE)
   - B. Transplantation procedures:
     - Umbilical cord stem-cell transplantation (SCT)
     - Bone marrow transplantation (BMT)
2. Malignancies treated with ovariotoxic radiotherapy or chemotherapy:
   - A. Adult cancers:
     - 1. Gynecologic cancers:
       - Cancer of the cervix
       - Breast cancer
     - 2. Non-gynecologic cancers:
       - Sarcomas
       - Lymphomas
       - Colorectal cancer
   - B. Childhood malignancies:
     - 1. Hematopoietic cancers:
       - Lymphomas
       - Leukemias
   - 2. Musculoskeletal cancers:
     - Ewing's sarcoma
     - Osteosarcoma
   - 3. Other cancers:
     - Wilms' tumor
     - Neuroblastomas
3. Bilateral oophorectomy for benign ovarian tumors, endometriosis, or prophylaxis.

has also been postulated.[44,45] However, theory and practice do not always meet. The few observational studies addressing this issue have come to conflicting conclusions. Blumenfeld and colleagues reported a diminished frequency of POF in patients who received a GnRH agonist prior to chemotherapy in their analysis of all studies on GnRH agonist use.[46] Most of those studies, however, were limited by short follow-up period in the GnRH group and the retrospective nature of the control groups.[46] Other investigators[47,48] have come to similar conclusions. When Demeestere et al. (2012) studied triptorelin, a GnRH agonist, for its ability to prevent chemotherapy-induced ovarian failure in patients with lymphoma, 20% of patients in both the control and treatment groups experienced POF during a 1-year follow-up.[49] Another recent study of 281 patients suggested that triptorelin-induced temporary ovarian suppression during chemotherapy in premenopausal patients with early-stage breast cancer reduced the occurrence of chemotherapy-induced early menopause.[50] On the other hand, a prospective controlled study found that GnRH analogs were not effective in the prevention of POF.[51] That particular study, however, was limited by a small sample size.

Patients and oncologists strongly advocate GnRH use; oncologists are satisfied with starting cancer therapy without avoidable delays caused by standard protocols of assisted reproductive technologies (ART) and patients find it simple. Alternatively, counter-arguments downplaying the use of GnRH agonists are centered on the fact that FSH suppression will not protect the primordial follicles constituting the ovarian reserve. Combining a GnRH antagonist with a GnRH agonist, which would add the quick onset of action of a GnRH antagonist to the long-lasting effects of a GnRH agonist, is being considered.[52,53] Because prospective randomized studies with statistically accurate numbers of patients and sufficient follow-up are few and showed contradictory results, the evidence of efficacy of GnRH agonists and their protective mechanisms remains lacking and the debate will continue.[49, 54-57] Empirical use of other suppressive drugs such as combined oral contraceptives (COCs) or progestins has not been successful in preventing chemotherapy/radiotherapy-induced ovarian damage.

Transposition of the Ovaries (Oophoropexy)

Another possible fertility preservation option for women scheduled to undergo sterilizing ovariotoxic radiotherapy is surgery, in which the ovaries are moved away from the intended irradiation field. In fact, robotic-assisted ovarian transposition is available.[58] Ovarian transposition helps curtail ovarian radiation exposure in patients with low intestinal and genitourinary malignancies and in those with Hodgkin's disease receiving pelvic irradiation. The radiation dose to the ovaries is reduced to approximately 5% to 10% following transposition.[59] Given an initial dose of 4,500 cGy, the dose to each transposed ovary is 126 cGy for intracavitary radiation, 135–190 cGy for external radiation therapy and 230–310 cGy with para-aortic lymph node inclusion in irradiation.[60] Lateral transposition of the ovaries was shown to be more effective than medial transposition—with the latter, the ovaries are sutured posteriorly to the uterus and shielded during treatment.[61,62]

Lateral ovarian transposition can be performed during staging laparotomy for Hodgkin's disease (which is not customary nowadays) and during radical hysterectomy for cervical cancer.[63] Laparoscopic ovarian transposition could be considered a valuable option before starting radiotherapy. Moreover, immediate postoperative radiotherapy could be initiated, which could furthermore help prevent POF if the ovaries were to migrate back to the irradiation field.[31,64,65] Additionally, the same anesthetic can be used for laparoscopic ovarian transposition as that used to insert a brachytherapy device in cases of cervical or vaginal cancers treated by brachytherapy.[66] It can also be performed on an outpatient basis in patients with Hodgkin's disease, leading to a better cosmetic effect and earlier recovery with minimal cost and discomfort.

Following laparoscopic ovarian transposition, almost all women with Hodgkin's disease (stage I and stage II) treated with radiation alone or with minimal chemotherapy retain their ovarian function and fertility.[31] Laparoscopic ovarian transposition is not a complication-free procedure, however. POF is still a concern, and symptomatic ovarian cysts may develop as well. There are many potential causes of ovarian failure following ovarian transposition[67] and they are summarized in **Table 2**. Although, COCs can help suppress cyst formation, the underlying etiology remains largely obscure.[68]

Assisted Reproductive Technologies

In patients, who wish to proceed to fertility preservation, ART are probably the most commonly adopted policy, as seen in **Table 3**.

TABLE 2 Potential causes of ovarian failure following ovarian transposition before radiotherapy
A. Vascular insult:
1. Jeopardizing ovarian vessels
2. Radiation-mediated injury of the vascular pedicle
B. Anatomically-mediated mechanisms:
1. Transposed ovaries not moved far enough
2. Ovarian migration back to original position following use of absorbable sutures

Oocyte Cryopreservation

In unmarried women and those without a male partner, freezing mature or immature oocytes may be the only practical option. For oocyte cryopreservation, the present rate of pregnancy after thawing, IVF and intrauterine transfer is 57% per embryo.[69] A multitude of factors come into play to determine the efficacy of oocyte cryopreservation, given the complex structural nature of the ovary. In contrast to pre-implantation embryos, subcellular organelles in the oocytes are far more complex and perhaps more sensitive to thermal injury.[70, 71] Oocytes can be cryopreserved for years and still retain their reproductive potential. Moreover, the duration of oocyte cryopreservation does not seem to interfere with oocyte survival; a number of pregnancies have been reported several years after oocyte cryopreservation using liquid nitrogen.[72]

Based on the evidence available in 2008, the ASRM practice committee concluded that, although no longer considered an experimental, oocyte cryopreservation is associated with a limited number of established pregnancies and deliveries resulting from cryopreserved oocytes.[73] However, no increases in chromosomal abnormalities, birth defects, or developmental deficits were noted among offspring at that time. In 2012, the ASRM practice committee released an evaluation of mature oocyte cryopreservation and found that vitrification for oocyte cryopreservation significantly improved oocyte survival and pregnancy rates.[74] Further, it stated that there is a decent amount of evidence that the fertilization and pregnancy rates of vitrified/warmed oocytes as a part of IVF/intracytoplasmic sperm injection (ICSI) in young patients was similar to that of IVF/ICSI with fresh oocytes. The practice committee cautioned, however, that the data was not necessarily generalizable because of reporting bias, the use of only healthy, young oocyte donors and the specific cryopreservation protocols used.

Successful human oocyte cryopreservation has recently become a reality. In fact, human GV oocytes also can be successfully cryopreserved after undergoing in vitro maturation (IVM).[75] The human oocyte is one of the largest cells in the body measuring approximately 130μm and has a low surface area to volume ratio.[76] This makes the oocyte more prone to water retention and damage caused by ice crystals. Avoidance of chilling injury is the most important goal to improve survival rates. Cryoprotectants protect the cells by forming hydrogen bonds with water molecules, hence eliminating ice formation and limiting damage caused by high salt concentration.

From 1986, when the first pregnancy using frozen oocytes was achieved by Chen until 1997 when ICSI was first used to fertilize frozen/thawed oocytes,[77] there have only been a few live births from frozen oocytes.[76] By 2004, only 100 births were recorded from frozen oocytes.[78, 79] By 2012, more than 1000 babies have been born following oocyte cryopreservation.[76,80]

To maintain the long-term viability after storage, living cells must be brought into a state of suspended animation in which they remain for indefinite periods of time.[76] The temperature of liquid nitrogen (–196°C) appears to be adequate for these purposes. At these temperatures, water exists in only a solid state and no biologic reactions occur. Human oocytes are viable at 37°C and inactive at –196°C. Therefore, the lapse time of major danger occurs during the temperature decreasing and the rewarming phases.[76]

TABLE 3 Live births after fertility preservation techniques. Modified from Yasmin E and Davies MC. Pregnancy after fertility preservation. In: Jauniaux E and Rizk B (Eds), pregnancy after assisted reproductive technology. Cambridge University Press; New York. 2012; Chapter 11:pp. 124-36

Method	*Evidence*	*Live Births*
Embryo cryopreservation	Wennerholm et al., 2009	>350,000**
Oocyte cryopreservation	Troukoudes et al., 2011 Grynberg et al., 2011	>500
Ovarian tissue cryopreservation and regrafting	Donnez et al., 2004, 2011 Meirow et al., 2005 Anderson et al., 2008 Silber et al., 2008 Sanchez Serrano et al., 2010	15 reported
Ovarian transposition and oophoropexy	Bisharah and Tulandi, 2003 Kuohung et al., 2008 Terenziani et al., 2009	Not quantified
Ovarian suppression with GnRH	Badaiwy et al., 2009 Guiseppe et al., 2007 Nitzschki et al., 2010	Not quantified

**p=0.01

Conventional slow freezing methods are associated with relatively low success rates, although survival rates are acceptable. Slow freezing methods need low initial cryoprotectant levels, which are associated with lower toxicity. Concentration increases only when the cells decrease their metabolism. At the temperature of -6°C, introducing a seed-ice crystal may be induced. The temperature is then slowly decreased up to -196°C. During thawing, a rapid transitional temperature is preferred to prevent recrystallization of water.

During the last decade, vitrification has been introduced whereby water is prevented from forming ice due to the viscosity of the highly protective cryoprotectant cooled at an extremely rapid rate. The recent advances in vitrification methods have increased oocyte survival to over 80%. Recent studies suggest that vitrification is the most efficient means of oocyte cryopreservation.

Recently, Noyes et al. (2009) published data regarding verified live-born infants after oocyte cryopreservation between 1986 and 2008.[80] The authors included 609 live-born babies; 308 from slow freezing, 289 from vitrification and 12 from both methods. An additional 327 live births were documented[76] (**Table 4, 5**). The rate of birth anomalies that resulted was 1.3%, which is comparable to that in spontaneous pregnancies.[81]

Chian et al. (2008) reported the obstetric and perinatal outcomes of 200 infants born in 165 pregnancies from oocyte vitrification at McGill University in Montreal, Canada.[82] The multiple birth rate was 17% (26 twins and 2 triplets). The cesarean section rate was 37% in singleton pregnancies and 96% in multiple pregnancies, whereas the mean birth weight was 2920 +/-37g for singletons and 2231 +/-55g for multiples. The incidence of congenital malformations was 2.5% (two ventricular septal defects, one biliary atresia, one clubfoot and one skin

TABLE 4 Data from oocyte cryopreservation births "series reports". Modified from Porcu and Bazzocchi, pregnancy outcome after oocyte and embryo cryopreservation. In: Jauniaux E and Rizk B (eds), pregnancy after assisted reproductive technology. Cambridge University Press; New York. 2012; Chapter 10:pp.108-23.

Parameter	***Cryopreservation method***		
	Slow-freezing	***Vitrification***	***Both***
Number of embryo transfers	1974	834	19
Number of oocytes thawed/warmed	11.890	5435	271
Number of oocytes that survived	8056	4392	244
% oocyte survival	68 (range: 22–90)	81 (range:69–99)	90
% of 2-pronucleate fertilization	73 (range:50-86	79 (range:59–93	81
Number of live-born babies	282	285	12
Baby gender (gender information available for 168 slow freezing, 189 vitrification, and 12 for both methods)	99 female, 69 male	86 female, 103 male	8 female, 4 male
Birth defects	1 ventricular septal defect, 1 choanal atresia, 1 Rubinstein-Taybi syndrome	2 ventricular septal defects, 1 biliary atresia, 1 clubfoot, 1 skin hemangioma	None

TABLE 5 Obstetric and perinatal outcomes and incidence of congenital malformations in children conceived after oocyte vitrification. Reproduced with permission from: Porcu and Bazzocchi, pregnancy outcome after oocyte and embryo cryopreservation. In: Jauniaux E and Rizk B (Eds), pregnancy after assisted reproductive technology. Cambridge University Press; New York. 2012; Chapter 10:pp.108-23.

Characteristics	***All pregnancies (n=165)***	***Singleton pregnancies (n=137)***	***Multiple gestation (n=28)***
(Mean gestational age (weeks + days)	37 + 1	37 + 3	35 + 5
Number of deliveries at 34–37 weeks (%)	46 (30)	30 (22)	16 (57)
Number of deliveries at <34 weeks	10 (6)	6 (4)	4 (14)
	All newborns (n=200)	Singleton newborns (n=141)	Multiple gestation newborns (n=59)
Birth weight (g) (Mean +/–SEM)	2784 +/–37	2920 +/–37	2231+/–55
Number of LBW (%)	68 (34)	24 (17)	44 (74)
Number of VLBW (%)	4 (2)	1 (0.7)	3 (5)
Median Apgar score at 1 min	8	9	8
Median Apgar score at 5 min	10	10	10
Incidence of congenital anomalies			
Biliary atresia	1	0	1
Club foot	1	1	0

hemangioma). Wennerholm et al. (2009) published data on 148 children born from oocyte slow-freezing and 221 children born after vitrification of oocytes.[83]

The obstetric and perinatal data on the outcome of children born after oocyte vitrification is of primary importance. In the United States, a national 5 year prospective multi-center observational study (HOPE) has been registered and its reports are awaited with interest.[84]

Embryo Cryopreservation

In 2005, embryo cryopreservation was described by the ASRM as the only established evidence-based and clinically valuable fertility preservation option for women with a male partner. There are two basic techniques employed for cooling of embryos: controlled slow freezing and ultra rapid vitrification.[85] Embryo cryopreservation is presumably the most effective means of fertility preservation in women undergoing ovarian stimulation regimens for IVF and it offers them a satisfactory chance of success. The delivery rate per embryo transfer has been reported by the Society for Assisted Reproduction Technology (SART), using cryopreserved embryos, to be 31.8% for women less than 35 years of age.[86] Post-thaw embryo survival rates range between 35% and 90% and implantation rates range between 8% and 30%; cumulative pregnancy rates have been reported to be more than 60%.[87,88]

Consequently, embryo cryopreservation is considered the fertility preservation option with the best outcome. Moreover, long-term follow-up data on the outcome of children born from these procedures are reassuring and confirm that the procedure is safe. A number of limitations do, however, exist. First, it is unsuitable for pre-pubertal or adolescent females and for women without a partner. Second, ovarian stimulation protocols in IVF inevitably lead to extremely high estradiol levels, which may be dangerous for women with estrogen-sensitive tumors such as breast cancer. The typical time interval between breast cancer surgery and initiation of chemotherapy is six weeks. In lieu of the standard protocol, a short flare protocol is adopted, which usually requires less time to achieve follicle recruitment.[89] Conventional controlled ovarian hyperstimulation (COH) produces exceptionally high levels of estrogen, potentially affecting the overall prognosis.[90] Therefore, some centers offer unstimulated natural-cycle IVF, where a single oocyte is aspirated. Cancellation rates are, however, high and pregnancy rates very low (7.2% per cycle and 15.8% per embryo transfer).[91, 92]

The nonsteroidal antiestrogen tamoxifen[92] and the aromatase P450 inhibitor letrozole[93] were used as potential alternatives for ovulation induction in the breast cancer patient. Oktay and colleagues reported, in their prospective controlled study comparing tamoxifen to letrozole as ovarian stimulation agents in breast cancer patients, that when combined with low-dose FSH, both drugs had a better outcome than when tamoxifen was used alone.[93] Letrozole was preferred to tamoxifen because its use was accompanied with significantly lower peak serum estradiol levels, which is a potential asset for breast cancer patients.[93] They further compared the safety and success of ovarian stimulation with letrozole and tamoxifen in breast cancer patients undergoing IVF to cryopreserve their embryos for fertility preservation and reported similar cancer recurrence rates between those who underwent COH and those who did not.[94] Because there are various ethical and legal issues associated with embryo cryopreservation, it is encouraged that these patients be cared for using a multidisciplinary approach, including both psychological and legal counseling.[95]

Cryopreservation and Ovarian Tissue Transplantation

Ovarian tissue cryopreservation and transplantation have emerged as promising experimental fertility preservation procedures in women at risk of losing their reproductive capacity. Given the fact that ovarian tissue transplantation is an auto-transplantation rather than transplantation between two genetically distinct humans, immunosuppression is unnecessary. In contrast, long-term immunosuppression is required after transplantation of reproductive organs between genetically distinct humans. Cryopreservation of ovarian tissue is, therefore, an indispensible prerequisite to the potential auto-transplantation process, allowing preserved germ cells to be replaced after completion of the ovariotoxic cancer therapy. Owing to their smaller size and lack of follicular fluid, better survival is expected to occur with primordial follicles occupying the ovarian cortical strips.[96] Moreover, the advantage of ovarian tissue harvesting is that it can be immediately performed laparoscopically and avoids exposing estrogen sensitive tumors to the higher estrogen levels associated with ovarian stimulation.[97]

Animal models have provided invaluable information about transfer methods. Sheep ovaries, which resemble human ovaries, have been used as a model for ovarian tissue cryopreservation and transplantation by Gosden and colleagues.[98] Survival and endocrine activity of the follicular apparatus as well as pregnancy and delivery after transplantation of cryopreserved-thawed ovarian cortical strips have been successfully reported.[98,99]

Minimizing Ischemic Damage in Ovarian Tissue Transplantation

In some human ovarian transplants, where non-vascularized grafts were used, an initial ischemic insult was noted, which was postulated to be, at least in part, responsible for the limited lifespan of ovarian function. Therefore, it is vital to reduce the duration of ischemia and provide immediate revascularization of the grafts to prolong their longevity and help preserve their function for as long a duration as possible. Thus, the subject of graft longevity as affected by graft ischemia time or by cryopreservation damage is now the subject of intense study.[100]

To minimize ischemic damage of the grafts, Almodin and associates described a novel technique in which frozen-thawed fragments of one ovary were injected into the cortex of the remaining sterile ovary.[101] In that experimental trial, radiotherapy was administered to ewes to induce ovarian failure in one ovary while fragments of the other ovary were kept frozen. Consequently, injection of the thawed fragments of the frozen ovary inside the cortex of the remaining irradiated ovary was carried out adopting a "sowing" procedure, which did require suturing. Rams were used to impregnate the ewes 6 months after grafting. By this novel procedure, they documented that prevention of ischemic damage was successful via intracortical grafting of the germinative ovarian tissue.[101] Transplantation of ovarian tissue into angiogenic granulation tissue during the process of wound healing was improvised to help prevent the initial ischemic insult to oocytes. The duration of ischemia was reduced by 24 hours, thereby significantly increasing the healthy primordial follicular pool and the reperfused area of the transplanted grafts. Two days after transplantation, the graft became revascularized (functional blood vessels were seen) and functional integrity returned.[102]

INTRODUCTION OF VASCULAR GRAFTS IN ANIMAL MODELS

As a potential way of avoiding ischemic damage to the graft, vascularized grafts have been successfully developed. With these grafts, there is immediate revascularization of the grafted ovarian tissue. The principle of vascularized grafting was challenging in two distinctive perspectives, despite its theoretical plausibility. First, the whole ovary along with the vascular pedicle must be cryopreserved, which is technically challenging. Second, the graft is reattached using microvascular anastomosis, which is a time-consuming and skill-demanding procedure. Reproductive surgeons are, therefore, required to be skillful at microvascular anastomosis; experience can readily be obtained from vascular and plastic surgeons with their vast experience in microsurgery on small vessels.

The 'ischemia time' is defined as the duration of time in which the grafted ovarian tissue can withstand ischemia without resultant ischemic tissue damage. Large ovarian cortical strips were reported to withstand an ischemic insult for variable durations[103] without inducing significant histological or molecular changes.[104] Transplanting an intact fresh ovary together with its vascular pedicle using microvascular reanastomosis has been successfully performed. As with other tissue grafting procedures, if the vascular graft was technically feasible and successful, survival of the ovarian graft was assured.[105]

Preservation of ovarian function after grafting is all important. Restoration of ovarian function after transplantation of a cryopreserved intact sheep ovary with its vascular pedicle has been documented.[106] Consequently, transplantation of fresh as well as cryopreserved-thawed (C-T) intact ovaries to heterotopic sites was established as a relatively simple, easily accessible and technically feasible procedure with a short operative time.[106] Moreover, the intricate procedure of orthotopic auto-transplantation of an intact frozen-thawed ovary to the upper genital tract using conventional microvascular principles has also been documented in rats.[107]

A number of different techniques of auto-transplantation of an intact fresh or frozen-thawed ovary together with its vascular pedicle using microvascular anastomosis in animal models were recently published.[108] Special attention was directed towards identifying potential heterotopic locations containing adequate blood vessels that can be used to host and vascularize human ovarian grafts. Moving one step further, contralateral orthotopic auto-transplantation of cryopreserved whole ovaries with microanastomosis of the ovarian vascular pedicle has been successfully performed with very promising results, emphasizing the feasibility, practicality and reproducibility of that principle. Intriguingly, luteal function was demonstrated in 4 sheep and delivery of a healthy lamb less than 2 years after transplantation following spontaneous intercourse has recently been reported. Unfortunately, histological verification of ovarian tissue 18 to 19 months after transplantation has shown that the life span of the graft was short and the follicular survival rate in the grafted ovaries was only 1.7% to 7.6%.[109] Despite a functioning vascular anastomosis and fertility, the grafts still had limited survival that could only be maintained for a finite length of time. Apart from decreased graft longevity, the concept of whole organ cryopreservation became established as a promising new fertility preserving option. In the same context, recent models for cryopreservation of an intact uterus[110] as well as a whole rabbit ovary have been documented.[111]

THE USE OF VASCULARIZED GRAFTS IN HUMAN TRIALS

A number of human trials using cryopreserved auto-transplanted ovarian cortical strips have been carried out, based on previous successes with animal models using C-T ovarian cortical strips with reported follicular survival, preservation of endocrine function as well as restoration of fertility.[98,99] The process of in vitro production of follicles from the cultured ovarian cortical strips, either in isolated fragments of cortex or after tridimensional reconstruction in alginate-based artificial follicles, is still unproven in humans.[112,113]

Many techniques can be adopted to make use of the cryopreserved ovarian tissue: transplantation back into the host, IVM of primordial follicles and xenografting into a host animal. Considering the first principle, cryopreserved ovarian tissue may be transplanted back into the patient, with the obvious limitation of reintroducing cancer in malignancies known to preferentially involve the ovaries such as leukemias and possibly breast cancer. Ovarian tissue strips are removed from the women and kept frozen in small strips prior to chemotherapy using novel techniques. When pregnancy is desired, the ovarian tissue strips are transplanted back into the patient in an orthotopic or heterotopic site. Given the fact that such ovarian tissue grafts are avascular, any ischemic insult to the transplanted tissue would invariably result in irreversible loss of the whole growing follicle population together, with a significant number of primordial follicles.

Three different surgical techniques of transplanting ovarian cortical strips have been improvised by Oktay and associates.[114] Those are orthotopic transplantation into the pelvis and heterotopic transplantation into either the arm or abdominal wall. In one study, the orthotopic transplant stopped functioning nine months after transplantation.[114] In the heterotopic transplant, however, function was preserved and resulted in the generation of a four-cell stage embryo that was transferred without pregnancy occurring. Multiple ovarian stimulation cycles were undertaken before this one embryo was obtained.[115]

Worldwide, 12 patients delivered 17 babies in eight centers from frozen ovarian cortex tissue transplants[116] (**Tables 6 and 7**). Donnez et al. (2004) reported the first live birth after orthotopic transplantation of cryopreserved ovarian tissue.[117]

A 32-year-old woman from Belgium treated for Hodgkin's lymphoma was reportedly the first lady to give birth to a baby after successful orthotopic auto-transplantation of cryopreserved ovarian tissue obtained prior to the start of ovariotoxic chemotherapy.[117] Despite developing chemotherapy-induced POF, the re-implantation of her ovarian tissue was successful in resuming ovulatory activity five months later. She became pregnant 11 months after re-transplantation by natural fertilization and gave birth to a healthy baby seven years after ovarian tissue banking.

Another pregnancy was reported in a woman with non-Hodgkin's lymphoma in which a refined IVF stimulation protocol was used following orthotopic auto-transplantation of cryopreserved-thawed ovarian cortical strips.[118] Some critics were doubtful as to the exact site of origin of the oocytes that resulted in the two pregnancies in the abovementioned reports. The reason for such skepticism was based on reports of documented spontaneous pregnancies in women with POF after repeated courses of ovariotoxic radiotherapy and/or chemotherapy and the fact that the tissue transplanted to the native ovary does not rule out the chance of resumption of native ovarian activity.[27]

A recognized complication of ovarian tissue cryopreservation and transplantation is loss of a considerable part of the follicular apparatus during the initial post-transplantation ischemic insult, which can seriously limit its use. After transplantation, almost 70% of follicles are lost. Freezing is not the major cause of such follicular loss, though.[98,119,120] Therefore, ovarian tissue freezing has been recommended only for women under the age of 35.[114] Proposed sites of ovarian tissue transplantation with and without vascular anastomosis were reported previously by us and others.

HETEROLOGOUS OVARIAN TRANSPLANTATION

Silber et al. (2005, 2007) reported on the success of ovarian transplantation from a healthy fertile 24-year-old woman to her monozygotic twin sister, who had suffered from POF at the young age of 14.[121,122] Monozygotic twins with discordant ovarian function have provided the basis of this work. Via mini-laparotomy, ovarian cortical tissue was transplanted from the fertile sister to her sterile twin sister. Resumption of normal menstrual cyclicity was witnessed 3 months after transplantation, with a consequent drop of serum gonadotropin levels back to normal levels. During the second cycle, she conceived and the pregnancy progressed uneventfully until delivery of a healthy female baby at 38 weeks' gestation.[121] Such an outstanding success only helps to emphasize the concept of transplanting large segments of ovarian tissue between monozygotic twins without the need for immunosuppression.

Silber (2012) recently reported on ovarian cortex transplantation in a cohort of nine sets of twins discordant for POF in which ovarian cortical tissue was transplanted from the twin with normal ovarian function to the sister with POF[116] (**Table 6**). Similar to their previous reports, folliculogenesis, hormonal functions and menses were restored in all recipients. Five spontaneous pregnancies were documented in this cohort.[122,123] Donnez and associates[124] have recently reported on a successful ovarian allograft between two non-identical twins. Ovarian cortical tissue from the donor sister who had already been the donor of bone marrow for a transplant was used. The recipient had received chemotherapy, total body radiation and bone marrow transplantation. The recipient developed spontaneous cycles after receiving the transplant. Moreover, two oocytes and two embryos were obtained.[123,124] However, in most patients with an intact immune system, the potential for acute graft rejection and risks of long-term immunosuppressive complications in the mother, such as infection and obstetrical complications may seriously limit its use.[123] Following documented ovarian function in a small number of cases following both orthotopic and heterotopic transplantation of thawed ovarian cortical strips, the ASRM practice committee recommended that the procedures of ovarian tissue cryopreservation or transplantation are to be regarded as experimental and performed only under IRB surveillance.[73]

Del Priore et al. performed uterine extirpation during a multi-organ retrieval from a cadaver and demonstrated the technical feasibility in 8 donors.[125] A number of vascular pedicles were utilized including the ovarian, uterine, or internal iliac vessels. Serial histology sections throughout the period of cold ischemia, taken every 15 to 30 minutes, showed no significant change over 12 hours of cold ischemia. They concluded that the human uterus can be obtained from local organ donor networks using existing protocols.[125] Since a multitude of methodological

TABLE 6 Summary table of worldwide frozen ovarian cortex tissue transplant pregnancies. Modified from Silber SJ. Pregnancy after ovarian transplantation. In: Jauniaux E and Rizk B (Eds), pregnancy after assisted reproductive technology. Cambridge University Press; New York. 2012; Chapter 12;pp.137-47.

Case	*Diagnosis*	*Babies*	*Where*
1	Hodgkins	1	Donnez
2	Neuro Tumor	1	Donnez
3	Non-Hodgkins	1	Meirow
4	Hodgkins	1	Demeestere
5	Ewings	3	Andersen
6	Hodgkins	1	Andersen
7	POF	1	Silber
8	Hodgkins	2	Silber
9	Polyangiitis	1	Piver
10	Breast Cancer	2	Pellicer
11	Sickle Cell	1	Piver
12	Hodgkins	2	Revel
Totals: 12 patients		17 Babies	8 Centers
Fresh + Frozen		28 Babies	Silber-14 Babies

and technical difficulties are associated with this procedure, the technique of human uterus transplantation is more experimental than practical at this point.

IN VITRO MATURATION OF OOCYTES

The rationale behind IVM is the fact that primordial follicles obtained from the frozen-thawed ovarian cortical strips can be allowed to mature in vitro. However, this procedure is still under investigation and will only become available in the future. In severe combined immune deficiency mice (SCID), transplantation studies demonstrated follicular maturation and completion of meiosis I in preparation for ovulation and potential fertilization.[126] Concerns have been raised pertaining to technical problems and potential viral infection transmission. To avoid spreading malignant cells, ovarian tissue culture with in vitro follicle maturation can be performed. Isolated follicle culture from the primordial stage has been tried, given the fact that the primordial cells represent >90% of the total follicular pool and by virtue of their ability to withstand cryoinjury.[127] However, isolated primordial follicles do not mature properly in culture.[128] Originally described for patients with polycystic ovary syndrome (PCOS), IVM of antral follicles may have applications for cancer patients. Unfortunately, its implementation is still being studied. IVM of oocytes could be considered a fertility preservation strategy as well; it is a safe and effective treatment offered in some fertility centers for assisted reproduction. Potential advantages include avoidance of ovarian stimulation with expensive, and at times, dangerous, gonadotropins, side effects of the medications and risks such as ovarian hyperstimulation syndrome (OHSS).

Although primary candidates for IVM of oocytes have classically been PCOS patients with multiple antral follicles, the spectrum of IVM indications is expanding to include women with primarily poor-quality embryos in repeated cycles and poor responders to stimulation. Two new applications for IVM, especially in women with cancer who are undergoing ovariotoxic therapy, are oocyte donation and fertility preservation. It is combined with oocyte vitrification in younger women without partners needing this treatment for fertility preservation. Clinical pregnancy rates per cycle in women choosing IVM are related to their age; approximately 38% for infertility treatment up to the age of 30 and around 50% in recipients of IVM egg donation. Moreover, in a study evaluation the incidence of chromosomal abnormality (CA) in embryos from IVM and IVF cycles, IVM embryos were similar to IVF embryos (58.7% versus 57.4%, respectively).[129] For embryos derived from oocytes that matured 48 hours after collection, a higher CA rate was observed as compared with embryos derived from in-vivo matured oocytes and to embryos derived from oocytes that matured in the first 24 hours after collection.

The issue of clinical applicability and practical value of IVM as a fertility preservation strategy is still unsettled.[130,131] Xu et al. improvised a method using tissue engineering principles for the culture of immature ovarian follicles followed by fertilization of oocytes in vitro).[132] This methodology is a great step forward in the search for new fertility preservation options in female cancer patients. [132-134] An additional strategy of fertility preservation, which combines ovarian tissue cryobanking with retrieval of immature oocytes from excised ovarian tissue followed by IVM and vitrification, has recently been described. [135] Recently, the first healthy baby was delivered following retrieval of immature oocytes in a natural menstrual cycle, followed by IVM and cryopreservation of the oocytes by vitrification.[136] This provides proof-of-principle

TABLE 7: Summary table of the ovarian transplant results with the first nine fresh and three frozen ovary transplants. Modified from Silber SJ. Pregnancy after ovarian transplantation. In: Jauniaux E and Rizk B (Eds), pregnancy after assisted reproductive technology. Cambridge University Press; New York. 2012;Chapter 12;pp.137-47.

Patient	*Age*	*Preop FSH*	*Postop FSH*	*Initial postop menses intervals*	*Pregnancy*	*Babies delivered*	*Years of graft function*
1	24	75	7.1	2nd baby: FROZEN	3	2	4
2	38	96	5.2	93, 42, 24, 27, 25	3	3	>7
3	25	112	6.8	76, 23, 30, 26, 25, 26, 21, 24, 27, 34, 25, 27, 51, 30, 27, 26, 28, 19	1	2	>6
4	34	58	9.4	81, 22, 47, 26, 21, 20, 27, 26	2	1	4
5	40	60	6.8	86, 29, 38, 34, 28, 28, 31, 35, 24, 28, 33, 35, 30	0	0	4
6	26	101	7.5	64, 20, 39, 40, 32, 26, 29, 26, 26, 41	1	1	2
7	34	86	4.4	83, 22, 29, 29	3	2	>6
8	37	86	7.4	100, 17, 39, 29, 27, 22, 23, 20, 34, 25, 26, 29	1	1	>4
9	35	54	4.2	128, 42, 18, 25	1	0	2
10	31	78	3.4	FROZEN	1	1	2
11	33	85	8.6	FROZEN	1	1	>1

evidence that the novel fertility preservation strategy of immature oocyte retrieval, IVM, and vitrification of oocytes can lead to a successful pregnancy and healthy live birth.[136]

CONCLUSION

Most of the currently available strategies to preserve fertility in women are still experimental and do not guarantee subsequent fertility. The only established method in women is IVF with oocyte or embryo cryopreservation prior to cancer therapy. Other proposed strategies to preserve fertility in women with cancer include: [a] storage of frozen embryos, [b] storage of frozen ovarian tissue or the whole ovary for future transplantation, [c] storage of isolated follicles for in vitro growth and maturation and [d] ovarian transposition before radiotherapy. The effectiveness of ovarian protection during chemotherapy with GnRH analogs is yet to be shown.

REFERENCES

1. Signorello LB, Cohen SS, Bosetti C, Stovall M, Kasper CE, Weathers RE, et al. Female survivors of childhood cancer: preterm birth and low birth weight among their children. J Natl Cancer Inst. 2006;98(20):1453-61.
2. Ethics Committee of the American Society for Reproductive Medicine. Fertility preservation and reproduction in cancer patients. Fertil Steril. 2005;83(6):1622-8.
3. Block E. A quantitative morphological investigation of the follicular system in newborn female infants. Acta Anat (Basel). 1953;17(3):201-6.
4. Forabosco A, Sforza C, De Pol A, Vizzotto L, Marzona L, FerrarioVF. Morphometric study of the human neonatal ovary. Anat Rec. 1991;231(2):201-8.
5. Gougeon A. Regulation of ovarian follicular development in primates: facts and hypotheses. Endocr Rev. 1996;17(2):121-55.
6. Fauser BC, Van Heusden AM. Manipulation of human ovarian function: physiological concepts and clinical consequences. Endocr Rev. 1997;18(1):71-106.
7. Wandji SA, Srsen V, Voss AK, Eppig JJ, Fortune JE. Initiation in vitro of growth of bovine primordial follicles. Biol Reprod. 1996;55(5):942-8.
8. Oktay K, Briggs D, Gosden RG. Ontogeny of follicle-stimulating hormone receptor gene expression in isolated human ovarian follicles. J Clin Endocrinol Metab. 1997;82(11):3748-51.
9. Ahmed CE, Dees WL, Ojeda SR. The immature rat ovary is innervated by vasoactive intestinal peptide (VIP)-containing fibers and responds to VIP with steroid secretion. Endocrinology. 1986;118(4):1682-9.
10. Ezoe K, Holmes SA, Ho L, et al. Novel mutations and deletions of the KIT (steel factor receptor) gene in human piebaldism. Am J Hum Genet. 1995;56(1):58-66.
11. Elvin JA, Clark AT, Wang P, Wolfman NM, Matzuk MM. Paracrine actions of growth differentiation factor-9 in the mammalian ovary. Mol Endocrinol. 1999;13(6):1035-48.
12. Dong J, Albertini DF, Nishimori K, Kumar TR, Lu N, Matzuk MM. Growth differentiation factor-9 is required during early ovarian folliculogenesis. Nature. 1996;383(6600):531-5.
13. Elvin JA, Yan C, Wang P, Nishimori K, Matzuk MM. Molecular characterization of the follicle defects in the growth differentiation factor 9-deficient ovary. Mol Endocrinol. 1999;13(6):1018-34.
14. Dube JL, Wang P, Elvin J, Lyons KM, Celeste AJ, Matzuk MM. The bone morphogenetic protein 15 gene is X-linked and expressed in oocytes. Mol Endocrinol. 1998;12(12):1809-17.
15. Anderson R, Wallace W. Fertility preservation in girls and young women. Clin Endocrinol. 2011;75(4): 409-19.
16. Johnson J, Canning J, Kaneko T, Pru JK, Tilly JL. Germline stem cells and follicular renewal in the postnatal mammalian ovary. Nature. 2004;428(6979):145-50.
17. Johnson J, Bagley J, Skaznik-Wikiel M, et al. Oocyte generation in adult mammalian ovaries by putative germ cells in bone marrow and peripheral blood. Cell. 2005;122(2):303-15.
18. Gosden RG. Germline stem cells in the postnatal ovary: is the ovary more like a testis? Hum Reprod Update. 2004;10(3):193-5.
19. Telfer EE. Germline stem cells in the postnatal mammalian ovary: a phenomenon of prosimian primates and mice? Reprod Biol Endocrinol. 2004;2:24.
20. Telfer EE, Gosden RG, Byskov AG, et al. On regenerating the ovary and generating controversy. Cell. 2005;122(6):821-2.
21. Chen H, Li J, Cui T, Hu L. Adjuvant gonadotropin-releasing hormone analogues for the prevention of chemotherapy induced premature ovarian failure in premenopausal women (Review). Cochrane Database Systematic Reviews. 2011, Issue 11. Art. No.: CD008018.
22. Blumenfeld Z. Chemotherapy and fertility. Best Pract Res Clin Obstet Gynaecol. 2012;26:379-90.
23. Manger K, Wildt L, Kalden JR, Manger B. Prevention of gonadal toxicity and preservation of gonadal function and fertility in young women with systemic lupus erythematosus treated by cyclophosphamide: the PREGO-Study. Autoimmun Rev. 2006;5(4):269-72.
24. Schilsky RL, Sherins RJ, Hubbard SM, Wesley MN, Young RC, DeVita VT. Long-term follow up of ovarian function in women treated with MOPP chemotherapy for Hodgkin's disease. Am J Med. 1981;71(4):552-6.
25. Blumenfeld Z, Avivi I, Linn S, Epelbaum R, Ben-Shahar M, Haim N. Prevention of irreversible chemotherapy-induced ovarian damage in young women with lymphoma by a gonadotropin-releasing hormone agonist in parallel to chemotherapy. Hum Reprod. 1996;11(8):1620-6.
26. BFS. MWGcbt. A strategy for fertility services for survivors of childhood cancer. Hum Fertil. 2003;6:A1-40.
27. Bath LE, Tydeman G, Critchley HO, Anderson RA, Baird DT, Wallace WH. Spontaneous conception in a young woman who had ovarian cortical tissue cryopreserved before chemotherapy and radiotherapy for a Ewing's sarcoma of the pelvis: case report. Hum Reprod. 2004;19(11):2569-72.
28. Meirow D, Nugent D. The effects of radiotherapy and chemotherapy on female reproduction. Hum Reprod Update. 2001;7(6):535-43.
29. Husseinzadeh N, Nahhas WA, Velkley DE, Whitney CW, Mortel R. The preservation of ovarian function in young women undergoing pelvic radiation therapy. Gynecol Oncol. 1984;18(3):373-9.
30. Gaetini A, De Simone M, Urgesi A, et al. Lateral high abdominal ovariopexy: an original surgical technique for protection of the ovaries during curative radiotherapy for Hodgkin's disease. J Surg Oncol. 1988;39(1):22-8.
31. Williams RS, Littell RD, Mendenhall NP. Laparoscopic oophoropexy and ovarian function in the treatment of Hodgkin disease. Cancer. 1999;86(10):2138-42.
32. Meirow D, Schenker JG, Rosler A. Ovarian hyperstimulation syndrome with low oestradiol in non-classical 17 alpha-hydroxylase,17,20-lyase deficiency: what is the role of oestrogens? Hum Reprod. 1996;11(10):2119-21.

33. Gosden RG, Wade JC, Fraser HM, Sandow J, Faddy MJ. Impact of congenital or experimental hypogonadotrophism on the radiation sensitivity of the mouse ovary. Hum Reprod. 1997;12(11):2483-8.
34. Wallace WH, Thomson AB, Kelsey TW. The radiosensitivity of the human oocyte. Hum Reprod. 2003;18(1):117-21.
35. Bath LE, Wallace WH, Shaw MP, Fitzpatrick C, Anderson RA.. Depletion of ovarian reserve in young women after treatment for cancer in childhood: detection by anti-Mullerian hormone, inhibin B and ovarian ultrasound. Hum Reprod. 2003;18(11):2368-74.
36. Crofton PM, Thomson AB, Evans AE, et al. Is inhibin B a potential marker of gonadotoxicity in prepubertal children treated for cancer? Clin Endocrinol (Oxf). 2003;58(3):296-301.
37. Su HI, Chung K, Sammel MD, et al. Antral follicle count provides additive information to hormone measures for determining ovarian function in breast cancer survivors. Fertil Steril. 2011; 95:1857-59.
38. Feyereisen E, Mendez Lozano DH, Taieb J, Hesters L, Frydman R, Fanchin R. Anti-Mullerian hormone: clinical insights into a promising biomarker of ovarian follicular status. Reprod Biomed Online. 2006;12(6):695-703.
39. Weir HK, Thun MJ, Hankey BF, et al. Annual report to the nation on the status of cancer, 1975-2000, featuring the uses of surveillance data for cancer prevention and control. J Natl Cancer Inst. 2003;95(17):1276-99.
40. Jemal A, Murray T, Samuels A, Ghafoor A, Ward E, Thun MJ. Cancer statistics, 2003. CA Cancer J Clin. 2003;53(1):5-26.
41. Rodriguez-Wallberg KA, Oktay K. Options on fertility preservation in female cancer patients. Cancer Treat Rev. 2012;38(5):354-61.
42. Waggoner SE. Cervical cancer. Lancet. 2003;361:2217-25.
43. Wallace WH, Barr RD. Fertility preservation for girls and young women with cancer: what are the remaining challenges? Human Reprod Update. 2010;16(6):614-6.
44. Chiarelli AM, Marrett LD, Darlington G. Early menopause and infertility in females after treatment for childhood cancer diagnosed in 1964-1988 in Ontario, Canada. Am J Epidemiol. 1999;150(3):245-54.
45. Tangir J, Zelterman D, Ma W, Schwartz PE. Reproductive function after conservative surgery and chemotherapy for malignant germ cell tumors of the ovary. Obstet Gynecol. 2003;101(2):251-7.
46. Blumenfeld Z, Dann E, Avivi I, Epelbaum R, Rowe JM. Fertility after treatment for Hodgkin's disease. Ann Oncol. 2002;13(Suppl.1):138-47.
47. Pereyra Pacheco B, Mendez Ribas JM, Milone G, et al. Use of GnRH analogs for functional protection of the ovary and preservation of fertility during cancer treatment in adolescents: a preliminary report. Gynecol Oncol. 2001;81(3):391-7.
48. Fox KR BJ, Mik R, Moore HC. Prevention of chemotherapy associated amenorrhea (CRA) with leuprolide in young women with early stage breast cancer (Abstract). Proc Ann Soc Clin Oncol. 2001(20):25a.
49. Demeestere I, Brice P, Peccatori FA, et al. Gonadotropin-Releasing Hormone Agonist for the Prevention of Chemotherapy-Induced Ovarian Failure in Patients With Lymphoma: 1-Year Follow-Up of a Prospective Randomized Trial. J Clin Oncol. 2013;31(7):903-9.
50. Mastro D, Boni L, Michelotti L, et al. Effect of the gonadotropin-releasing hormone analogue triptorelin on the occurrence of chemotherapy-induced early menopause in premenopausal women with breast cancer: a randomized trial. JAMA. 2011;3:312-4.
51. Waxman JH, Ahmed R, Smith D, et al. Failure to preserve fertility in patients with Hodgkin's disease. Cancer Chemother Pharmacol. 1987;19(2):159-62.
52. Von Wolff M, Kämmerer U, Kollmann Z, et al. Combination of gonadotropin-releasing hormone (GnRH) agonists with GnRH antagonists before chemotherapy reduce but does not completely prevent a follicle-stimulating hormone flare-up. Fertil Steril. 2011;95:452-4.
53. Elgindy E, El-Haieg D, Khorshid O, et al. Gonadatropin Suppression to Prevent Chemotherapy-Induced Ovarian Damage. A Randomized Controlled Trial. Obstet Gynecol. 2013;121(1):78-86.
54. Del Mastro L, Boni L, Michelotti A, et al. Effect of the gonadotropin-releasing hormone analogue triptorelin on the occurrence of chemotherapy-induced early menopause in premenopausal women with breast cancer: a randomized trial. JAMA. 2011; 306: 269-76.
55. Gerber B, von Minckwitz G, Stehle H, et al. Effect of luteinizing hormone-releasing hormone agonist on ovarian function after modern adjuvant breast cancer chemotherapy: the GBG 37 ZORO study. J Clin Oncol. 2011; 29: 2334-41.
56. Behringer K, Wildt L, Mueller H, et al. No protection of the ovarian follicle pool with the use of GnRH-analogues or oral contraceptives in young women treated with escalated BEACOPP for advanced-stage Hodgkin lymphoma. Final results of a phase II trial from the German Hodgkin Study Group. Ann Oncol. 2010; 21: 2052-60.
57. Kim SS, Donnez J, Barri P, et al. Recommendations for fertility preservation in patients with lymphoma, leukemia, and breast cancer. J Assisted Reprod Genetics. 2012; 29: 465-8.
58. Al-Badawi I, Al-Aker M, Tulandi T. Robotic-Assisted Ovarian Transposition Before radiation. Sur Technol Int. 2010;19:141-3.
59. Howell SJ, Shalet SM. Fertility preservation and management of gonadal failure associated with lymphoma therapy. Curr Oncol Rep. 2002;4(5):443-52.
60. Covens AL, van der Putten HW, Fyles AW, et al. Laparoscopic ovarian transposition. Eur J Gynaecol Oncol. 1996;17(3):177-82.
61. Hadar H, Loven D, Herskovitz P, Bairey O, Yagoda A, Levavi H. An evaluation of lateral and medial transposition of the ovaries out of radiation fields. Cancer. 1994;74(2):774-9.
62. Howard FM. Laparoscopic lateral ovarian transposition before radiation treatment of Hodgkin disease. J Am Assoc Gynecol Laparosc. 1997;4(5):601-4
63. Anderson B, LaPolla J, Turner D, Chapman G, Buller R. Ovarian transposition in cervical cancer. Gynecol Oncol. 1993;49(2):206-14.
64. Treissman MJ, Miller D, McComb PF. Laparoscopic lateral ovarian transposition. Fertil Steril. 1996;65(6):1229-31.
65. Yarali H, Demirol A, Bukulmez O, Coskun F, Gurgan T. Laparoscopic high lateral transposition of both ovaries before pelvic irradiation. J Am Assoc Gynecol Laparosc. 2000;7(2):237-9.
66. Clough KB, Goffinet F, Labib A, et al. Laparoscopic unilateral ovarian transposition prior to irradiation: prospective study of 20 cases. Cancer. 1996;77(12):2638-45.
67. Feeney DD, Moore DH, Look KY, Stehman FB, Sutton GP. The fate of the ovaries after radical hysterectomy and ovarian transposition. Gynecol Oncol. 1995;56(1):3-7.
68. Chambers SK, Chambers JT, Holm C, Peschel RE, Schwartz PE. Sequelae of lateral ovarian transposition in unirradiated cervical cancer patients. Gynecol Oncol. 1990;39(2):155-9.
69. Grifo JA, Noyes N. Delivery rate using cryopreserved oocytes is comparable to conventional in vitro fertilization using fresh oocytes: potential fertility preservation for female cancer patients. Fertil Steril. 2010; 93(2): 391-6.
70. Magistrini M, Szollosi D. Effects of cold and of isopropyl-Nphenylcarbamate on the second meiotic spindle of mouse oocytes. Eur J Cell Biol. 1980;22(2):699-707.
71. Stachecki JJ, Cohen J, Willadsen S. Detrimental effects of sodium during mouse oocyte cryopreservation. Biol Reprod. 1998;59(2):395-400.
72. Porcu E, Fabbri R, Damiano G, Fratto R, Giunchi S, Venturoli S. Oocyte cryopreservation in oncological patients. Eur J Obstet Gynecol Reprod Biol. 2004;113 (Suppl. 1):S14-16.
73. Practice Committee of The American Society of Reproductive Medicine; Practice Committee of the Society for Assisted Reproductive Technology. Ovarian tissue and oocyte cryopreservation. Fertil Steril. 2008;90:S241-6.
74. Practice Committee of The American Society of Reproductive Medicine; Practice Committee of the Society for Assisted

Reproductive Technology. Mature oocyte cryopreservation: a guideline. Fertil Steril. 2013;99(1):37-43.
75. Chian RC, Gilbert L, Huang JY, et al. Live birth after vitrification of in vitro matured human oocytes. Fertil Steril. 2009; 91(2): 372-6.
76. Porcu E, Bazzocchi A. Pregnancy outcome after oocyte and embryo cryopreservation. In: Jauniaux ERM, Rizk B (Eds). Pregnancy after Assisted Reproductive Technology. Cambridge: Cambridge University Press. 2012;10:108-23.
77. Porcu E, Fabbri R, Seracchioli R, et al. Birth of a healthy female after intracytoplasmic sperm injection of cryopreserved human oocytes. Fertil Steril. 1997; 68:724-6.
78. Stachecki JJ, Cohen J. An overview of oocyte cryopreservation. Reprod Biomed Online. 2004;9:152-63.
79. Yasmin E, Davies M. Pregnancy after fertility preservation. In: Jauniaux ERM, Rizk B (Eds). Pregnancy after Assisted Reproductive Technology. Cambridge: Cambridge University Press. 2012;11:124-36.
80. Noyes N, Porcu E, Borini A. Over 900 oocyte cryopreservation babies born with no apparent increase in congenital anomalies. Reprod Biomed Online. 2009;18:769-76.
81. Porcu E, Fabbri R, Seracchioli R, et al. Obstetric, perinatal outcome and follow up of children conceived from cryopreserved oocytes. Fertil Steril. 2000;74:S48.
82. Chian RC, Huang JY, Tan SL, et al. Obstetric and perinatal outcome in 200 infants conceived from vitrified oocytes. Reprod Biomed Online. 2008;16:608-10.
83. Wennerholm UB, Söderström-Anttila V, Bergh C, et al. Children born after cryopreservation of embryos or oocytes: a systematic review of outcome data. Hum Reprod. 2009; 24:2158-72.
84. Ezcurra D, Rangnow J, Craig M, Schertz J. The Human Oocyte Preservation Experience (HOPE): a phase IV, prospective, multicenter, observational oocyte cryopreservation registry. Reprod Biol Endocrinol. 2009;7:53.
85. Ata B, Chian RC, Tan SL. Cryopreservation of oocytes and embryos for fertility preservation for female cancer patients. Best Pract Res Clin Obstet Gynaecol. 2010;24(1):101-12.
86. Assisted reproductive technology in the United States: 1998 results generated from the American Society for Reproductive Medicine/ Society for Assisted Reproductive Technology Registry. Fertil Steril. 2002;77(1):18-31.
87. Wang JX, Yap YY, Matthews CD. Frozen-thawed embryo transfer: influence of clinical factors on implantation rate and risk of multiple conception. Hum Reprod. 2001;16(11):2316-19.
88. Son WY, Yoon SH, Yoon HJ, Lee SM, Lim JH. Pregnancy outcome following transfer of human blastocysts vitrified on electron microscopy grids after induced collapse of the blastocoele. Hum Reprod. 2003;18(1):137-9.
89. Meniru GI, Craft I. In vitro fertilization and embryo cryopreservation prior to hysterectomy for cervical cancer. Int J Gynaecol Obstet. 1997;56(1):69-70.
90. Pena JE, Chang PL, Chan LK, Zeitoun K, Thornton MH2nd, Sauer MV. Supraphysiological estradiol levels do not affect oocyte and embryo quality in oocyte donation cycles. Hum Reprod. 2002;17(1):83-7.
91. Pelinck MJ, Hoek A, Simons AH, Heineman MJ. Efficacy of natural cycle IVF: a review of the literature. Hum Reprod Update. 2002;8(2):129-39.
92. Oktay K, Buyuk E, Davis O, Yermakova I, Veeck L, Rosenwaks Z. Fertility preservation in breast cancer patients: IVF and embryo cryopreservation after ovarian stimulation with tamoxifen. Hum Reprod. 2003;18(1):90-5.
93. Oktay K, Buyuk E, Akar Z, Rosenwaks N, Libertella N. Fertility preservation in breast cancer patients: a prospective controlled comparison of ovarian stimulation with tamoxifen and letrozole for embryo cryopreservation. Fertil Steril. 2004;82(2):s1(Abstract).
94. Oktay K. Further evidence on the safety and success of ovarian stimulation with letrozole and tamoxifen in breast cancer patients undergoing in vitro fertilization to cryopreserve their embryos for fertility preservation. J Clin Oncol. 2005;23(16):3858-9.
95. Seli E, Agarwal A Fertility Preservation. Emerging Technologies and Clinical applications. New York: Springer. 2012:424 pages.
96. Mazur P. The role of intracellular freezing in the death of cells cooled at supraoptimal rates. Cryobiology. 1977;14(3):251-72.
97. Telfer EE, McLaughlin M. In vitro development of ovarian follicles. Semin Reprod Med. 2011;29(1):15-23.
98. Gosden RG, Baird DT, Wade JC, Webb R. Restoration of fertility to oophorectomized sheep by ovarian autografts stored at -196 degrees C. Hum Reprod. 1994;9(4):597-603.
99. Baird DT, Webb R, Campbell BK, Harkness LM, Gosden RG. Long-term ovarian function in sheep after ovariectomy and transplantation of autografts stored at 196°C. Endocrinology. 1999;140(1):462-71.
100. Silber S, Kagawa N, Kuwayama M, Gosden R. Duration of fertility after fresh and frozen ovary transplantation. Fertil Steril. 2010;94(6):2191-6.
101. Almodin CG, Minguetti-Camara VC, Meister H, Ceschin AP, Kriger E, Ferreira JO. Recovery of natural fertility after grafting of cryopreserved germinative tissue in ewes subjected to radiotherapy. Fertil Steril. 2004;81(1):160-4.
102. Israely T, Nevo N, Harmelin A, Neeman M, Tsafriri A. Reducing ischaemic damage in rodent ovarian xenografts transplanted into granulation tissue. Hum Reprod. 2006;21(6):1368-79.
103. Jeremias E, Bedaiwy MA, Nelson D, Biscotti CV, Falcone T. Assessment of tissue injury in cryopreserved ovarian tissue. Fertil Steril. 2003;79(3):651-3.
104. Hussein MR, Bedaiwy MA, Falcone T. Analysis of apoptotic cell death, Bcl-2, and p53 protein expression in freshly fixed and cryopreserved ovarian tissue after exposure to warm ischemia. Fertil Steril. 2006;85 (Suppl. 1):1082-92.
105. Jeremias E, Bedaiwy MA, Gurunluoglu R, Biscotti CV, Siemionow M, Falcone T. Heterotopic autotransplantation of the ovary with microvascular anastomosis: a novel surgical technique. Fertil Steril. 2002;77(6):1278-82.
106. Bedaiwy MA, Jeremias E, Gurunluoglu R, et al. Restoration of ovarian function after autotransplantation of intact frozen-thawed sheep ovaries with microvascular anastomosis. Fertil Steril. 2003;79(3): 594-602.
107. Wang X, Chen H, Yin H, Kim SS, Lin Tan S, Gosden RG. Fertility after intact ovary transplantation. Nature. 2002;415(6870):385.
108. Bedaiwy MA, Falcone T. Harvesting and autotransplantation of vascularized ovarian grafts: approaches and techniques. RBM Online. 2007; 14(3):360-71.
109. Imhof M, Bergmeister H, Lipovac M, Rudas M, Hofstetter G, Huber J. Orthotopic microvascular reanastomosis of whole cryopreserved ovine ovaries resulting in pregnancy and live birth. Fertil Steril. 2006;85(Suppl. 1):1208-15.
110. Dittrich R, Maltaris T, Mueller A, et al. Successful uterus cryopreservation in an animal model. Horm Metab Res. 2006;38(3):141-5.
111. Chen CH, Chen SG, Wu GJ, Wang J, Yu CP, Liu JY. Autologous heterotopic transplantation of intact rabbit ovary after frozen banking at 196 degrees C. Fertil Steril. 2006;86(Suppl. 4):1059-66.
112. Johnson J, Patrizio P. Ovarian cryopreservation strategies and the fine control of ovarian follicle development in vitro. Annals New York Academy Sciences. 2011;1221:40-46.
113. Smitz J, Dolmans MM, Donnez J, et al. Current achievements and future research directions in ovarian tissue culture, in vitro follicle development and transplantation: Implications for fertility preservation. Human Reprod Update. 2010;16(4): 395-414.
114. Sonmezer M, Oktay K. Fertility preservation in female patients. Hum Reprod Update. 2004;10(3):251-66.
115. Oktay K, Buyuk E, Veeck L, et al. Embryo development after heterotopic transplantation of cryopreserved ovarian tissue. Lancet. 2004;363(9412):837-40.

116. Silber SJ. Pregnancy after ovarian transplantation. In: Jauniaux ERM, Rizk B (Eds). Pregnancy after Assisted Reproductive Technology. Cambridge: Cambridge University Press. 2012; 12: 137-48.
117. Donnez J, Dolmans MM, Demylle D, et al. Livebirth after orthotopic transplantation of cryopreserved ovarian tissue. Lancet. 2004;364(9443): 1405-10.
118. Meirow D, Levron J, Eldar-Geva T, et al. Pregnancy after transplantation of cryopreserved ovarian tissue in a patient with ovarian failure after chemotherapy. N Engl J Med. 2005;353(3):318-21.
119. Oktay K, Nugent D, Newton H, Salha O, Chatterjee P, Gosden RG. Isolation and characterization of primordial follicles from fresh and cryopreserved human ovarian tissue. Fertil Steril. 1997;67(3):481-6.
120. Aubard Y. Ovarian tissue graft: from animal experiment to practice in the human. Eur J Obstet Gynecol Reprod Biol. 1999;86(1):1-3.
121. a) Silber SJ, Lenahan KM, Levine DJ, et al. Ovarian transplantation between monozygotic twins discordant for premature ovarian failure. N Engl J Med. 2005;353(1):58-63.
b) Silber SJ, De Rosa M, Pineda J, et al. A series of monozygotic twins discordant for ovarian failure: ovary transplantation (cortical versus microvascular) and cryopreservation. Hum Reprod. 2008;23: 1531-37.
c) Silber SJ, Grudzinskas G, Gosden RG. Successful pregnancy after microsurgical transplantation of an intact ovary. N Eng J Med. 2008;359:2617-8.
122. Bedaiwy MA, Shahin AY, Falcone T. Reproductive organ transplantation: advances and controversies. Fertil Steril. 2008;90(6):2031-55.
123. Silber SJ, Gosden RG. Ovarian transplantation in a series of monozygotic twins discordant for ovarian failure. N Engl J Med. 2007;356:1382-4.
124. Donnez J, Dolmans MM, Pirard C, Langendonckt AV, Demylle D, Jadoul P, Squifflet J. Allograft of ovarian cortex between two genetically non-identical sisters: Case Report. Hum Reprod. 2007;22(10):2653-9.
125. Del Priore G, Stega J, Sieunarine K, Ungar L, Smith JR. Human uterus retrieval from a multi-organ donor. Obstet Gynecol. 2007;109(1): 101-4.
126. Gook DA, Edgar DH, Borg J, Archer J, Lutjen PJ, McBain JC. Oocyte maturation, follicle rupture and luteinization in human cryopreserved ovarian tissue following xenografting. Hum Reprod. 2003;18(9):1772-81.
127. Smitz JE, Cortvrindt RG. The earliest stages of folliculogenesis in vitro. Reproduction. 2002;123(2):185-202.
128. Abir R, Fisch B, Nitke S, Okon E, Raz A, Ben Rafael Z. Morphological study of fully and partially isolated early human follicles. Fertil Steril. 2001;75(1):141-6.
129. Zhang XY, Ata B, Son WY, et al. Chromosome abnormality rates in human embryos obtained from in-vitro maturation and IVF treatment cycles. Reprod Biomed Online. 2010;21:552-9.
130. Rao GD, Chian RC, Son WS, Gilbert L, Tan SL. Fertility preservation in women undergoing cancer treatment. Lancet. 2004;363(9423): 1829-30.
131. Rao GD, Tan SL. In vitro maturation of oocytes. Semin Reprod Med. 2005;23(3):242-7.
132. Xu M, Kreeger PK, Shea LD, Woodruff TK. Tissue-engineered follicles produce live, fertile offspring. Tissue Eng. 2006;12:2739-46.
133. Brännström M, Milenkovic M . Advances in fertility preservation for female cancer survivors. Nat Med. 2008;14:1182-4.
134. Kim SS. Fertility preservation in female cancer patients: current developments and future directions. Fertil Steril. 2006;85:1-11.
135. Huang JY, Tulandi T, Holzer H, Tan SL, Chian RC. Combining ovarian tissue cryobanking with retrieval of immature oocytes followed by in vitro maturation and vitrification: an additional strategy of fertility preservation. Fertil Steril. 2008;89:567-72.
136. Chian RC, Gilbert L, Huang JY, Demirtas E, Holzer H, Benjamin A, Buckett WM, Tulandi T, Tan SL. Live birth after vitrification of in vitro matured human oocytes. Fertil Steril. 2009;91:372-6.

Fertility Preservation in Cancer and Noncancer Patients

2

Demeestere Isabelle, Englert Yvon

CHAPTER OUTLINE

INTRODUCTION

During the last two decades, the rapid increase in the number of patients diagnosed with cancer, as well as, the growing number of successfully cured patients, highlights, the importance of managing the long-term side effects of cancer treatments. The risk of gonadal failure has become a major issue for both oncologists and young patients as it dramatically affects the quality of life.

Fertility is associated with happiness, family and it gives meaning to life. Depending on one's current phase of life, the inability to procreate is a source of distress and family disorder.[1] This is especially true for women. Balancing the importance of fertility, cancer is a life-threatening disease. It suddenly evokes the possibility of death. Patients are also worried about pain, the physical impact of the treatment and the socio-economic consequences of the disease. In addition to this life altering better phrase diagnosis, there are the risks of physical and emotional changes associated with gonadal failure, disturbance of sexual functioning and fear of loss of fertility. With this unfavorable psychological context, the risk of infertility is a major issue for young patients.[1] Many studies have addressed the importance of giving accurate information and offering adequate options to patients to preserve fertility.[1] By addressing the issue of fertility preservation, patients are encouraged to think about their future, which positively boosts their feelings towards the disease. While cancer is the major indication for fertility preservation, non-cancer patients, including those affected by autoimmune diseases, hemoglobinopathies, or genetic diseases, may also benefit from these techniques.

Whatever the indication, the risk of infertility must be anticipated at the time of diagnosis, before the initiation of the treatment. Indeed, if gonadal failure is only confirmed after patients have recovered from their cancer treatment and when they then attempt pregnancy, it is too late for medically assisted procreation techniques, leaving only egg donation or adoption as the remaining options.

Despite the strong recommendation for fertility preservation with many indications and the growing number of centers around the world offering this service, access to the information and/or to adapted fertility services is still limited. A recent review reported that 34% to 72% of cancer survivors recalled being counselled by a health provider about the impact of cancer treatments on fertility.[1] Not all health professionals have, however, specific knowledge, enough time and accurate access to fertility preservation techniques to advise patients in an efficient and supportive manner. For adult men, sperm banking is easily available, but is often introduced just as another part of the process. Many men express that they do not have information about the reality of infertility risk and about what they could expect in the future from their cryopreserved gametes. For women, methods of fertility preservation are more expensive, less well validated, more invasive and require more time. The management of this complex issue cannot be effective without specialized education and well-established organizations.

A consequence of the lack of information is that some patients may develop independent opinions. They may choose an inappropriate option to preserve their fertility, leading to a hostile relationship with the oncological team. In an extreme situation, patients may even refuse to start cancer treatment. Not all fertility preservation options are in the best interest of all patients; it is, the diagnosis however, essential that the patients understand and accept the diagnosis. On the contrary, they may wrongly assume that the oncological treatment will definitively render them infertile. These patients may become unexpectedly pregnant after treatment.

The challenge of a fertility preservation program is to provide information and counseling that is easily understood, which helps patients in their decision and offers the most efficient and accurate options according to individualized infertility risk, age and disease. Furthermore, the bioethical rules for each patient, according to his or her cultural or religious background, should also be taken into consideration during fertility preservation counseling.

WHO IS A CANDIDATE FOR FERTILITY PRESERVATION?

Cancer Patients

In the United Kingdom, approximately 1 in 10 of all cancers occur in adults aged 15 to 49 years (Cancer Research UK statistics, http://info.cancerresearchuk.org/) and 1 out of 715 adults today is a survivor of childhood cancer.[2] Major improvements in the treatment and the diagnosis of cancer result in a marked increase in the survival rate, particularly for children. As a result of advances in treatment, almost 80% of children and adolescents who receive a diagnosis of cancer become long-term survivors.[2] For a large majority of these patients or their parents, preservation of fertility is an important issue.

Both radiotherapy and chemotherapy, including alkylating agents, deplete the ovarian reserve and damage spermatogenic stem cells, leading to temporary or permanent gonadal failure. The incidence of subsequent permanent infertility depends on the age of the patient and the type, dose and duration of the treatment. Radiation that includes the gonads in the field or high-dose chemotherapy with bone-marrow transplantation as consolidation are considered the most gonadotoxic, inducing permanent infertility in more than 90% of patients. Less than 1% of patients conceived after stem cell transplantation.[3] In contrast, other oncological treatments such as vincristine or fluorouracil present a negligible risk of infertility.[4]

Giving an accurate estimate of the risk of gonadal damage constitutes an essential step in the management of cancer patients. It is, however, often difficult to evaluate, as other factors may influence the risk of infertility. Moreover, the treatment may change if the patient relapses after the first line therapy, modifying the initial estimation. Furthermore, the disease itself may affect gonadal function. It has been reported that more than 70% of patients with Hodgkin's lymphoma have impaired semen quality before any treatment, including 11% with azoospermia.[5] Spermatogenesis is also impaired in men with testicular cancer before orchiectomy.[6] In women, one study suggests that malignancy may also affect oocyte quality,[7] but this result is not supported by other studies.[8] After estimating the infertility risk, the decision for fertility preservation must be made rapidly as the oncologists usually have to start the cancer treatment without delay. The best option takes into consideration many factors such as the health status of the patient, the disease itself and other associated co-morbidities that may contraindicate some of the approaches (**Flow chart 1**).

Counseling for fertility preservation not only informs the patients about the infertility risk and the options available, but also addresses the particular concerns expressed by cancer patients regarding the impact of pregnancy on the disease outcome and the potential for birth defects among offspring conceived after mutagenic drug exposure. To date, none of the largest studies evaluating the incidence of cancers or malformations in the offspring of childhood cancer survivors, excluding hereditary disorders, revealed an increased risk compared to control populations. Sperm DNA damage remains, however, up to 24 months after the completion of the chemotherapy in men treated for Hodgkin's lymphoma or testicular cancer.[9] Because the potential negative consequences of this sperm abnormality on reproductive outcomes and on the offspring are still unknown, fertility preservation should be offered before the initiation of the therapy.

Other long-term side effects of chemotherapy may increase the risk of adverse obstetrical and perinatal outcomes, compromising the health of both mother and offspring. Higher-risk pregnant survivors who were treated with anthracycline or >30 Gy of mediastinal radiation should have their cardiac status monitored for peripartum cardiomyopathy. The risk, however, of peripartum anthracycline-induced clinical heart failure appears to be relatively low; in a cohort of 53 childhood cancer survivors, none of them developed this complication.[10] Recent studies also showed a higher risk of preterm delivery and low birth weight in the population of female cancer survivors compared with their siblings, but the perinatal mortality is not increased.[11]

The success of the fertility preservation for cancer patients relies on an efficient collaboration between oncologists and gynecologists from the fertility unit, who must be able to offer counseling and options on a very short delay. Each situation must be carefully analyzed, taking into consideration all of the factors that might affect the decision to proceed with fertility preservation before the initiation of treatment and subsequently, re-evaluating the plan depending on the evolution of the disease. Cancer patients represent the large majority of those counseled in the fertility preservation program and they rely on the well-integrated interaction of both departments.

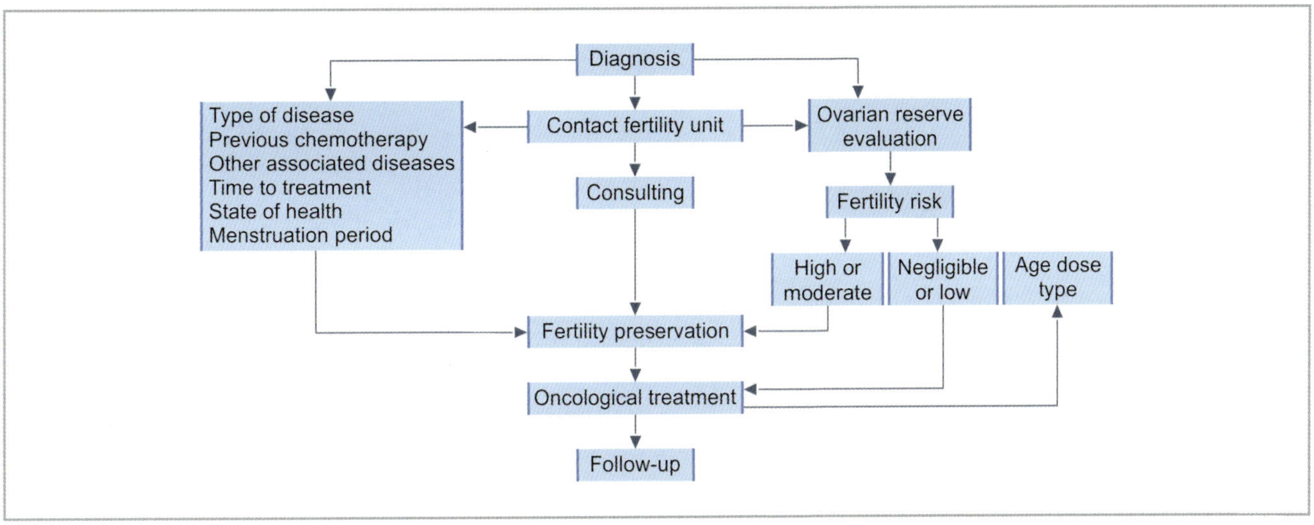

FLOW CHART 1 Counseling strategies for fertility preservation.

Table 1 summarizes the major indications for fertility preservation in both adults and children. All cancer patients requiring high risk infertility related therapy constitute an indication for fertility preservation. The limitations come, however, from patients with terminal disease or very poor prognosis, who present a complex situation that involves specific ethical issues.

Children and Teenagers

Forty-five percent of all cancers during childhood and early adolescence consist of leukemia or lymphoma.[12] Severe hematological malignancies represent 38% of the requests for fertility preservation in our cohort of 47 patients under the age of 19 years, due to the high risk of gonadal damage associated with bone marrow transplantation conditioning regimens or high dose alkylating agent based therapy (**Figure 1**). The therapy may also include irradiation, which is highly gonadotoxic, especially if the testes or pelvis are included in the field. In men, a radiation dose over 4Gy induces permanent gonadal damage.[13] This dose is largely surpassed in the case of testis infiltration by leukemia or when total body irradiation is needed. The somatic compartment of the testis is, however, more resistant and the production of testosterone by Leydig cells is usually not affected with a dose <20Gy. In women, a radiation dose of less than 2Gy has been estimated to destroy half of the ovarian reserve (LD50).[14] Furthermore, the effect of radiation on the uterus during childhood may also dramatically affect pregnancy outcomes.[15]

Advanced stage disease, such as stage IV soft-tissue sarcoma, pelvic rhabdomyosarcoma, metastatic Ewing's sarcoma, or osteosarcoma, which require combined intensive chemotherapy regimens or pelvic radiation, may induce premature ovarian failure in more than 80% of patients.[2] The Ewing family of tumors represents the second most common osseous malignancy in children and young adults. The 5-year overall survival rate reaches 75% for localized tumors, but may require multimodal therapies, including for some patients, sterilizing surgery. Though spontaneous pregnancies have been reported in female

TABLE 1 Major indications of fertility preservation for adults and children

Adults	*Children and teenagers*
Malignancies	Malignancies
Breast Cancer	**Hematologic malignancies**
Testicular cancer	Leukemia
Hematologic malignancies	Lymphoma (Hodgkin's and non-Hodgkin's)
Leukemia	Sarcoma
Lymphoma (Hodgkin's and non-Hodgkin's)	Pelvic osteosarcoma
Gynecologic malignancies	Ewing's sarcoma
Borderline tumors	Soft tissue sarcoma (pelvis)
Early stage cervical/vaginal cancer	Other solid tumors
Early stage endometrial cancer	Brain tumor (with cranial irradiation)
Other solid tumors	Neuroblastoma
Colo-rectal adenocarcinoma	Hepatoblastoma
Brain tumor	Wilms tumor
Neuroblastoma	
Sarcoma	
Melanoma	
Benign Diseases	*Benign diseases*
Gynecologic benign disorders	**Gynecologic benign disorders**
Endometriosis	Recurrent ovarian cyst (Dysgerminoma)
Recurrent ovarian cyst	Ovarian/testis torsion
Autoimmune Diseases	**Bone Marrow Transplantation:**
SLE	Drepanocytosis
Hashimoto's thyroiditis	Thalassemia
Churg-Strauss Syndrome	Aplastic/Fanconi Anaemia
Wegener granulomatosis	Juvenile SLE
Multiple sclerosis	Juvenile idiopathic arthritis
Behcet's disease	**Radiotherapy**
Pemphigus vulgaris	Benign bone tumor (sacrum)
Rheumatoid arthritis	**Genetic disorders**
Genetic disorders	Turner's Syndrome
BRCA1 mutation carries	Klinefelter's Syndrome
Family history of POF	Mucopolysaccharidosis (Hurler Syndrome)
	Osteopetrosis

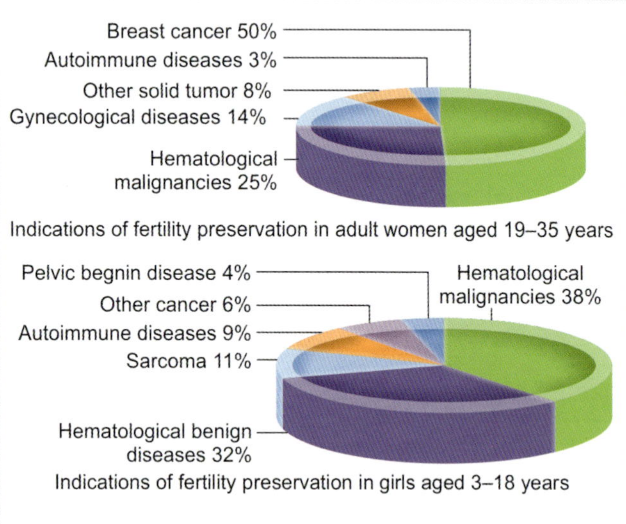

FIGURE 1 Indications of fertility preservation in a cohort of 193 patients who underwent ovarian tissue cryopreservation in Erasme Hospital (Brussels, Belgium) between 1999 and 2010.

survivors, they have a 35% less likelihood of becoming pregnant compared to their siblings.[16] Furthermore, among Ewing's sarcoma survivors, nearly 80% of these patients face at least one chronic health condition. Even if some may require particular obstetrical care, most osteosarcoma survivors have the capacity to bear children.[17] For all of these childhood malignancies with a high-risk of infertility, fertility preservation is thus highly recommended after an appropriate discussion with the patient's parents, who must give consent for their child.

For medium risk pathologies such as neuroblastoma, non-Hodgkin's lymphoma or acute myeloblastic leukemia (AML), it often remains difficult to predict each individual's risk of ovarian failure.[2] Advanced disease needs intensified regimens, which are associated with a poor recovery rate of gonadal function. AML is rare in children and only half of the patients are cured of their disease. That said, the cure rate for acute lymphoblastic leukemia (ALL) is >80%. The treatment usually includes intensive chemotherapy regimens based on cytarabin and anthracycline, frequently followed by stem cell transplantation (SCT). Most patients receiving chemotherapy alone preserve their fertility, while almost all of those patients treated with SCT face gonadal failure.[18] In cases of brain tumors or medulloblastoma, craniospinal irradiation itself does not compromise future testicular function, but adjuvant chemotherapy regimens including alkylating agents may induce permanent testicular dysfunction.[19] Ovarian damage, however, has been reported to occur in 64% of girls receiving craniospinal radiation for brain tumors with or without chemotherapy.[19] In female patients, localization of the ovaries before craniospinal irradiation should be performed to offer fertility preservation in cases in which the ovaries are included in the irradiation field.

Furthermore, the correlation between the age of the patient and the risk of ovarian failure has been clearly established. However, the restoration of ovarian function does not necessarily guarantee future fertility. The risk of premature ovarian failure increases by a factor of 27 among women between 21–25 years old treated for cancer during childhood. Forty-two percent of survivors of childhood and adolescent cancer who were still menstruating at the age of 21 face premature ovarian failure by the age of 31.[20] Because estimating infertility risk is often difficult, the most important consideration is to perform conservative surgery when fertility preservation is offered.[21]

Finally, many first-line chemotherapy regimens for common pediatric cancers, such as retinoblastoma, brain tumor (with cranial irradiation <24Gy), Wilm's tumor, or ALL, present a low risk of future infertility (<20%).[13] Fertility preservation is not systematically offered before the initiation of treatment in the low infertility risk groups, but could be proposed if more intensive therapy is required.

Fertility preservation is also recommended in cases of solid ovarian tumors. Germinal and stromal tumors, such as Stage IA dysgerminoma of the ovary, occur most commonly in young women and children. These tumors are usually managed with conservative surgery and have a 5-year survival rate over 95%. Fertility preservation may be offered in cases of bilaterality, high risk of disease relapse, or radiotherapy.

The particularly complex situation of childhood cancer emphasizes the importance of appropriate counselling with parents. A recent study by Goodwin et al. reveals that 64.3% of the pediatric health professionals reported difficulties accessing fertility centers.[22] In contrast, the majority of parents are clearly concerned about fertility-related side effects of the treatment and seek accurate information and options.

Adults

Breast cancer is the most common malignancy in women, with a life-time risk of developing breast cancer of 1 in 9 for women in the United Kingdom. Breast cancer accounts for nearly half of all cancers diagnosed in women aged 25–49 years (Cancer Research UK, 2010, http://info.cancerresearchuk.org/). Most young patients receive adjuvant therapy. After classical therapy of cyclophosphamide, methotrexate and 5-fluorouracil (CMF) or cyclophosphamide, epirubicin and 5-fluorouracil (CEF) regimens, 30–50% of premenopausal women <40-years-old will face premature ovarian failure after one year of follow-up. However, around 95% of the patients less than 35-years-old recovered menstrual cycles regardless of the chemotherapy type.[23] Unfortunately, many studies evaluated menstruation recovery rate and may have underestimated the real infertility risk. In a study reported by Schmidt et al., 5 out of 8 women with breast cancer who were treated with CMF or CEF had undetectable inhibin B levels despite reporting menstrual periods.[24]

The disease by itself has profound medical and psychological impact on treatment-related infertility. Breast cancer is a source of great distress in young women who fear losing their femininity. This issue contributes to an increase in the importance of fertility preservation in these young patients. Breast cancer has become the major indication in adult women, reaching nearly 50% of the requests in our institution (**Figure 2**). On the other hand, many concerns about safety and pregnancy outcomes after breast cancer represent additional sources of anxiety for patients. Recurrent questions involve the risk of disease relapse associated with pregnancy and the genetic risks for the baby. To date, all retrospective studies are reassuring and even suggest a "healthy mother effect," as women who are able to have a pregnancy are less likely to develop a recurrence.[25] The common recommendation for patients treated for breast cancer is to wait for 2 to 5 years before attempting conception. This delay, suggested as a guide and not based on strong clinical evidence, allows the completion of the therapy and prevents pregnancy in women who may relapse early and have a poor prognosis. For 90% of women having localized and good prognosis disease, conception six months after treatment is unlikely to reduce survival.[26]

Patients also seek information about the genetic risk for their offspring. Mutation of the *BRCA1* or *BRCA2* genes is associated with a high susceptibility of developing breast or ovarian cancer. While the carrier incidence is low in the general population (0.1%), it is much higher in the group of women with breast cancer being counseled for fertility preservation. Thirteen to 30 percent of these young women are positive for one of the two mutations.[27,28] At the time of fertility preservation, however, genetic testing is usually not available and is not part of the decision.

In men, testicular cancer reaches a peak between ages 30–39, with an incidence of 15 per 100,000. While it is the most common cancer in men between ages 15 and 45, it is also the more curable, with a 5-year disease survival rate over 96%.[29] Classical therapy combines surgery with cisplatin-based chemotherapy and radiotherapy. Transient high-grade oligo-azoospermia and hormonal dysfunction is usually observed after the treatment, with gradual recovery for 50–70% of patients, leading to a restoration of fertility for most men.[30] Approximately 70–80% of the testicular cancer survivors who attempt to conceive succeed.[31] Extensive surgery may, however, lead to "dry ejaculation" and severely compromised future fertility. Furthermore, testicular irradiation over 2 Gy frequently causes prolonged azoospermia.[32] The patients should be counseled before treatment and referred for sperm cryobanking, despite the usual low quality of semen at the time of diagnosis.

For both men and women, hematologic diseases constitute the second most frequent indication for fertility preservation. Patients with leukemia and lymphoma represent 25% of those seeking ovarian tissue cryopreservation in Erasme Hospital (**Figure 2**). As with children, spontaneous restoration of fertility is unlikely to occur in patients requiring conditioning treatment for SCT, though pregnancies have been reported after this treatment.[33] In both women and men with Hodgkin's lymphoma, chemotherapy regimens containing procarbazine as COPP, MOPP, MVPP, ChIVPP, ChIVPP/EVA, or BEACCOP lead to gonadal dysfunction in more than 80% of patients.[34] The incidence of gonadal failure is higher in high-stage Hodgkin's lymphoma than in non-Hodgkin's lymphoma patients, probably due to the procarbazine therapy and the adjuvant infradiaphragmatic irradiation. For early-stage Hodgkin's lymphoma, chemotherapy regimens, including ABVD (doxorubicin, bleomycin, vinblastin, dacarbazin), allow for the preservation of fertility in almost all young patients.[35]

Conservative surgery has become an established approach for preserving fertility in young women with early-stage gynecological cancer, such as endometrial adenocarcinoma, cervical or vaginal carcinoma and in some cases of unilateral ovarian cancer.[36] Fertility preservation may be proposed only when adjuvant therapy with local irradiation or alkylating agent based chemotherapy are required. Borderline ovarian tumor frequently affects young women. Management of this tumor has also changed from radical surgery to fertility-sparing therapy. Recurrence occurs, however, in 11% to 56% of patients treated with conservative surgery, but the survival remains excellent.[37,38] To avoid the risk of infertility related to a second surgery for disease relapse, a fragment of ovarian tissue from the remaining healthy ovary could be cryopreserved at the time of the oophorectomy.

Finally, any solid tumors such as colorectal carcinoma and brain cancer, treated with alkylant-based therapy or radiotherapy that includes the gonads in the irradiation field, constitutes an indication for fertility preservation counseling.

Noncancer Patients

Approximately 12% of the requests for fertility preservation in our institution originate from noncancer patients affected by immunological disease, benign hematological disorders, or solid tumors (**Figure 2**). Immunosuppressive therapy with cyclophosphamide remains a classic treatment for severe autoimmune diseases, such as systemic lupus erythematosis (SLE), Churg-Strauss Syndrome, Wegener's granulomatosis, Behcet's disease, inflammatory bowel disease or pemphigus vulgaris, in both adults and children. Juvenile SLE represents 15–20% of all the SLE cases reported. Even in the absence of gonadotoxic therapy, gonadal function may be impaired through organ specific involvement in autoimmune disease. More than 60% of female juvenile SLE patients reported abnormalities in their menstrual cycles.[39] Boumpas et al. analyzed the risk of amenorrhea in a cohort of 39 patients (mean age 27 years old) treated with cyclophosphamide for severe SLE. After a minimum of four years follow-up, 28% of the patients faced sustained amenorrhea.[40] More recently, permanent amenorrhea was described in 40% of patients treated with monthly pulsed cyclophosphamide.[41] Severe sperm abnormalities associated with Sertoli cell dysfunction have also been described in male SLE patients. Post-pubertal cyclophosphamide therapy is identified as the major factor in permanent damage to the testis.[42]

Fertility preservation is thus particularly recommended in both men and women affected by severe immunological diseases treated with immunosuppressive therapy.

Allogeneic SCT is curative in children and even adults with hematological disorders such as sickle cell disease, thalassemia, aplastic anemia or Fanconi anemia. Some rare, severe forms of inherited metabolic disease, such as mucopolysaccharidosis or congenital skeletal disorders like osteopetrosis, also require allogeneic SCT to improve survival and quality of life, particularly when performed early in the course of the disease.[43] Fertility preservation is crucial in these circumstances due to the high risk of gonadal damage. However, the potential pre-existent reduction of gonadal function related to long-term therapy, or to the disease itself, must be taken into consideration at the time of evaluation.

Fertility preservation has also been proposed for patients at high risk of premature ovarian failure due to genetic disease. Turner's Syndrome is one of the most common genetic diseases affecting 1 in 2000 girls. The patients usually face gonadal failure at puberty, but follicles have been described in the ovaries of Turner's Syndrome patients up to age 17, suggesting the possibility of fertility preservation.[44] Descriptions of spontaneous pregnancy in these women are limited to case reports and these patients usually require oocyte donation. Ovarian tissue or oocyte cryopreservation at an early age has been recently proposed to preserve their fertility. Genetic analysis of the oocytes provides reassurance of the efficacy of this approach, but must be confirmed in a larger population.[45]

Fertility preservation may also be offered in *BRCA1* mutation positive patients who wish to delay childbearing.[46] Recently, Oktay et al. reported a a response 38 times lower to ovarian stimulation of patients compared to controls, suggesting an occult primary ovarian insufficiency.[27] Furthermore, the cumulative lifetime risk of developing ovarian cancer is approximately 60%, justifying a prophylactic oophorectomy by age 35–40.

In men, fertility preservation has also been offered for patients with Klinefelter's Syndrome (KS). KS is the most common sex chromosomal disorder and it is characterized by hypogonadism and infertility. Although the great majority of children born by intracytoplasmic sperm injection from men with KS are chromosomally normal, the risk of producing offspring with chromosome aneuploidies is significant.[47]

Whatever the type of genetic disorder, the consequences and risks of future pregnancy for the mother and the child should always be discussed.

Finally, some benign ovarian diseases need repeated surgeries or may be progressive, leading to reduced ovarian reserve. Mature teratoma, the most frequently encountered ovarian cyst in pre-pubertal girls, may recur in 15% of cases, requiring repeat surgery. In the management of endometriosis, oophorectomy is occasionally needed in cases of both medical and conservative surgical failure. At the time of oophorectomy, part of the healthy ovarian cortex can be dissected and cryopreserved if recurrence of the disease is of concern. Ovarian torsion, even without an underlying cyst, may also occur with an increased risk of recurrence and irreversible necrosis.[12] Fertility preservation can also be proposed in these situations. In men, cryopreservation of sperm has been recently proposed in cases of testicular torsion with severe ischemic injury.[48]

Progressively, fertility preservation is becoming an option for a larger number of noncancer indications (**Table 1**). Social issues also evolve and proposing fertility preservation for women who have chosen to delay childbearing beyond age 35 for personal reasons may be acceptable in many clinics around the world.

OPTION TO PRESERVE FERTILITY

Women and Girls

Several options are now available to preserve fertility in women, and remarkable progress has been made in the last decade in this field (**Flow chart 2**). The decision to choose one or a combined procedure depends on several factors, including the previous

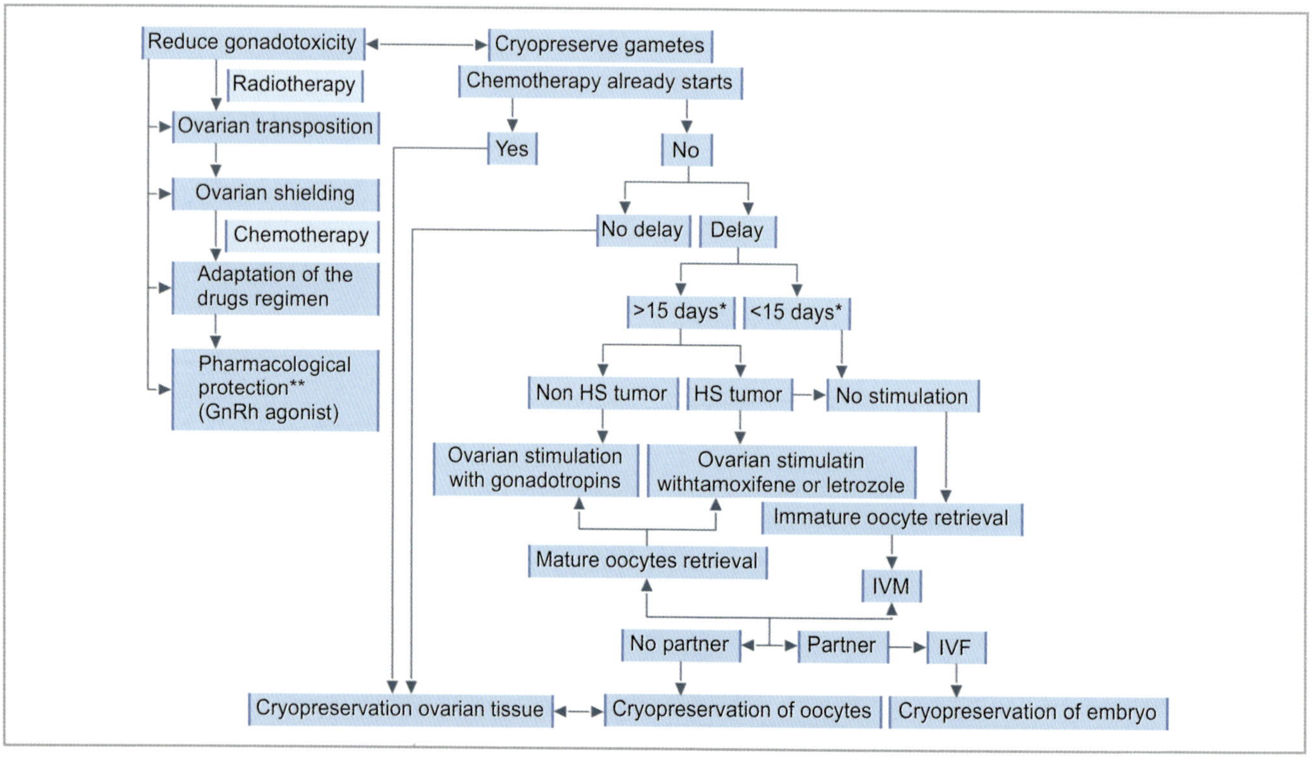

FLOW CHART 2 Strategies to preserve fertility of women.
*approximate evaluation, varied according to the menstrual cycle
** experimental option, long-term prospective randomized studies needed to confirm the efficiency
HS: hormone-sensitive

chemotherapy, the urgency to treat, the health status of the patient, the disease and the patient's age.

The best option is to reduce the gonadotoxicity of the oncological treatment with the intention of preserving ovarian function and future natural fertility. The introduction of non-alkylating therapy, such as ABVD, has substantially improved the fertility prognosis of young patients with early-stage Hodgkin's lymphoma.[49]

For early-stage gynecological cancer, surgical advances have led to more conservative therapy in women who desire preservation of fertility. This approach also includes ovarian transposition in the case of pelvic or craniospinal irradiation for both adults and girls. By moving the ovaries behind the uterus or laterally away from the field of radiation, ovarian function is preserved in more than 80% of cases.[50]

This effective procedure has been performed before radiation for Hodgkin's disease, cervical or rectal cancers, Ewing's sarcoma and medulloblastoma. The possibility of minimizing gonadal damage by the administration of protective therapy is another attractive option. Based on promising results from animal studies, concomitant administration of a gonadotropin-releasing hormone (GnRH) agonist during treatment with alkylating agents has also been tested. The efficacy of GnRH agonists to prevent chemotherapy-induced ovarian failure in humans has been debated for the past 15 years in the literature and the question is still unresolved.[51] Prospective randomized study, with statistically accurate numbers of patients and sufficient follow-up are limited and showed contradictory results.[52-55]

Evidence of the efficacy of GnRH agonists and of their protective mechanisms are therefore still lacking.[56] Large prospective randomized studies are ongoing and results of long-term follow-up should be available in the near future.[53] Recently, new experimental "fertoprotective adjuvant therapy" is being investigated in animals and it is a promising approach for using chemotherapy without harming the resting germ cell.[57]

The second option is to use cryopreserved oocytes or embryos in order to later restore fertility. An average of 15 mature oocytes can be harvested from young patients with cancer after pituitary down-regulation followed by ovarian stimulation with gonadotropins.[58] Embryo cryopreservation is an efficient and established procedure routinely performed in in vitro fertilization (IVF) clinics. The disadvantages of this technique in a fertility preservation program relate to the delay between evaluation and oocyte retrieval (2–3 weeks) and the need of a partner to fertilize the oocytes.

Over the last few years, progress in cryobiology has led to the development of a vitrification protocol for both embryos and oocytes. Vitrification results in survival rates as high as 89% to 100% and many successful live births worldwide. Vitrification of unfertilized oocytes has become an acceptable and equally viable alternative for preserving fertility in single women.

In the case of hormonally sensitive tumors, alternatives to the gonadotropin ovarian stimulation protocol can be proposed. Gonadotropin stimulation, inducing a 10 to 15 fold increase of the estradiol level, is typically avoided in patients with breast cancer, even though this is a precaution and not a clinical, evidence-based practice. New strategies for safe multi-follicular growth induction using tamoxifen or aromatase inhibitors have been successfully developed.[59]

Immature oocytes can also be retrieved without previous ovarian stimulation, followed by in vitro maturation (IVM) and vitrification. This last procedure has the advantage of shortening the time to oocyte retrieval and avoiding ovarian stimulation. In a recent study, on average, 7.9 oocytes per patient with breast cancer were vitrified after an unstimulated IVM cycle. The median duration from the first evaluation to oocyte retrieval was 13 days.[60] However, the implantation rate following this procedure remains significantly lower than after vitrification of in vivo matured oocytes.

Regardless of the protocol, cryopreservation of oocytes or embryos cannot be performed when the patient has already received chemotherapy. The efficacy of IVF procedures is dramatically reduced after a single chemotherapy regimen.[61] Potential DNA damage induced by cytotoxic agents on growing oocytes represents an additional concern, reinforcing the fact that this procedure should not be offered in this situation. Finally, cryopreservation of oocytes and embryos is not available for pre-pubertal patients.

Alternative strategies for preserving fertility include the cryopreservation of ovarian tissue.[62] Cryopreservation of ovarian tissue has the following advantages: (a) it allows the storage of a large number of primordial follicles; (b) it can be performed at any period of the menstrual cycle without delay; and (c) it is available for pre-pubertal patients. Ovarian tissue cryopreservation is considered experimental, although many studies have reported high survival rates after thawing. The challenge at present remains the restoration of ovarian function using frozen-thawed ovarian tissue. Options for restoring fertility include follicular *in vitro* culture and ovarian tissue transplantation. The development of *in vitro* culture systems supporting primordial follicular growth in humans will probably not be available for some years.

Transplantation of cryopreserved ovarian tissue has been recently performed successfully in humans.[63,64] Several women reported in the literature underwent cryopreserved ovarian tissue transplantation, leading to the restoration of spontaneous menstrual cycles for several months in almost all cases. Around the world, 20 healthy babies have been born following this procedure, either by spontaneous pregnancy or with the additional help of assisted reproduction technology. Ovarian stimulation for IVF lead to a very low number of oocytes collected (mean 1.3/cycle), giving an implantation rate around 5%.[65] Overall, success rate of the procedure in terms of pregnancies has been estimated to be 25% and some women even obtained successive pregnancies and births from the same graft.[66-68] A successful, large series of fresh tissue transplantation between monozygotic twins discordant for ovarian failure has also been reported.[63]

Despite these encouraging results, some important issues still limit the application of the procedure.[69] For cancer patients, the possible involvement of the ovarian cortex by the tumor cells at the time of diagnosis leads some patients to avoid transplantation because of high risks of disease relapse. Most of the malignant diseases diagnosed during childhood or the reproductive age have a low risk of ovarian involvement, with the exception of leukemia, neuroblastoma and Burkett's lymphoma.[70] Despite the high probability of avoiding transplantation in these patients, cryopreservation of ovarian tissue is still offered.

That said, alternative strategies are being investigated in many research centers and may be available for clinical application in the future when the patients wish to conceive. Combined procedures linking cryopreservation of ovarian tissue and oocyte vitrification after IVM could also optimize the efficiency of fertility preservation and offer an alternative to transplantation.[71] These patients, however, must be clearly informed about this issue during fertility preservation counselling. In Hodgkin's lymphoma patients, including those with stage IV disease, histological evaluation of the ovarian cortex was reassuring in confirming the safety of ovarian tissue transplantation for this indication.[72] In breast cancer, occult ovarian metastases are rare and mainly belong to the infiltrating lobular histological subtype. Transplantation of cryopreserved ovarian tissue is conceivable for almost all women treated for early-stage breast cancer.[59]

Although the concern for reintroducing cancer cells by ovarian transplantation is low for most patients, careful histological evaluation of an ovarian tissue sample should be systematically performed before transplantation for all cancer survivors. When available, high sensitivity methods to detect minimal residual disease by PCR reaction are indicated and should be developed, although the clinical significance of these tests must be further investigated.[72]

Surgical contraindications may compromise cryopreservation of ovarian tissue. Additionally, the procedure is sometimes postponed until after the first course of chemotherapy. In our series of 260 patients eligible for ovarian tissue cryopreservation in Erasme Hospital, only seven patients did not undergo the procedure for reasons of surgical contraindications. Other limitations are ovarian infiltration by the malignancy, the refusal of the patient, or poor prognosis.

Men and Boys

Differentiating spermatogonia proliferate rapidly and are the first target of cytotoxic agents. Consequently, temporary impairment of sperm quality is commonly observed during treatment with various chemotherapeutic agents. Abnormalities in semen may remain upto two years after the completion of treatment and depend on the ability of the surviving stem spermatogonia to restore spermatogenesis. While these cells are less susceptible to cytotoxic drugs or irradiation than differentiating spermatogonia, the stem cell pool may be severely depleted, leading to permanent azoospermia. As with women, high dose alkylating agents and irradiation that includes the testes in the field are both associated with the development of permanent infertility in male patients. Conditioning therapy for SCT is the most gonadotoxic, with 85% of the patients found to be azoospermic after treatment. Any regimen containing procarbazine or high dose cyclophosphamide used to treat Hodgkin's lymphoma, neuroblastoma, sarcoma or acute lymphoblastic leukemia, as well as testes irradiation (over 2.5 Gy in men and over 6.5 Gy in boys) presents a high risk of prolonged azoospermia.[34]

As with women, reducing the gonadotoxicity of the oncological treatment, either by adaptation of the chemotherapy or by in vivo pharmacological protection, constitutes the best option. Limited radiation by shielding or removing the testes from the irradiation field is also effective whenever appropriate. There is insufficient evidence to suggest that hormonal suppression during chemotherapy with GnRH agonists is effective in preventing sperm damage from alkylating agents. This procedure is not recommended in men.[73]

Cryopreservation of sperm is the most reliable and efficient procedure for preserving fertility in men. For 64% of men with cancer, alteration of sperm quality occurs before any treatment due to disease infiltration in the central nervous system, in the testes, or to the poor health status of the patients at the time of diagnosis. Even poor sperm quality, however, could lead to successful fatherhood, due to the development of intracytoplasmic sperm injection technologies. Unsuccessful procedures may also occur due to unfavorable psychological conditions and illnesses, rendering ejaculation difficult to perform. More invasive alternatives, such as epididymal sperm aspiration, testicular sperm extraction (TESE), or electro-ejaculation, can be proposed to obtain a sperm sample when masturbation fails. TESE has also been considered for patients with Hodgkin's lymphoma who failed sperm banking before chemotherapy because of disease induced azoospermia.[74]

Despite the fact that preservation of sperm is a simple and rapid procedure, many oncologists are not routinely providing information on or referrals for sperm banking, particularly for young teenagers. Studies show that less than 20% of eligible adolescent male patients successfully banked sperm.[75] Both oncologists and parents should encourage the teenagers to cryopreserve sperm, despite the psychological barriers related to their young age.

For pre-pubertal boys, sperm banking is not feasible and an alternative approach must be developed. At present, there is no established option for preserving fertility in pre-pubertal boys. Testicular tissue cryopreservation before the initiation of the gonadotoxic treatment is being offered as a promising experimental procedure in some centers. The restoration of testicular function after cure by autologous intratesticular stem cell transplantation is a hypothetical option that is currently being successfully investigated in animal studies.[76]

As with women there is concern regarding the risk of reintroduction of malignant cells to the patients with autologous transplantation. For high-risk cancer patients, isolation of spermatogonial stem cells before transplantation or *in vitro* culture of spermatogonia may be alternative options, but important technical obstacles have yet to be resolved.[43]

While none of these applications is feasible at the present time in humans, testicular tissue banking in pre-pubertal boys offers the prospect of fertility restoration in the decades to come. The patients and their parents, however, must be carefully informed about the experimental nature of the procedure and the absence of guarantees that the tissue can be used in the future.

CONCLUSION

For a decade, counseling about the risk of gonadal damage and the options to preserve fertility has become an essential part of the overall management of most young patients and children with cancer. Non-cancer patients with autosomal disease, gynecological disorders, or genetic disorders are also concerned. Many international organizations have published fertility-preservation guidelines, stressing the importance of managing this issue with multidisciplinary teams and offering the most appropriate option to each patient.

REFERENCES

1. Tschudin S, Bitzer J. Psychological aspects of fertility preservation in men and women affected by cancer and other life-threatening diseases. Human Reprod Update. 2009;15:587-97.
2. Brougham MF, Wallace WH. Subfertility in children and young people treated for solid and haematological malignancies. Br J Haematology. 2005;131:143-55.
3. Salooja N, Szydlo RM, Socie G, et al. Pregnancy outcomes after peripheral blood or bone marrow transplantation: a retrospective survey. Lancet. 2001;358:271-6.
4. Levine J, Canada A, Stern CJ. Fertility Preservation in Adolescents and Young Adults With Cancer. J Clin Oncol. 2010;28(32):4831-41.
5. Sieniawski M, Reineke T, Josting A, et al. Assessment of male fertility in patients with Hodgkin's lymphoma treated in the German Hodgkin Study Group (GHSG) clinical trials. Ann Oncol. 2008;19:1795-801.
6. Petersen PM, Skakkebaek NE, Vistisen K, et al. Semen quality and reproductive hormones before orchiectomy in men with testicular cancer. J Clin Oncol. 1999;17:941-7.
7. Pal L, Leykin L, Schifren JL, et al. Malignancy may adversely influence the quality and behaviour of oocytes. Human Reprod (Oxford, England). 1998;13:1837-40.
8. Robertson AD, Missmer SA, Ginsburg ES. Embryo yield after in vitro fertilization in women undergoing embryo banking for fertility preservation before chemotherapy. Fertil Steril. 2011 Feb;95(2):588-91.
9. O'Flaherty C, Hales BF, Chan P, et al. Impact of chemotherapeutics and advanced testicular cancer or Hodgkin lymphoma on sperm deoxyribonucleic acid integrity. Fertil Steril. 2010;94:1374-9.
10. van Dalen EC, van der Pal HJ, van den Bos C, et al. Clinical heart failure during pregnancy and delivery in a cohort of female childhood cancer survivors treated with anthracyclines. Eur J Cancer. 2006;42:2549-53.
11. Fossa SD, Magelssen H, Melve K, et al. Parenthood in survivors after adulthood cancer and perinatal health in their offspring: a preliminary report. J Natl Cancer Inst. 2005;77-82.
12. Jadoul P, Dolmans MM, Donnez J. Fertility preservation in girls during childhood: is it feasible, efficient and safe and to whom should it be proposed? Human Reprod Update. 2010;16(6):617-30.
13. Wallace WH, Anderson RA, Irvine DS. Fertility preservation for young patients with cancer: who is at risk and what can be offered? Lancet Oncology. 2005;6:209-18.
14. Wallace WH, Thomson AB, Kelsey TW. The radiosensitivity of the human oocyte. Human Reprod (Oxford, England). 2003;18:117-21.
15. Sanders JE, Hawley J, Levy W, et al. Pregnancies following high-dose cyclophosphamide with or without high-dose busulfan or total-body irradiation and bone marrow transplantation. Blood. 1996;87:3045-52.
16. Ginsberg JP, Goodman P, Leisenring W, et al. Long-term survivors of childhood Ewing sarcoma: report from the childhood cancer survivor study. J Natl Cancer Instit. 2010;102:1272-83.
17. Greenberg DB, Goorin A, Gebhardt MC, et al. Quality of life in osteosarcoma survivors. Oncology (Williston Park, NY). 1994;8:19-25; discussion -6, 32, 5.
18. Leung W, Hudson MM, Strickland DK, et al. Late effects of treatment in survivors of childhood acute myeloid leukemia. J Clin Oncol. 2000;18:3273-9.
19. Livesey EA, Brook CG. Gonadal dysfunction after treatment of intracranial tumours. Archives of Disease in Childhood. 1988; 63:495-500.
20. Byrne J, Fears TR, Gail MH, et al. Early menopause in long-term survivors of cancer during adolescence. Am J Obstet Gynecol. 1992;166:788-93.
21. Wallace WH, Barr RD. Fertility preservation for girls and young women with cancer: what are the remaining challenges? Human Reprod Update. 2010;16(6):614-6.
22. Goodwin T, Elizabeth Oosterhuis B, Kiernan M, et al. Attitudes and practices of pediatric oncology providers regarding fertility issues. Pediatric Blood Cancer. 2007;48:80-5.
23. Sukumvanich P, Case LD, Van Zee K, et al. Incidence and time course of bleeding after long-term amenorrhea after breast cancer treatment: a prospective study. Cancer. 2010;116:3102-11.
24. Schmidt KL, Andersen CY, Loft A, et al. Follow-up of ovarian function post-chemotherapy following ovarian cryopreservation and transplantation. Human Reprod (Oxford, England). 2005;20:3539-46.
25. Partridge AH, Ruddy KJ. Fertility and adjuvant treatment in young women with breast cancer. Breast (Edinburgh, Scotland). 2007;16 Suppl 2:S175-81.
26. Ives A, Saunders C, Bulsara M, et al. Pregnancy after breast cancer: population based study. BMJ (Clinical research ed.). 2007;334:194.
27. Oktay K, Kim JY, Barad D, et al. Association of BRCA1 mutations with occult primary ovarian insufficiency: a possible explanation for the link between infertility and breast/ovarian cancer risks. J Clin Oncol. 2010;28:240-4.
28. Lee S, Ozkavukcu S, Heytens E, et al. Value of Early Referral to Fertility Preservation in Young Women With Breast Cancer. J Clin Oncol. 2010;28(31):4683-6.
29. McGlynn KA, Devesa SS, Sigurdson AJ, et al. Trends in the incidence of testicular germ cell tumors in the United States. Cancer. 2003;97:63-70.
30. Fossa SD, Magelssen H. Fertility and reproduction after chemotherapy of adult cancer patients: malignant lymphoma and testicular cancer. Ann Oncol. 2004; 15 Suppl 4: iv259-65.
31. Huddart RA, Norman A, Moynihan C, et al. Fertility, gonadal and sexual function in survivors of testicular cancer. Br J Cancer. 2005;93:200-7.
32. Lee SJ. Preservation of fertility in patients with cancer. New England J Med 2009; 360: 2680; author reply 2-3.
33. Gulati SC, Van Poznak C. Pregnancy after bone marrow transplantation. J Clin Oncol. 1998;16:1978-85.
34. Levine J, Canada A, Stern CJ. Fertility Preservation in Adolescents and Young Adults With Cancer. J Clin Oncol. 2010;28(32):4831-41.
35. Brusamolino E, Lunghi F, Orlandi E, et al. Treatment of early-stage Hodgkin's disease with four cycles of ABVD followed by adjuvant radio-therapy: analysis of efficacy and long-term toxicity. Haematologica. 2000;85:1032-9.
36. Donnez J, Martinez-Madrid B, Jadoul P, et al. Ovarian tissue cryopreservation and transplantation: a review. Human Reprod Update. 2006;12:519-35.
37. Uzan C, Kane A, Rey A, et al. Outcomes after conservative treatment of advanced-stage serous borderline tumors of the ovary. Ann Oncol. 2010;21:55-60.

38. Suh-Burgmann E. Long-term outcomes following conservative surgery for borderline tumor of the ovary: a large population-based study. Gynecol Oncol. 2006;103:841-7.
39. Medeiros PB, Febronio MV, Bonfa E, et al. Menstrual and hormonal alterations in juvenile systemic lupus erythematosus. Lupus. 2009;18: 38-43.
40. Boumpas DT, Austin HA, 3rd, Vaughan EM, et al. Risk for sustained amenorrhea in patients with systemic lupus erythematosus receiving intermittent pulse cyclophosphamide therapy. Ann Int Med. 1993;119:366-9.
41. Katsifis GE, Tzioufas AG. Ovarian failure in systemic lupus erythematosus patients treated with pulsed intravenous cyclophosphamide. Lupus. 2004;13:673-8.
42. Suehiro RM, Borba EF, Bonfa E, et al. Testicular Sertoli cell function in male systemic lupus erythematosus. Rheumatology (Oxford, England). 2008; 47:1692-7.
43. Wyns C, Curaba M, Vanabelle B, et al. Options for fertility preservation in prepubertal boys. Human Reprod Update. 2010;16:312-28.
44. Hreinsson JG, Otala M, Fridstrom M, et al. Follicles are found in the ovaries of adolescent girls with Turner's syndrome. J Clin Endocrinol Metabol. 2002;87:3618-23.
45. Balen AH, Harris SE, Chambers EL, et al. Conservation of fertility and oocyte genetics in a young woman with mosaic Turner syndrome. BJOG 2010;117:238-42.
46. Sonmezer M, Oktay K. Fertility preservation in female patients. Human Reprod Update. 2004;10:251-66.
47. Paduch DA, Bolyakov A, Cohen P, et al. Reproduction in men with Klinefelter syndrome: the past, the present, and the future. Seminars Reprod Med. 2009;27:137-48.
48. Woodruff DY, Horwitz G, Weigel J, et al. Fertility preservation following torsion and severe ischemic injury of a solitary testis. Fertil Steril. 2010;94:352 e4-5.
49. Hodgson DC, Pintilie M, Gitterman L, et al. Fertility among female hodgkin lymphoma survivors attempting pregnancy following ABVD chemotherapy. Hematological Oncol. 2007;25:11-5.
50. Bisharah M, Tulandi T. Laparoscopic preservation of ovarian function: an underused procedure. Am J Obstet Gynecol. 2003;188:367-70.
51. Beck-Fruchter R, Weiss A, Shalev E. GnRH agonist therapy as ovarian protectants in female patients undergoing chemotherapy: a review of the clinical data. Human Reprod Update. 2008;14:553-61.
52. Del Mastro L, Boni L, Michelotti A, et al. Effect of the gonadotropin-releasing hormone analogue triptorelin on the occurrence of chemotherapy-induced early menopause in premenopausal women with breast cancer: a randomized trial. JAMA. 2011;306:269-76.
53. Demeestere I, Brice P, Peccatori FA, et al. Gonadotropin-Releasing Hormone Agonist for the Prevention of Chemotherapy-Induced Ovarian Failure in Patients With Lymphoma: 1-Year Follow-Up of a Prospective Randomized Trial. J Clin Oncol. 2013;31(7):903-9.
54. Gerber B, von Minckwitz G, Stehle H, et al. Effect of luteinizing hormone-releasing hormone agonist on ovarian function after modern adjuvant breast cancer chemotherapy: the GBG 37 ZORO study. J Clin Oncol. 2011;29:2334-41.
55. Behringer K, Wildt L, Mueller H, et al. No protection of the ovarian follicle pool with the use of GnRH-analogues or oral contraceptives in young women treated with escalated BEACOPP for advanced-stage Hodgkin lymphoma. Final results of a phase II trial from the German Hodgkin Study Group. Ann Oncol. 2010;21:2052-60.
56. Kim SS, Donnez J, Barri P, et al. Recommendations for fertility preservation in patients with lymphoma, leukemia, and breast cancer. J Assisted Reprod Genetics. 2012;29:465-8.
57. Gonfloni S, Di Tella L, Caldarola S, et al. Inhibition of the c-Abl-TAp63 pathway protects mouse oocytes from chemotherapy-induced death. Nature Med. 2009;15:1179-85.
58. Noyes N, Labella PA, Grifo J, et al. Oocyte cryopreservation: a feasible fertility preservation option for reproductive age cancer survivors. J Assisted Reprod Genetics. 2010;27:495-9.
59. Sonmezer M, Oktay K. Fertility preservation in young women undergoing breast cancer therapy. Oncologist. 2006;11:422-34.
60. Shalom-Paz E, Almog B, Shehata F, et al. Fertility preservation for breast-cancer patients using IVM followed by oocyte or embryo vitrification. Reprod Biomed Online. 2010;21:566-71.
61. Dolmans MM, Demylle D, Martinez-Madrid B, et al. Efficacy of in vitro fertilization after chemotherapy. Fertil Steril. 2005;83:897-901.
62. Demeestere I, Simon P, Englert Y, et al. Preliminary experience of ovarian tissue cryopreservation procedure: alternatives, perspectives and feasibility. Reprod Biomed Online. 2003;7:572-9.
63. Bedaiwy MA, El-Nashar SA, El Saman AM, et al. Reproductive outcome after transplantation of ovarian tissue: a systematic review. Human Reprod (Oxford, England). 2008;23:2709-17.
64. Donnez J, Silber S, Andersen CY, et al. Children born after autotransplantation of cryopreserved ovarian tissue. a review of 13 live births. Ann. Med. 2011;43:437-50.
65. Schmidt KT, Rosendahl M, Ernst E, et al. Autotransplantation of cryopreserved ovarian tissue in 12 women with chemotherapy-induced premature ovarian failure: the Danish experience. Fertil Steril. 2011;95:695-701.
66. Demeestere I, Simon P, Moffa F, et al. Birth of a second healthy girl more than 3 years after cryopreserved ovarian graft. Human Reprod (Oxford, England). 2010;25:1590-1.
67. Demeestere I, Simon P, Emiliani S, et al. Fertility preservation: successful transplantation of cryopreserved ovarian tissue in a young patient previously treated for Hodgkin's disease. Oncologist. 2007;12:1437-42.
68. Ernst E, Bergholdt S, Jorgensen JS, et al. The first woman to give birth to two children following transplantation of frozen/thawed ovarian tissue. Human Reprod (Oxford, England). 2010;25:1280-1.
69. Demeestere I, Simon P, Emiliani S, et al. Orthotopic and heterotopic ovarian tissue transplantation. Human Reprod Update. 2009;15:649-65.
70. Oktay K. Ovarian tissue cryopreservation and transplantation: preliminary findings and implications for cancer patients. Human Reprod Update. 2001;7:526-34.
71. Fasano G, Demeestere I, Moffa F, et al. In vitro maturation and vitrification of immature oocytes combined with ovarian tissue cryopreservation: a new strategy for fertility preservation. *CRYO Congress* Valencia 2010.
72. Meirow D, Hardan I, Dor J, et al. Searching for evidence of disease and malignant cell contamination in ovarian tissue stored from hematologic cancer patients. Human Reprod (Oxford, England). 2008;23:1007-13.
73. Waxman JH, Ahmed R, Smith D, et al. Failure to preserve fertility in patients with Hodgkin's disease. Cancer chemotherapy pharmacology. 1987;19:159-62.
74. Schrader M, Muller M, Sofikitis N, et al. Testicular sperm extraction prior to treatment in azoospermic patients with Hodgkin's disease. Ann Oncol. 2002;13:333.
75. Chong AL, Gupta A, Punnett A, et al. A cross Canada survey of sperm banking practices in pediatric oncology centers. Pediatr Blood Cancer. 2010;55(7):1356-61.
76. Geens M, Goossens E, De Block G, et al. Autologous spermatogonial stem cell transplantation in man: current obstacles for a future clinical application. Human Reprod Update. 2008;14:121-30.

3 Reproductive Implications of Chemotherapy and Radiotherapy

Mohamed A Bedaiwy, Drisana Henry, Candice P Holliday, Botros RMB Rizk

CHAPTER OUTLINE

- Chemotherapy
  - Chemotherapeutic Agents
  - Chemotherapy Protocols
- Radiotherapy
  - Radiation Dose
  - Radiation Field
  - Patient Age
- Protective and Preventive Measures

INTRODUCTION

Although the incidence of childhood and reproductive age cancers is rare, the consequences of a cancer diagnosis and/or treatment can be long lasting. The National Cancer Institute indicated that as of January 2012, 13.7 million Americans were living with a history of cancer.[1] It has also been projected that childhood cancer survivors will, by 2010, comprise 1 in 250 young adults in the industrialized world.[2] For most childhood cancers, the five year survival rate is greater than 70%.[3] Given the improved modalities of early detection of malignancies and more aggressive treatment to optimize survival, the overall relative 5-year survival rate improved from 56% to 64% in women and from 56% to 75% children.

The overall most common malignancy in women is breast cancer. Advances in early breast cancer diagnosis and treatment have contributed to an increase in survival rates in the United States. Twenty-five percent of breast cancers are diagnosed in premenopausal women.[3] One of the greatest concerns of women cancer survivors is fertility, since infertility and early menopause can result from chemotherapy. Early onset menopause results in osteoporosis, heart disease, depression and an overall decreased quality of life. Five to 10% of reproductive age breast cancer patients become pregnant, annually.[4] In these cases, assisted reproductive technology (ART) is increasingly being used. Fifty percent of women over age 25 and 25% of women under age 25 will develop primary ovarian insufficiency (POI) after being treated with mechloroethamine, vincristine, procarbazine and prednisone.[5]

The modern advances in the management of cancer have not only given new hope for survival, but also improved quality of life. Reports describing the birth of children from ovarian tissue transplantation have attached a clinical relevance to a previously academic discussion.[6-9] Reproductive organ loss or damage includes ovarian insufficiency due to premature failure, exposure to radiotherapy and/or chemotherapy and systemic and genital tract malignancies that result in organ removal.

The ovary is particularly susceptible to permanent or transient damage from a variety of medical, radiological and surgical treatments. This peculiarity stems from the fact that there is a limited endowment of follicles in the ovary at birth, which declines naturally over time.[10] POI, also known as premature ovarian failure (POF), is defined as the spontaneous and irreversible cessation of menses before 40 years of age. It is caused by a depletion of functional ovarian follicles, resulting in amenorrhea.[3] The number of patients facing the risk of POI or loss of their uteri who are seeking help in preserving their fertility has increased dramatically. This incremental increase is in part due to cancer treatment regimens that have proven successful because of their aggressive nature. Furthermore, because many women are delaying childbearing, there is a higher probability of encountering patients with a malignancy who have no children and require treatment that is potentially sterilizing.

A wide variety of etiologies of POI include abnormal karyotype, translocations, point mutations, ovarian autoimmunity, pelvic infection, cytotoxic drugs, radiotherapy and ovarian surgery. These etiologies can lead to the failure of follicles to reach maturity, either by depletion of the store of primordial follicles or making them refractory to growth stimuli.[11] The deterioration of ovarian follicular endowment is accelerated by exposure to alkylating agents and ionizing radiation. When given to premenopausal breast cancer patients, cyclophosphamide, methotrexate and 5-fluorouracil (CMF) resulted in ovarian failure with no effect on pituitary and adrenal functions.[12]

In addition to the direct effects of chemotherapy, radiotherapy and surgery, the increased catabolic state and malnutrition associated with systemic malignancies result in weight loss and other metabolic abnormalities of the endocrine system. Hypothalamic dysfunction secondary to weight loss causes pituitary gonadotropin levels to drop.[13] Stress hormones that bring about a rise in prolactin and opiate secretion[12] can also disrupt the hypothalamic pituitary ovarian axis. However, these abnormalities usually may be reversible with a return to a healthy state. The reproductive failure associated with the treatment of malignancies is often not reversible.

CHEMOTHERAPY

Chemotherapy has been used widely to treat malignant and non-malignant conditions. The probability of POI after chemotherapy is influenced by the type of chemotherapeutic agents (**Table 1**), cell cycle-specificity (**Figure 1**), the cumulative dose of the cytotoxic drugs and the patient's age at the time of exposure. The type and dose of chemotherapeutic agent influences the progression to ovarian failure, with alkylating agents increasing the risk of POI by a factor of 9.[14] POI rates range from 10–100%.[5] The outcome of the deleterious sterilizing effect of these agents is age-sensitive. Growing follicles are more susceptible to cytotoxic agents than are primordial follicles. Once all primordial follicles in the ovary are destroyed, permanent ovarian failure sets in. Using a mathematical model, Faddy and Gosden[15] predicted that POI would set in by the age 27 if the germ cell population was reduced by 90% before the age of 14.

Alkylating agents are very ovariotoxic and cyclophosphamide is the agent most commonly implicated in damaging oocytes and granulosa cells in a dose-dependent manner.[16-19] One study showed that 42% of women treated with alkylating agents experienced POI, while those treated with other agents (plant alkaloids, platinum agents) did not have an increased risk of POI.[3] A dose of 5, 9 and 20 g can cause complete amenorrhea in women over 40, 30–40 years and 20–30 years of age, respectively.[20] Women under the age of 20 treated with alkylating agents were 9 times more likely than controls to experience premature menopause.[3] There was a 4-fold increased risk of POI in teenagers treated for cancer with an alkylating agent and this risk increased by a factor of 27 in women between the ages of 21 and 25.[21] Approximately, 60–80% of women treated with CMF will undergo POI.[3] Sanders et al.[17] reported that no pregnancies occurred after hematopoietic cell transplantation in a group pretreated with busulfan in combination with

TABLE 1 Gonadotoxicity chemotherapeutic agents*

High toxicity	***Alkylating agents (Cell cycle phase nonspecific)***			***Methylhydrazine derivative (Cell cycle phase nonspecific)***	
	Nitrogen mustards • Cyclophosphamide • Melphalan • Chlorambucil • Mechlorethamine	Nitrosoureas • Carmustine • Lomustine	Alkyl sulfonates • Busulfan	• Procarbazine (N-methylhydrazine-MIH)	
Intermediate toxicity	Platinum coordination complexes (Cell cycle phase nonspecific)		Antibiotics (Cell cycle phase nonspecific)		
	• Cisplatinum • Carboplatinum		• Doxorubicin		
Low Toxicity	Folic acid analogs (Cell cycle phase specific)	Pyrimidine analogs (Cell cycle phase specific)	Antibiotics (Cell cycle phase nonspecific)		Vinca alkaloids (Cell cycle phase specific)
	• Methotrexate	• Fluorouracil	• Bleomycin • Dactinomycin (actinomycin D)		• Vincristine • Vinblastin

*Female gonads; male gonads may have different sensitivity. Many drugs have unknown risks

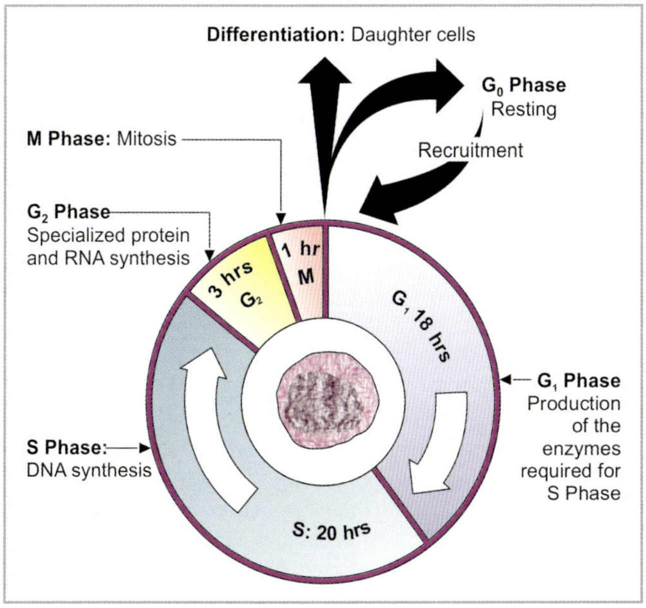

FIGURE 1 Schematic representation of the cell cycle. The relative gonadotoxicity and cell cycle specificity of the different chemotherapeutic agents are: Agents with phase specificity: M Phase: A—Podophyllotoxins as etoposide and teniposide. B—Taxanes as Docetaxel and Paclitaxel. C—Vinca Alkaloids as vinblastine, vincristine. G2 Phase: Bleomycin. S Phase: A—Antimetabolites as A—Anitfolates: methotrexate, Antipurines: mercaptopurine, thioguanine, B—Antinpyrimidines: cytarabine, fluorouracil, azacitidine and C—Miscellaneous: hydroxyurea, procarbazine, cisplatin and carboplatin. G_0 Phase: Nitrosoure as carmustine, lomustine, semustine. G1 Phase: As paraginase as Diglycoaldehyde and Steroids. Agents without phase specificity: A—Alkylating Agents as bulsulfan, chlorambucil, cyclophosphamide, mechlorethamine, melphalan. B—Anthracycline Antibiotics: doxorubicin, daunomycin, rubidazone, dactinomycin. C-Miscellaneous: DTIC, cisplatin, carboplatin and D—Nitrosoureas—also acts in G_0 Phase

cytoxan. Combined chemotherapeutic regimens like MOPP/ABV (chlormethamine, vincristine, procarbazine, prednisone, doxorubicin, bleomycin, vinblastine) induced an age-related, gradual ovarian failure.[22]

Age is an important factor in determining one's risk of POI. Older women have a higher incidence of acute POI, which is most likely due to their limited follicular reserve prior to treatment. However, anti-Müllerian hormone (AMH), a hormone produced by the granulosa cells, reflects growing follicles and is used to estimate the number of primordial follicles. AMH levels decrease during chemotherapy in women of all ages. A multivariate analysis showed that AMH was a better predictor than age in determining ovarian reserve. AMH is significantly lower in women undergoing aggressive chemotherapy protocols.

Chemotherapy has both immediate and long-term effects on the ovary. Immediate effects include amenorrhea induced by the loss of growing follicles. Menses typically resumes once this population is replenished. POI is a later effect resulting from loss of the primordial follicle pool. Transient amenorrhea is an indicator for early menopause,[3] but there is not yet longitudinal data demonstrating the likelihood of undergoing POI in women who resume normal menses.

Chemotherapy drugs are cytotoxic to dividing cells. Different cells have different sensitivities to these drugs since they vary in characteristics. While oocytes rapidly develop during the follicular stage, they are non-dividing once this is complete. Somatic cells, on the other hand, proliferate quickly. Chemotherapy depletes primordial follicles directly and indirectly. These drugs may either directly target these follicles, or indirectly target them by depleting activated, growing follicles. Growing follicles secrete AMH, which again is a hormone that plays an important role in regulating the growth of primordial follicles. Loss of growing follicles leads to dysregulation of primordial follicles, increased recruitment of primordial follicles into the growing pool and a reduction of the primordial follicle pool. Decreased levels of inhibin B and AMH during chemotherapy suggests a loss of follicles during the pre-antral and early antral stages.

It is suggested that the mitotically active ovarian somatic cells are the target of chemotherapeutic drugs, rather than the meiotically-arrested oocytes within immature follicles. Granulosa cells proliferate during maturation and can be damaged during chemotherapy, resulting in damage to the oocyte. Ovarian stromal tissue has shown fibrosis and capillary changes in children who had undergone chemotherapy for leukemia.

Chemotherapeutic Agents

Mechanisms of cell death in response to chemotherapy are apoptosis and necrosis. Different agents act on different players in the cell signaling pathway and these are explored below.

Doxorubicin

Doxorubicin is an anthracycline that works by intercalating DNA and inhibiting replication. It can be used to treat leukemias, lymphomas and sarcomas. This drug can induce caspase c, upregulate p53 expression and induce apoptosis. It causes double strand breaks in DNA and activates ataxia telangectasia mutated protein kinase (ATM), a protein that induces apoptosis in the presence of DNA damage.

Other than this drug's ability to induce apoptosis in ovulated murine oocytes, its actions on immature oocytes has not yet been elucidated. In vitro, doxorubicin has been shown to induce apoptosis and DNA damage in oocytes and granulosa of human primordial follicles. Though both types of cells are damaged, granulosa cells are thought to be the primary target.[3]

Cyclophosphamide

Cyclophosphamide is a drug that works by inducing intra- and inter-strand cross-linking, which ultimately inhibits cell division. It causes accumulation of cytochrome *c* in mitochondrial cytosol, which activates caspases and apoptosis. It also upregulates *Bax*, a proapoptotoic protein. In vitro human ovarian slices, as well *in vivo* ovarian samples, treated with this agent exhibit damaged follicular basement membranes and granulosa cell nuclei.[3]

Cisplatin

Cisplatin is a platinum-containing compound that works by inducing inter- and intra-strand adducts, which interfere with cellular replication. Cisplatin causes an accumulation of Abl (tyrosine kinase) and TAp63-a (p53 homologue), leading to oocyte death. This drug also induces apoptosis via the caspase *c* pathway. The primary cell targeted by this drug is the oocyte. Through its actions on the mitochondria, germ and somatic cells are also damaged.[3]

Irinotecan and Etoposide

These drugs are both topoisomerase inhibitors. They prevent DNA from being able to unwind during replication. Irinotecan induces Fas ligand in granulosa cells, resulting in activation of p53 and upregulation of *Bax* and caspase 9, leading to apoptosis. Granulosa cells are the preferential target for these Irinotecan. Etoposide, on the other hand, induces apoptosis by activating ATM and primarily targets the oocyte.[3]

Chemotherapy Protocols

The rate of POI after chemotherapy for Hodgkin's lymphoma ranged from 0%–50%, depending on age as well as protocol. The chlormethamine, oncovin, procarbazine and prednisone combined with adriamycin, bleomycin, vinblastine, dacarbazine (MOPP-ABV[D]) protocol was older and resulted in a POI rate of up to 50%. The newer adriamycin bleomycin vinblastine dacarbazine (ABVD) protocol, however, results in a POI rate of less than 10%. Another protocol combined bleomycin, etoposide, adriamycin, cyclophosphamide, oncovin, procarbazine and prednisone (BEACOPP) and resulted in POI in all women over 30 and 50% of women under 30 when 8 cycles were given. Two cycles of escalated BEACOPP combined with ABVD (or conventional BEACOPP alone), however, result in lower rates of POI.[5]

A higher risk of POI is associated with an escalated BEACOPP regimen, age over 30, advanced Hodgkin's lymphoma and no birth control pills. Cyclophosphamide has been shown to have detrimental ovarian effects at the following cumulative doses: 5g at 40 years, 9g at 30 years and 20g at 20 years. Four percent of women under 30 and 12.2% of women over 30, experience POI after 2 cycles of cyclophosphamide, oncovin, procarbazine and prednisolone (COPP) and ABVD. Four cycles of the same regimen, however, leads to POI in 23.5% of women under 30 and 53.3% in women over 30.[5] Eight cycles results in POI in 40.4% and over 70% in women under and over 30, respectively.

Cyclophosphamide, adriamycin, oncovin and prednisone (CHOP) protocol (or mega-CHOP) is often used in women with non-Hodgkin's lymphoma. This protocol has a lower incidence of POI with only 10% experiencing POI.

Women who have leukemia and undergo bone marrow transplantation experience the highest rates of POI. Women treated for breast cancer have a POI rate between 0–70%. After undergoing the CMF protocol, 45–68% of premenopausal women experience POI compared to those undergoing the adriamycin/cyclosphosphamide (AC) protocol (15%). Of all women under the age of 35, who underwent the CMF protocol or the cyclophosphamide, adriamycin, 5-fluorouracil (CAF) protocol, only 0–28% experienced POI. This is in contrast to the 45–68% of women over 35 who experienced POI with the CMF (or similar) protocol.[5] With regard to the AC protocol, 4 cycles will induce POI in 20% of women under 40. Of treated women over 40, 20–80% have been shown to suffer permanent hypergonadotropic amenorrhea and menopause.

Over 80% of women treated with the CMF or CAF protocols experienced POI. Women aged 30–39 will experience a POI rate of 20-80% and those under 30 will experience a rate of under 20%.

Chemotherapy induces acute follicular damage, reducing the number of follicles and leading to chronic follicular damage as they easily undergo atresia. Features of early atresia include intracytoplasmic vacuoles, multivesicular bodies, altered mitochondria and myelinic-like structures, which have been demonstrated in primordial follicles by electron microscopy studies after chemotherapy.[23]

Granulosa cells are highly involved in the process of apoptosis, which is triggered by chemotherapy. The end result is the eventual destruction of primordial follicles.[24-26] High-dose chemotherapy and/or total body irradiation before bone marrow transplantation (BMT) present the greatest risk of POI in almost all cases, regardless of patient age.[17,26,27]

RADIOTHERAPY

Radiotherapy regimens affect both ovarian and uterine function. The mechanism by which radiation causes damage is through an ionization process. Electrons are released and damage important components such as DNA, resulting in cell disruption.[28] The risk of ovarian damage after radiotherapy is related to the patient's age, treatment field, total dose, and number of doses (**Table 2**).

Radiation Dose

The relative risk of developing POI and infertility after radiation increases as the dose of abdominal radiation increases. The radiation doses used with standard pelvic radiation therapy will uniformly induce ovarian failure and doses even as low as 0.01–0.99 can induce POI.[28] The risk of POI is increased with combined radio and chemotherapy.[29,30] The combination of abdominal ionizing radiation with alkylating agents often induces POI, rendering patients infertile in almost 100% of cases. A dose of 5 Gy to 20 Gy administered to the ovary is sufficient to completely impair gonadal function at any age.[31] Less than 2 Gy destroys 50% of the oocyte reserve.[32] Single-dose radiation is more toxic than fractionated regimens.[26] The break point for radiation-induced ovarian failure is approximately 300 cGy to the ovaries, whereas only 11% to 13% experience ovarian failure below 300 cGy and 60% to 63% experience ovarian failure above this threshold value.[33] Uterine dysfunction has been also reported to follow radiation doses between 14 and 30 Gy.[31,34,35] Uterine irradiation at a young age reduces adult uterine volume.[36]

TABLE 2 Determinants of radiation induced gonadal failure

- Age of patient
- Cumulative dose to the ovary
  - Direct or scatter radiation
- Concomitant chemotherapy

Radiation Field

Mantle-field radiotherapy is administered above the diaphragm and delivers a 0.1% scattered radiation dose to the ovaries. Total body and below-diaphragm irradiation will lead to infertility in most women with rates being directly correlated with age.[5] Total-body irradiation results in a 90% POI rate.[17] Rates may be as high as 97% in abdominal radiation.[37] Similarly, pelvic irradiation results in significant damage to ovarian functions.

Patient Age

Women under the age of 40 are less sensitive to ovarian damage from radiation compared to older women. It is estimated that 20 Gy can produce permanent ovarian failure in the former group whereas only 6 Gy are required to produce this outcome in women over 40. In women receiving total abdominal pelvic radiation, the relative risk of developing POI was 1.02, 1.37 and 3.27 for radiation doses of <20 Gy, 20–35 Gy and >35 Gy, respectively. Twenty-two percent of women receiving 20–35 Gy of treatment experienced POI, compared to 32% of women receiving >35 Gy).[38]

Radiation has also been shown to have adverse effects on the uterus. Spontaneous miscarriages, infertility and intrauterine growth retardation have been caused by radiation.[32] Irreversible damage can include changes in uterine musculature, blood flow, and hormone-resistant endometrial insufficiency. Damage to uterine vasculature inhibits cytotrophoblast radiation, which decreases fetal-placental blood flow and leads to restricted fetal growth.[39]

Radiation can lead to myometrial fibrosis and a reduction in uterine elasticity and volume, resulting in preterm labor. There is also a reduction in uterine weight and length.[40] In young patients, treatment with sex steroids may improve uterine damage.[31] The mean uterine length in radiation-treated patients was 4.1 cm, compared to controls who had a mean length of 7.3 cm.[34]

A decrease in endometrial thickness that is not responsive to sex steroid replacement has also been observed in these patients. Though a later study showed improvement in endometrial thickness with sex steroid replacement,[35] radiation still results in some degree of irreversible damage. Damaged endometrium inhibits normal decidualization and prevents normal placental attachment, leading to placenta accreta and percreta.[39,41]

Obstetric complications can also result from radiation. Compared to the general population, women who have received radiation experience more spontaneous abortions (38% versus 12%), preterm labor (62% versus 9%) and low birth weight infants (62% versus 6%). [39] Fenig et al.[42] observed an increase in the incidence of spontaneous abortions and low birth weight infants in women conceiving less than a year after radiation treatment.

Radiation can impact reproduction through its effects on the hypothalamus-pituitary axis (HPA). Damage to the hypothalamus and pituitary gland occur frequently after high-dose cranial radiation. Cranial irradiation can result in amenorrhea and infertility. Dysregulation of the hypothalamus or pituitary gland leads to hormonal dysfunction. In a study of patients treated with cranial irradiation for primary brain tumors (not involving the HPA), 70% of post-pubertal, premenopausal women developed oligomenorrhea and 50% had low serum estradiol concentrations and mild hyperprolactinemia. Primary hypothalamic dysfunction was suggested from this study.[43]

Pre-pubertal girls with leukemia who receive prophylactic cranial irradiation (PCI) may be at an increased risk of POI and early pregnancy loss.[44] One study showed that women who received PCI doses of 18 Gy and 24 Gy during childhood, all had a significantly lower rate of first births than controls.[45] Other studies have shown that cranial irradiation can cause precocious puberty, resulting in cortical disinhibition of the hypothalamus.[44]

PROTECTIVE AND PREVENTIVE MEASURES

There has been a growing interest in strategies that can be used to protect ovaries from the effects of chemotherapy. Triptorelin, a gonadotropin-releasing hormone agonist, was tested for its ability to prevent chemotherapy-induced ovarian failure in patients with lymphoma.[46] However, 20% of patients in both the control and treatment groups experienced POI during a 1-year follow-up. Though this drug is ineffective in decreasing the risk of POI, it may potentially protect ovarian reserve in those individuals who recover ovarian function after chemotherapy. The only approved strategy for fertility preservation by the American Society for Reproductive Medicine (ASRM) is embryo cryopreservation. Strategies like oocyte, in vitro maturation of oocytes and ovarian tissue cryopreservation are considered experimental. Ovarian transposition is a unique surgical intervention that could protect the ovaries from radiotherapy induced damage where ovaries with (**Figure 2**) or without Fallopian tubes are moved away from the irradiation field. Oftentimes, radiopaque surgical clips are placed next to the ovaries as markers to track the ovaries radiologically in order to discover early if the ovaries migrated back to their original positions (**Figure 3**). These modalities will be discussed in their respective chapters.

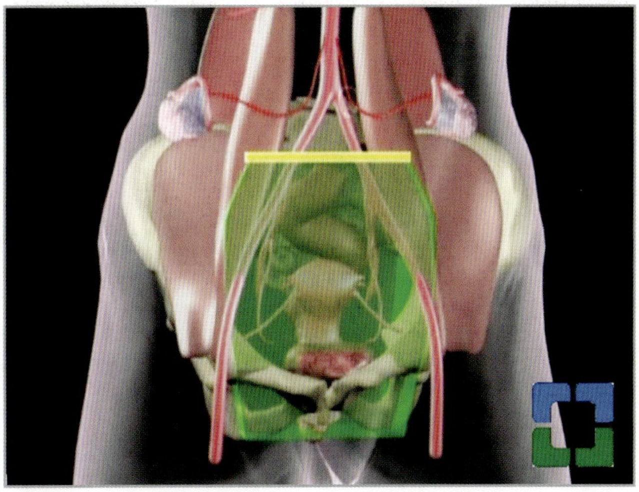

FIGURE 2 Pelvic irradiation field with the ovaries moved away. This schematic representation showed that the irradiation field is highlighted with the green color and the adnexa were moved outside the field of irradiation.

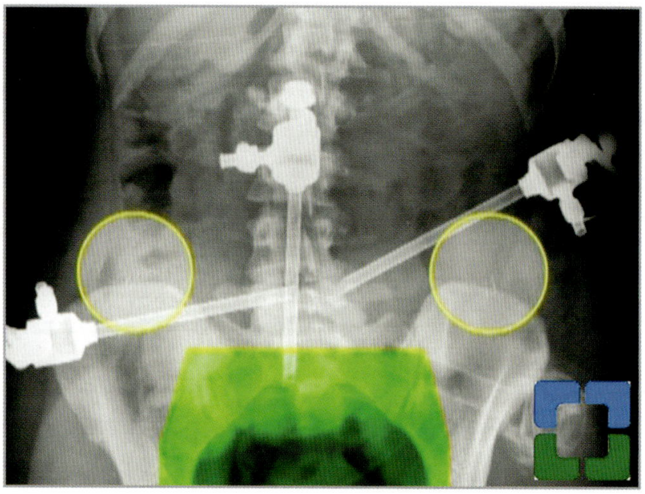

FIGURE 3 Plain X-ray of the abdomen at the completion of the laparoscopic ovarian suspension showing a midline umbilical trocar and lateral trocars. The irradiation field is highlighted with green color. The 2 yellow captions are showing the ovaries in their new position. Each ovary is marked with 2 radiopaquesurgical clips to facilitate subsequent follow up and exclude postoperative migration of the ovaries to their original location.

REFERENCES

1. Society AC. Cancer Treatment & Survivorship Facts & Figures. In. Vol. 2012, 2012.
2. Blatt J. Pregnancy outcome in long-term survivors of childhood cancer. Med Pediatr Oncol. 1999;33:29-33.
3. Morgan S, Anderson RA, Gourley C, et al. How do chemotherapeutic agents damage the ovary? Hum Reprod Update. 2012;18:525-35.
4. Bernik SF, Bernik TR, Whooley BP, Wallack MK. Carcinoma of the breast during pregnancy: a review and update on treatment options. Surg Oncol. 1998;7:45-9.
5. Blumenfeld Z. Chemotherapy and fertility. Best Pract Res Clin Obstet Gynaecol. 2012;26:379-90.
6. Meirow D, Levron J, Eldar-Geva T, et al. Ovarian Tissue Storing for Fertility Preservation in Clinical Practice: Successful Pregnancy, Technology, and Risk Assessment. Fertil Steril. 2005;84 (Suppl 1): S2.
7. Morishita S, Imai A, Kawabata I, Tamaya T. Acute myelogenous leukemia in pregnancy: fetal blood sampling and early effects of chemotherapy. Int J Gynaecol Obstet. 1994;44:273-7.
8. Silber SJ, Gosden RG. Ovarian transplantation in a series of monozygotic twins discordant for ovarian failure. N Engl J Med. 2007;356:1382-4.
9. Donnez J, Dolmans MM, Demylle D, et al. Livebirth after orthotopic transplantation of cryopreserved ovarian tissue. Lancet. 2004;364: 1405-10.
10. Faddy MJ, Gosden RG, Gougeon A, et al. Accelerated disappearance of ovarian follicles in mid-life: implications for forecasting menopause. Hum Reprod. 1992;7:1342-6.
11. Gosden RG, Faddy MJ. Biological bases of premature ovarian failure. Reprod Fertil Dev. 1998;10:73-8.
12. Bhatavdekar JM, Shah NG, Patel DD, et al. Endocrine function in premenopausal and postmenopausal advanced breast cancer patients treated with CMF or tamoxifen. Neoplasma. 1992;39:123-7.
13. Vigersky RA, Andersen AE, Thompson RH, Loriaux DL. Hypothalamic dysfunction in secondary amenorrhea associated with simple weight loss. N Engl J Med. 1977;297:1141-5.
14. Byrne J, Fears TR, Gail MH, et al. Early menopause in long-term survivors of cancer during adolescence. Am J Obstet Gynecol. 1992;166:788-93.
15. Faddy MJ, Gosden RG. A mathematical model of follicle dynamics in the human ovary. Hum Reprod. 1995;10:770-5.
16. Warne GL, Fairley KF, Hobbs JB, Martin FI. Cyclophosphamide-induced ovarian failure. N Engl J Med. 1973;289:1159-62.
17. Sanders JE, Hawley J, Levy W, et al. Pregnancies following high-dose cyclophosphamide with or without high-dose busulfan or total-body irradiation and bone marrow transplantation. Blood. 1996;87:3045-52.
18. Meirow D, Lewis H, Nugent D, Epstein M. Subclinical depletion of primordial follicular reserve in mice treated with cyclophosphamide: clinical importance and proposed accurate investigative tool. Hum Reprod. 1999;14:1903-7.
19. Kenney LB, Laufer MR, Grant FD, et al. High risk of infertility and long term gonadal damage in males treated with high dose cyclophosphamide for sarcoma during childhood. Cancer. 2001;91:613-21.
20. Shalet SM. Effects of cancer chemotherapy on gonadal function of patients. Cancer Treat Rev. 1980;7:141-52.
21. Larsen EC, Müller J, Schmiegelow K, et al. Reduced ovarian function in long-term survivors of radiation- and chemotherapy-treated childhood cancer. J Clin Endocrinol Metab. 2003;88:5307-14.
22. Schilsky RL, Sherins RJ, Hubbard SM, et al. Long-term follow up of ovarian function in women treated with MOPP chemotherapy for Hodgkin's disease. Am J Med. 1981;71:552-6.
23. Familiari G, Caggiati A, Nottola SA, et al. Ultrastructure of human ovarian primordial follicles after combination chemotherapy for Hodgkin's disease. Hum Reprod. 1993;8:2080-7.
24. Tilly JL, Kolesnick RN. Sphingolipids, apoptosis, cancer treatments and the ovary: investigating a crime against female fertility. Biochim Biophys Acta. 2002;1585:135-8.
25. Morita Y, Perez GI, Paris F, et al. Oocyte apoptosis is suppressed by disruption of the acid sphingomyelinase gene or by sphingosine-1-phosphate therapy. Nat Med. 2000;6:1109-14.

26. Meirow D, Nugent D. The effects of radiotherapy and chemotherapy on female reproduction. Hum Reprod Update. 2001;7:535-43.
27. Lobo RA. Potential options for preservation of fertility in women. N Engl J Med. 2005;353:64-73.
28. Cohen LE. Cancer treatment and the ovary: the effects of chemotherapy and radiation. Ann N Y Acad Sci. 2008;1135:123-5.
29. Gaetini A, De Simone M, Urgesi A, et al. Lateral high abdominal ovariopexy: an original surgical technique for protection of the ovaries during curative radiotherapy for Hodgkin's disease. J Surg Oncol. 1988;39:22-8.
30. Williams RS, Littell RD, Mendenhall NP. Laparoscopic oophoropexy and ovarian function in the treatment of Hodgkin disease. Cancer. 1999;86:2138-42.
31. Critchley HO, Wallace WH. Impact of cancer treatment on uterine function. J Natl Cancer Inst Monogr. 2005:64-8.
32. Wallace WH, Thomson AB. Preservation of fertility in children treated for cancer. Arch Dis Child. 2003;88:493-6.
33. Husseinzadeh N, Nahhas WA, Velkley DE, et al. The preservation of ovarian function in young women undergoing pelvic radiation therapy. Gynecol Oncol. 1984;18:373-9.
34. Critchley HO, Wallace WH, Shalet SM, et al. Abdominal irradiation in childhood; the potential for pregnancy. Br J Obstet Gynaecol. 1992;99:392-4.
35. Bath LE, Critchley HO, Chambers SE, et al. Ovarian and uterine characteristics after total body irradiation in childhood and adolescence: response to sex steroid replacement. Br J Obstet Gynaecol. 1999;106:1265-72.
36. Larsen E, Schmiegelow K, Rechnitzer C, et al Radiotherapy at a young age reduces uterine volume of childhood cancer survivors. Acta Obstet Gynecol Scand. 2004;83:96-102.
37. Wallace WH, Shalet SM, Crowne EC, et al. Ovarian failure following abdominal irradiation in childhood: natural history and prognosis. Clin Oncol (R Coll Radiol). 1989;1:75-9.
38. Maltaris T, Seufert R, Fischl F, et al. The effect of cancer treatment on female fertility and strategies for preserving fertility. Eur J Obstet Gynecol Reprod Biol. 2007;130:148-55.
39. Hawkins MM, Smith RA. Pregnancy outcomes in childhood cancer survivors: probable effects of abdominal irradiation. Int J Cancer. 1989;43:399-402.
40. Meirow D, Biederman H, Anderson RA, Wallace WH. Toxicity of chemotherapy and radiation on female reproduction. Clin Obstet Gynecol. 2010;53:727-39.
41. Critchley HO, Bath LE, Wallace WH. Radiation damage to the uterus -- review of the effects of treatment of childhood cancer. Hum Fertil (Camb). 2002;5:61-6.
42. Fenig E, Mishaeli M, Kalish Y, Lishner M. Pregnancy and radiation. Cancer Treat Rev. 2001;27:1-7.
43. Constine LS, Woolf PD, Cann D, et al. Hypothalamic-pituitary dysfunction after radiation for brain tumors. N Engl J Med. 1993;328:87-94.
44. Wo JY, Viswanathan AN. Impact of radiotherapy on fertility, pregnancy, and neonatal outcomes in female cancer patients. Int J Radiat Oncol Biol Phys. 2009;73:1304-12.
45. Nygaard R, Clausen N, Siimes MA, et al. Reproduction following treatment for childhood leukemia: a population-based prospective cohort study of fertility and offspring. Med Pediatr Oncol. 1991;19: 459-66.
46. Demeestere I, Brice P, Peccatori FA, et al. Gonadotropin-Releasing Hormone Agonist for the Prevention of Chemotherapy-Induced Ovarian Failure in Patients With Lymphoma: 1-Year Follow-Up of a Prospective Randomized Trial. J Clin Oncol. 2013;31(7):903-9.

4

Ovarian Reserve Testing for Cancer Patients

Luciano G Nardo, Lamiya Mohiyiddeen

CHAPTER OUTLINE

INTRODUCTION

Women undergoing cancer treatment are at greater risk of ovarian failure and subsequent infertility. Both the age of the woman and the type and dose of the chemo-radiotherapy influence the progression to ovarian failure. The gonadotoxic effect of chemotherapeutic agents is well-documented. Alkylating agents such as cyclophosphamide that are non-cell cycle specific are more cytotoxic to the ovaries than cell cycle-specific agents such as methotrexate and fluorouracil, whose major effect is on ovarian follicle growth and maturation[1]. Ovarian damage following chemotherapy can present with a variety of symptoms that reflect varying degrees of damage, culminating in premature ovarian failure (POF).

Those patients who are not immediately rendered infertile are still likely to suffer with infertility and develop POF. Approximately, 50% of patients under age 35 resume normal menses after completion of cytotoxic chemotherapy, and are therefore potentially capable of becoming pregnant spontaneously or through assisted conception treatment.[2] Although a regular menstrual cycle may serve as a convenient marker for satisfactory ovarian function, a normal menstrual cycle is not synonymous with satisfactory fertility. Similarly, irregular menses or amenorrhea does not always imply infertility. Because of the possibility of spontaneous recovery, it has been suggested that ovarian function be reassessed periodically in patients with chemotherapy-induced gonadal damage.[3]

Bone marrow transplantation (BMT, with its associated treatments) carries the worst prognosis, even when it is performed at a very young age. Only 19% of children treated with BMT have normal ovarian function, whereas in older women ovarian failure is virtually universal.[4] Pelvic irradiation by itself has significant consequences. It has been estimated that a total radiation exposure of 20 Gy fractionated over six weeks in younger women and children produces sterility with 95% confidence.[5]

So far, long-term follow-up studies have assessed ovarian function after cancer treatment using parameters such as follicle stimulating hormone (FSH) serum levels or clinical end-points such as cycle length or pregnancy rates. Despite the presence of high FSH levels and amenorrhea after chemotherapy, pregnancies in childhood cancer survivors have been reported as well. Hence, FSH levels or menstrual cyclicity after cancer treatment do not seem to be predictive of the chance to conceive.[6] A recent report on gonadal function in childhood cancer survivors showed that in patients with regular menstrual cycles following treatment with chemotherapy and cranial radiotherapy, ovarian reserve was compromised when assessed by serum anti-Müllerian hormone (AMH) concentrations.[7] Serum AMH levels, antral follicle count (AFC) and ovarian volume are more reliable predictors of ovarian function in cancer patients compared to FSH levels.

The increasing number of young survivors of cancer with favorable outcomes is defining the need for a more comprehensive approach that will improve the quality of life after cancer, including the preservation of fertility.

EFFECT OF CHEMOTHERAPY ON THE OVARY

The fact that ovaries of young girls contain a higher number of follicles than ovaries from older women makes them more resistant to chemotherapy. Thus, young girls tolerate higher doses of chemotherapy before entering POF. However, chemotherapeutic agents differ in relation to their toxicity on ovarian function. Cyclophosphamide and busulfan, which have frequently been used in the treatment of childhood cancer, are far more gonadotoxic than other agents [1]. Chemotherapy disrupts ovarian function by depleting the primordial follicle pool in a drug- and dose-dependent manner. Analysis of ovarian function after cancer therapy have mostly described the prevalence of ovarian failure after treatment, although follicular depletion may occur despite maintenance of regular menstrual cycles.

EFFECT OF RADIOTHERAPY ON THE OVARY

Despite the fact that radiotherapy interrupts the normal cellular proliferation cycle, causing extensive cell damage and that postnatal oocytes are mitotically inactive, they are still highly susceptible to the damage caused by radiotherapy. This is probably because of the risk of undergoing induced apoptosis. The high number of follicles in the pre-pubertal ovary makes it less vulnerable than the ovary of women in late reproductive life. That said the risk of primary ovarian failure after abdominal radiotherapy is still high. Complete ovarian failure occurs with a dose of 20 Gy in women under 40 years of age and with only 6 Gy in older women.[8] The uterus is extremely vulnerable to irradiation and decreases in volume by 40%. It has been suggested that if pregnancy occurs, problems may ensue that are related to abnormalities in uterine function.

ROLE OF OVARIAN RESERVE TESTS (ORT) IN CANCER PATIENTS

The natural fecundity and pregnancy rates decrease with increasing age, however, it is established that chronological age and menstrual characteristics are unreliable in predicting reproductive age. Several models have now been described that accurately chart the progressive decline of primordial follicles in the ovary with the woman's chronological age. The most important aspect of diminished ovarian reserve and the associated decline in reproductive potential is that its onset is highly variable. The continual decline in follicle number and quality is a dynamic process.

Treatment with chemo-therapeutic agents may not only have an immediate effect, but may cause a significant reduction in the ovarian reserve in the long term. Ovarian reserve markers can help identify the women who are at risk of this. These patients can be advised at an early age against postponing childbearing too long, as their reproductive career may be shorter than they expect.

The ability to predict a woman's reproductive potential would be of considerable value for many young cancer survivors for their treatment decision-making, family planning and contraception concerns. Women interested in future fertility should be able to undergo ovarian reserve testing before and upon completion of cancer therapy.

OVARIAN RESERVE TESTS

Follicle Stimulating Hormone

Biochemical markers like basal serum FSH is considered an indirect estimate of ovarian reserve and depends on the presence of an intact hypothalamus-pituitary-ovarian axis. It is one of the most established parameters for estimating ovarian performance. The values of FSH usually maintain within normal ranges and tend to rise only when ovarian function is deeply compromised.

Some studies suggest that young age exerts a protective effect over the deleterious effects of reduced ovarian reserve, while others reveal no difference in outcome between younger and older women with elevated FSH. Threshold levels for baseline FSH are also an issue. In one study, which is unique for its duration of follow-up, ongoing pregnancy was seen in as much as 28% of regularly cycling women with FSH levels of 15–20 IU/L. Only when the FSH level was >20 IU/L was there a clear fall in ongoing pregnancy rate regardless of age.[9] Others have shown elevated FSH to be of limited value in patients with regular cycles. Questions remain regarding the reproducibility of FSH measurements. One of its main limitations is the significant intercycle variability of FSH, hence limiting the usefulness of a normal value.

Most of the data regarding the performance of FSH in predicting ovarian reserve comes from studies in *in vitro* fertilization (IVF) populations. Information pertaining to the general sub-fertile population and cancer patients is lacking, but a case-control study revealed no statistically significant difference in cumulative pregnancy rates between patients with elevated FSH levels and controls. On day 3 of the menstrual cycle, serum FSH levels are usually less than 10 IU/L in most assays. FSH levels that are more than 15 IU/L on day 3 suggest a decreased ovarian reserve and a reduced probability of pregnancy; if values exceed 20 IU/L, the probability of pregnancy is extremely low.[10]

The establishment of threshold values within individual assay systems is also important to prevent errors in interpretation of results. This is more likely to happen in institutions where the clinical volume of patients is insufficient to allow these threshold values to be established. Other reasons for an elevated baseline FSH should be considered. Laboratory errors can occur in the presence of heterophilic antibodies, which can interfere with the FSH immunoassay.[10] FSH receptor variants have now been identified.[11] This may cause slightly diminished receptor function, resulting in higher levels of FSH to achieve adequate receptor response, whilst not necessarily affecting ovarian reserve.

Although basal FSH remains a frequently used marker of ovarian reserve in any level of fertility care, the controversies surrounding its use as a predictor of ovarian reserve and the fact that FSH is not a direct reflection of selectable ovarian follicles makes it a less reliable marker.

Anti-Müllerian Hormone

Serum AMH has emerged as a valuable marker of ovarian reserve in women of reproductive age. AMH is secreted by ovarian granulosa cells of primordial, preantral and small antral follicles. After puberty and before perimenopause, the AMH level remains stable in healthy women. Serum levels of AMH represent the quantity of the ovarian follicle pool, whilst the relationship with the quality has not yet been confirmed. AMH was found to be a more sensitive predictor of ovarian reserve than other markers.[12] AMH is relatively convenient to determine, especially as it seems to exhibit a relatively stable expression during the menstrual cycle, making it an attractive determinant of ovarian reserve.

A study in cancer patients showed that AMH levels were lower in the patients compared to controls, even though the latter group was older. This indicates that ovarian reserve in patients with cancer was already compromised before any therapy was initiated. Remarkably, all patients who developed POF after gonadotoxic chemotherapy had pre-treatment AMH levels lower than the 10th percentile of AMH levels in age-matched controls. However, not all patients with pre-treatment AMH below this threshold point developed POF. In this study, AMH levels prior to treatment were not predictive for ovarian reserve after treatment.[13]

Following chemotherapy, the decrease in AMH levels per year was not significantly different from that of controls. This suggests that ovarian damage after gonadotoxic therapy is due to a diminished primordial follicle pool rather than to an increased rate of follicle loss.

In a study of childhood cancer survivors including 185 patients, serum AMH levels were significantly lower in survivors who received radiotherapy of the abdomen, pelvis, sacrum or their total body than in controls, whereas survivors irradiated on other parts of their body had normal AMH levels.[7] There were no differences in AMH levels in subgroups classified according to disease. Survivors treated with three or more procarbazine containing chemotherapy cycles had significantly lower AMH levels than controls. The decrease in AMH levels was noted to precede changes in conventional parameters associated with perimenopausal status, such as FSH, inhibin B and estradiol.

Recently, AMH was measured in survivors of childhood Hodgkin's lymphoma, hematological malignancies and solid tumors. These studies confirmed that, in childhood cancer survivors with regular menstrual cycles, serum AMH levels were indicative of limited ovarian reserve, whereas FSH, estradiol and inhibin B levels were not different from healthy controls.[14,15] It may be premature to apply a cut-off value since this has not been validated in the population under study.

Although the secretory function of the ovary may recover to some extent and menses may return after the completion of chemotherapy treatment, ovarian reserve remains persistently affected. Neither baseline nor change in AMH predicts return of menstrual function, suggesting that ovarian reserve and endocrine function may be affected differently or may recover differently from chemotherapy.[7]

Antral Follicle Count

AFC is usually defined as the number of follicles measuring between 2–10mm in diameter detected by ultrasound scan in the early follicular phase. Studies in women with proven fertility reveal a continual decline of AFC with age. Additionally, AFC shows a better correlation with chronological age than other hormonal and ultrasound markers.

Reproducibility has been addressed and described as being moderate, with decreasing agreement at higher AFC. Intercycle variability has also been described as moderate in a fertile population. A more recent analysis, which studied infertile patients, showed that intercycle variability was greater than interobserver variations, suggesting a biological variation of AFC from cycle to cycle. AFC < 5 is predictive of poor ovarian reserve.[16]

A lower level of AMH appears to be the best serum predictor of diminished AFC, which is thought to reflect reduced likelihood of future pregnancy. Because AMH is a serologic test that does not fluctuate with the menstrual cycle, assessment of AMH may be a more practical factor for the measurement of fertility potential than AFC, which requires transvaginal scan.

Inhibin B

Inhibins are secreted by the ovarian granulosa and luteal cells during the menstrual cycle. Inhibins are a part of the hypothalamus-pituitary-ovarian axis, specifically having an inhibitory effect on pituitary FSH synthesis and secretion. Serum inhibin B is regarded as a direct measure of ovarian reserve as it is mainly secreted by antral follicles. Inhibin B rises from early in the follicular phase to reach a peak coincident with the onset of the mid-follicular phase decline in FSH concentrations. It then declines during the luteal phase apart from a periovular peak.

Inhibin B has also been shown to respond to exogenous FSH administration in the follicular phase. Studies in older women reveal significantly lower levels of inhibin B in women aged 40–50 years with raised FSH compared to women with normal FSH. Concentrations of inhibin B have been shown to be lower in women with elevated FSH and regular menstrual cycles. Decreased inhibin B was found in women with normal FSH levels, implying that decreased inhibin B precedes a rise in FSH.[17] Inhibin B has been evaluated in predicting response as a component of dynamic testing. These include the clomiphene citrate challenge test (CCCT), GnRH agonist test (GAST) and the exogenous FSH ovarian reserve test (EFORT). In a prospective study, the inhibin B response to exogenous FSH correlated well with AFC and the number of oocytes retrieved.[18] Given the expense of performing the test, further prospective evaluation and confirmation of its predictive capacity is required before inhibin B can assume a routine place in the clinical assessment of women with reduced ovarian reserve.

Ovarian Volume

The human ovary is a dynamic organ which changes in size and activity throughout its lifetime. Mean ovarian volume increases from 0.7 cm^3 at age 10 years to 5.8 cm^3 at age 17 years. Estimation of the mean primordial follicle population in women aged 25–51 years can be made using the Faddy-Gosden equation[19] and correlating it with mean ovarian volume at each chronological age.[20] This model makes a critical assumption that primordial follicle populations are fixed at birth, a notion that has recently been challenged. Whether or not ovarian volume can accurately reflect primordial follicle numbers or indeed follicle quality is questionable. The latter may be more important if reproductive age is to be correlated with fertility outcome. Ovarian volume estimation using conventional ultrasound is inexpensive and relatively easy to perform. Intra- and inter-observer variations are small, ensuring reproducibility. Its main limitation at present is the lack of data regarding ovarian volume measurements in the general population, both fertile and infertile, across different age cohorts.

Estradiol (E2)

The condensed follicular phase length in older women may be as a result of a more advanced follicular recruitment by cycle day 3. This early dominant follicle selection is expressed by high serum E2 concentrations. It has been shown in an assisted reproduction treatment population (where GnRH analogs were not administered) that increasing day 3 estradiol concentrations are associated with decreasing oocyte numbers and pregnancy rates. The predictive ability of E2 is improved in patients of advanced reproductive age, especially when combined with FSH.[21] No data are currently available regarding basal E2 levels in the general population. Further studies including data on day 3 estradiol values and fecundity in spontaneous cycles are required before evaluating this parameter further in cancer patients.

Dynamic Ovarian Reserve Tests

The recognized limitations of biochemical markers of ovarian reserve led to the development of a number of dynamic ovarian tests in an attempt to 'unmask' patients whose diminished ovarian reserve may have been missed using these markers.

The GAST (or G-test) evaluates the E2 serum concentration change from cycle day 2 to day 3 after administration of a GnRH agonist, the latter causing a temporary increase in pituitary secretion of gonadotropins. Early studies were able to show a limited ability for the early rise in E2 concentrations to differentiate between normal and reduced ovarian reserve, with different threshold values. Inhibin B is considered a direct marker of ovarian reserve. Combining Inhibin B with the GAST may have improved the predictive value of the test.[22] The GAST appears to have much promise as a dynamic test of ovarian reserve, but has not yet been validated outside an assisted reproductive setting. Furthermore, the cost of performing the test has limited its acceptability.

The CCCT involves the administration of 100 mg clomiphene citrate on cycle days 5-9 and the determination of FSH concentrations on days 3 and 10. In women with normal ovarian reserve, the overall increase in E2 and inhibin production by the developing follicles should be able to overcome the estrogen antagonist effect of clomiphene on the hypothalamus-pituitary-ovarian axis and suppress FSH levels back into the normal range by day 10. The CCCT may be more indicative of oocyte quality than quantity. Nevertheless, a quantitative relationship between the CCCT and follicle density has been shown.[23] Correlation with other biophysical markers of ovarian reserve (ovarian volume and AFC) has been shown in an infertile population.

The EFORT combines FSH with the rise in E2 over a 24 hour period after administration of a standardized dose (300 IU) of purified FSH on day 3. A randomized, prospective study in which basal and dynamic tests of ovarian reserve were compared revealed the EFORT as being the best predictor of ovarian reserve.[24] Further prospective evaluation is required to validate this test properly.

FERTILITY PRESERVATION

Hormonal Suppression

Gonadotropin releasing hormone analogs (GnRH-a) have been utilized during chemotherapy to suppress ovarian cycling and induce a temporary medical menopause. The action of GnRH-as are not clearly understood because primordial and primary follicles do not have GnRH receptors and it is possible that GnRH-a preserve those follicles that have already initiated growth. It has also been speculated that the hypo-estrogenic state caused by GnRH-a may decrease utero-ovarian perfusion, resulting in a decreased total cumulative exposure of the ovaries to the chemotherapeutic insult. Several studies in animals have suggested that protection may be offered by use of GnRH-a, however, the benefit in human therapy remains debatable.

A recent prospective, randomized, controlled study was published analyzing a group of 80 breast cancer patients younger than 40 years of age. The cancer patients were randomized to either co-treatment with GnRH-a (Zoladex, 3.6 mg subcutaneously) during chemotherapy (study group, n = 39) or treated with chemotherapy alone (control group, n = 39), with one dropout in each group.[25] Eighty-nine percent in the study group resumed menses and 69% resumed spontaneous ovulation, as compared with 33.3% and 25.6%, respectively, in the control group ($P < 0.01$). Median FSH and luteinizing hormone (LH) concentrations were significantly lower in the study group compared with the control group ($P <0.01$), suggesting a better ovarian reserve in the study group.

A recent trial of 281 patients suggested that the use of triptorelin-induced temporary ovarian suppression during chemotherapy in pre-menopausal patients with early-stage breast cancer reduced the occurrence of chemotherapy-induced early menopause.[26] Collectively, the few available studies suggest that there may be some degree of protection with GnRH-a. Before puberty, concomitant use of GnRH-a are not recommended. The human studies presently available are limited in design and lack long-term follow-up.

Transposition of the Ovaries (also known as Oophoropexy)

The aim of this approach is to surgically remove the ovaries from the direct field of radiation. The technique was first applied to women with cervical cancer in the 1950s. In many clinics, oophoropexy is now standard procedure in women suffering from cancers that require pelvic irradiation. Although the ovaries may be out of the field of direct radiation, the scatter dose may cause significant ovarian damage. In a review, it was found that women receiving pelvic irradiation after oophoropexy still experienced ovarian failure in 50–90% of the cases.[27] Complications to the procedure include chronic pelvic pain, vascular injury, fallopian tube infarction and ovarian migration—although all occurred rarely. Another aspect to be considered is the accessibility of the ovaries for oocyte collection if IVF becomes necessary. It is very likely that a transposed ovary located in the paracolic gutter may be inaccessible for safe oocyte retrieval.

Oophoropexy could be considered in cases of abdominal irradiation, either unilaterally or bilaterally, but the long-term effect remains uncertain. It may protect the ovarian function in <50% of cases in adults, but further clinical data providing good evidence for this approach is required.

Cryopreservation of Oocytes

The first report of a live birth originating from human cryopreserved oocytes appeared in 1986. The technique involves stimulation of the ovaries and harvesting of eggs followed by freezing. Stored eggs can later be thawed and IVF techniques with intracytoplasmic sperm injection (ICSI) can be employed. Oocytes are much more sensitive to damage from cryopreservation than embryos (probably secondary to spindle damage from ice crystal formation). The formation of ice crystal and the attendant cellular damage during freezing can potentially be avoided by vitrification.

An alternative approach could be the collection of immature oocytes that are subsequently put through *in vitro* maturation (IVM). When using this technique, oocytes can be collected at any time during the cycle (stimulated or unstimulated), or can even be retrieved from excised ovarian tissue in conjunction with cryopreservation of gonadal tissue. Since the first report of a birth from a frozen oocyte, the results of this procedure worldwide have been variable with a reported success rate of 2% per oocyte retrieved, despite the improved success rate when combined with ICSI.

Cryopreservation of Embryos

This is a very well-established technique in cancer patients. It involves controlled ovarian stimulation using exogenous gonadotropins, generating multiple follicular development so that several oocytes can be collected. This technique requires 2–4 weeks for completion and therefore can delay the antineoplastic treatment. In cancer patients, the fresh embryos are not replaced and are cryopreserved for later use. Recently, a protocol has been described in which ovarian stimulation may start even during the luteal phase in cancer patients, thus requiring a maximum of 2 weeks before oocyte collection. The stimulation of the ovaries using gonadotropins results in high estrogen levels, and certainly this raises concerns for some steroid sensitive tumors. It is still unclear what the risks of such techniques are in terms of tumor progression or relapse in a hormone dependent cancer. This risk has been addressed by using tamoxifen or letrozole alone or in combination with standard IVF stimulation for women with breast cancer or endometrial cancer. This is an established method available in clinical practice to preserve fertility in women being treated for cancer.

Cryopreservation of Ovarian Tissue

This is a technique that can be used for adults and for children, but at present it is still regarded as experimental due to the lack of large longitudinal follow up studies. An entire ovary, or part of it, is removed surgically, often during laparoscopy or in conjunction with an operation for the disease. The cortex, which is the site of the primordial follicles, is isolated 1–2 mm in thickness and cut into strips or fragments. The tissue can be kept indefinitely in liquid nitrogen at –196°C. After the patient is cured, some of the cryopreserved tissue can be transplanted back in to the pelvis, and follicular growth, endogenous hormone production and ovulation may resume. Optimal treatment benefit can only be expected in the presence of a healthy ovarian reserve. As such, it is less likely to be beneficial for older women and those with a suboptimal ovarian performance. Donnez and colleagues reported in 2004 a live birth after transplanting cryopreserved ovarian tissue back into the pelvis of a woman following treatment for stage 4 non-Hodgkin's lymphoma.[28] All the cases of successful post-implantation pregnancy reported to date have utilized the whole cortical ovarian tissue. The risk of re-implanting tissue with occult cancer, while small, remains a matter of concern and ongoing research. Only patients with cancer associated with low risk of ovarian metastasis, such as squamous cell carcinoma of the cervix, Wilm's tumor, Hodgkin and non-Hodgkin's lymphoma, should be considered for future auto-transplantation. On the contrary, women with moderate and high risk of ovarian primary or secondary involvement should not be offered this fertility preservation option.

CONCLUSION

Chemotherapy decreases ovarian reserve rapidly and significantly. Although the secretory function of the ovary may recover to some extent and menses may return after completion of chemotherapy treatment, ovarian reserve remains persistently affected. Chronological age remains an important factor for the recovery of endocrine function after chemotherapy and potentially for fertility. For young women looking for fertility preservation before the start of chemotherapy, the most reliable and successful method to date is embryo freezing, although other options can be offered. Oocytes or ovarian tissue cryopreservation and GnRH agonist or antagonist therapy in conjunction with chemotherapy are all active areas of research. Oktay and colleagues reported using a combined letrozole-FSH protocol for ovulation induction in cancer patients that produced results comparable to those of standard IVF without a significant increase in E2 levels.[29]

Some studies have shown that female cancer survivors with regular menses and normal serum FSH levels had significantly smaller ovaries along with a lower AFC as compared to age-matched controls. These observations indicate that parameters such as cycle length and FSH serum levels are not accurate markers of ovarian function. Serum AMH levels, AFC and ovarian volume appear to be more reliable predictors. Neither baseline nor change in AMH concentrations was seen to predict return of menstrual function, suggesting that ovarian reserve and endocrine function may be affected differently or may recover differently from chemotherapy.

The relationship between AMH and other markers of ovarian reserve has been assessed, where AMH was found to be a more sensitive predictor of ovarian reserve than the other markers. AMH is relatively convenient to determine, especially as it seems to exhibit a relatively stable expression during the menstrual cycle, making it an attractive determinant of ovarian reserve. More prospective large studies are required to validate ovarian reserve markers in cancer patients in order to determine cut off levels to accurately predict the possible reproductive outcome in this cohort of women.

REFERENCES

1. Hensley ML, Reichman BS. Fertility and pregnancy after adjuvant chemotherapy for breast cancer. Crit Rev Oncol Hematol. 1998; 28:121-8.
2. Parker SL, Tong T, Bolden S, Wingo PA. Cancer statistics, 1997. CA Cancer J Clin. 1997;47:5-27.
3. Singh KL, Davies M, Chatterjee R. Fertility in female cancer survivors: Pathophysiology preservation and the role of ovarian reserve testing. Hum Reprod Update. 2005;11:69-89.
4. Barrett A, Nicholls J, Gibson B. Late effects of total body irradiation. Radiother Oncol. 1987;9:131-5.
5. Locatelli F, Giorgiani G, Pession A, Bozzola M. Late effects in children after bone marrow transplantation: a review. Haematologica. 1993;78:319-28.
6. Sklar C. Maintenance of ovarian function and risk of premature menopause related to cancer treatment. J Natl Cancer Inst Monogr. 2005;34:25-7.
7. Fong SL, Laven JSE, Hakvoort-Cammel FGAJ, et al. Assessment of ovarian reserve in adult childhood cancer survivors using anti-Mullerian hormone. Hum Reprod. 2009;24:982-90.
8. Wallace WHB, Thomson AB, Saran F, Kelsey TW. Predicting age of ovarian failure after radiation to a field that includes the ovaries. Int J Radiat Oncol Biol Phys. 2005;62:738-44.
9. van Rooij IA, de Jong E, Broekmans FJ, et al. High follicle-stimulating hormone levels should not necessarily lead to the exclusion of subfertile patients from treatment. Fertil Steril. 2004;81:1478-85.
10. Scott RT Jr. Diminished ovarian reserve and access to care. Fertil Steril. 2004;81:1489-92.
11. Perez MM, Gromoll J, Behre HM, et al. Ovarian response to follicle-stimulating hormone (FSH) stimulation depends on the FSH receptor genotype. J Clin Endocrinol Metab. 2000; 85:3365-69.
12. Nardo LG, Gelbaya TA, Wilkinson H, et al. Circulating basal anti-Müllerian hormone levels as predictor of ovarian response in women undergoing ovarian stimulation for in vitro fertilization. Fertil Steril. 2009;92:1586-93.
13. Lie Fong S, Lugtenburg PJ, Schipper I, et al. Anti-mullerian hormone as a marker of ovarian function in women after chemotherapy and radiotherapy for haematological malignancies. Hum Reprod. 2008;23:674-8.
14. Bath LE, Wallace WH, Shaw MP, et al. Depletion of ovarian reserve in young women after treatment for cancer in childhood: detection by anti-Mullerian hormone, inhibin B and ovarian ultrasound. Hum Reprod. 2003;18:2368-74.
15. van Beek RD, van den Heuvel Eibrink MM, Laven JSE, et al. Anti-Mullerian hormone is a sensitive serum marker for gonadal function in women treated for Hodgkin's lymphoma during childhood. J Clin Endocrinol Metab. 2007;92:3869-74.
16. Su HI, Chung K, Sammel MD, et al. antral follicle count provides additive information to hormone measures for determining ovarian function in breast cancer survivors. Fertil Steril. 2011;95:1857-59.
17. de Koning CH, Popp-Snijders C, Schoemaker J, et al. Elevated FSH concentrations in imminent ovarian failure are associated with higher FSH and LH pulse amplitude, response to GnRH. Hum Reprod. 2000;15:1452-56.
18. Yong PY, Baird DT, Thong KJ, et al. Prospective analysis of the relationships between the ovarian follicle cohort and basal FSH concentration, the inhibin response to exogenous FSH and ovarian follicle number at different stages of the normal menstrual cycle and after pituitary down-regulation. Hum Reprod. 2003;18:35-44.
19. Faddy MJ, Gosden RG. A model conforming the decline in follicle numbers to the age of menopause in women. Hum Reprod. 1996;11:1484-86.
20. Wallace WH, Kelsey TW. Ovarian reserve and reproductive age may be determined from measurement of ovarian volume by transvaginal sonography. Hum Reprod. 2004;19:1612-17.
21. Buyalos RP, Daneshmand S, Brzechffa PR. Basal estradiol and follicle-stimulating hormone predict fecundity in women of advanced reproductive age undergoing ovulation induction therapy. Fertil Steril. 1997;68:272-7.
22. Ravhon A, Lavery S, Michael S, et al. Dynamic assays of inhibin B and oestradiol following buserelin acetate administration as predictors of ovarian response in IVF. Hum Reprod. 2000;15:2297-301.
23. Hofmann GE, Sosnowski J, Scott RT, et al. Efficacy of selection criteria for ovarian reserve screening using the clomiphene citrate challenge test in a tertiary fertility center population. Fertil Steril. 1996;66:49-53.
24. Kwee J, Elting MW, Schats R, et al. Comparison of endocrine tests with respect to their predictive value on the outcome of

ovarian hyperstimulation in IVF treatment: results of a prospective randomized study. Hum Reprod. 2003;18:1422–27.
25. Badawy A, Elnashar A, El-Ashry M, et al. Gonadotropin-releasing hormone agonists for prevention of chemotherapy-induced ovarian damage: prospective randomized study. Fertil Steril. 2009;91:694–7.
26. Mastro D, Boni L, Michelotti L, et al. Effect of the gonadotropin-releasing hormone analogue triptorelin on the occurrence of chemotherapy-induced early menopause in premenopausal women with breast cancer: a randomized trial. JAMA 2011;3:312-4.
27. Wo JY, Viswanathan AN. Impact of radiotherapy on fertility, pregnancy, and neonatal outcomes in female cancer patients. Int J Radiat Oncol Biol Phys. 2009;73:1304-12.
28. Donnez J, Dolmans MM, Demylle D, et al. Livebirth after orthotopic transplantation of cryopreserved ovarian tissue. Lancet. 2004;364:1405-10.
29. Oktay K, Buyuk E, Libertella N, et al. Fertility Preservation in Breast Cancer Patients: A Prospective Controlled Comparison of Ovarian Stimulation with Tamoxifen and Letrozole for Embryo Cryopreservation. Journ of Clin Oncol. 2005;23:4347-53.

Medical Approaches for Fertility Preservation in Female Cancer Patients

5

Eman Elgindy, Mohamed A Bedaiwy

CHAPTER OUTLINE

Fertility preservation is a newly developed branch of reproductive medicine aiming to preserve the potential for genetic parenthood in adults of reproductive age or in children, who are at risk of sterility before undergoing anti-cancer treatments.[1] There is a growing recognition of the fertility threats associated with these treatments and the past few years have witnessed a remarkable alignment between oncologists and fertility specialists to overcome this problem. Different approaches have been suggested and in the current chapter, we will review the medical approaches for fertility preservation.

THE NEED FOR FERTILITY PRESERVATION

Cancer is a major health problem in many parts of the world. Treatment innovations and developments in cytotoxic treatment have contributed to reduced mortality rates, with marked parallel improvement in survival. Death rates from all cancer types decreased among men by 21.0% from the year 1999 to 2006. For women, a 12.3% decrease in cancer death rates occurred between the years 1991 to 2006. Therefore, there was an avoidance of approximately 767,000 deaths from cancer over these 16 years.[2] In parallel, recent years have also witnessed a growing recognition of the importance of the survivor's life quality following cancer treatment.

There have been significant adverse effects of cancer treatment, of which gonadal toxicity is a major concern. Cancer treatment usually involves aggressive chemotherapy and/or radiotherapy, which may have permanent adverse impact on reproductive function.[3-5]

Indeed, iatrogenic infertility is a distressing complication for many survivors and their families.[6,7] In young women, reproductive issues are increasingly shown to have an important role in decision-making regarding their cancer treatment. Infertility concerns had influenced treatment decisions of 29% of women, according to a web-based survey study.[8] Many young cancer survivors stated that their cancer physicians did not inform them adequately about the gonadotoxic effect of their cancer treatment.[9,10] The American Society of Clinical Oncology (ASCO) 2006 has emphasized that patients must be informed about the risk of cancer treatment on their fertility.[11]

Currently, there is rising interest among oncologists and reproductive consultants for integration of fertility preservation in the plan for cancer treatment. This interest has been driven by the development of a number of distinct strategies to preserve fertility. ASCO 2006 has, however, underscored the need to start the approaches of fertility preservation as early as possible during the planning of treatment.[11]

DEVELOPMENT OF GONADAL DYSFUNCTION FOLLOWING CYTOTOXIC TREATMENT

Normal Physiological Considerations

The number and quality of follicles present in the ovary constitute the ovarian reserve (OR).[12,13] Approximately 90% of the total follicle pool is formed from non-growing primordial follicles (PMF).[14,15] Each day, some of these follicles enter the growth phase, which takes several months and the follicles become increasingly gonadotropin-dependent (**Figure 1**).[16] This process involves proliferation of the steroidogenic theca and granulosa cells around the growing oocyte, which has been in an arrested stage of meiosis since before birth.[14] Resumption of meiosis does not occur until just before ovulation.[16] Indeed, the dynamic nature of folliculogenesis makes it a principal target for the cytotoxic treatment.[17] Still, what is pivotally important for future reproduction is the effect on the stock of PMF.

The Impact of Cytotoxic Treatment on Ovarian Function

Both chemotherapy and radiotherapy, with a field that includes the pelvis, are potentially gonadotoxic.[18] The gonadotoxic effect of radiotherapy depends on the total dose, field of treatment,

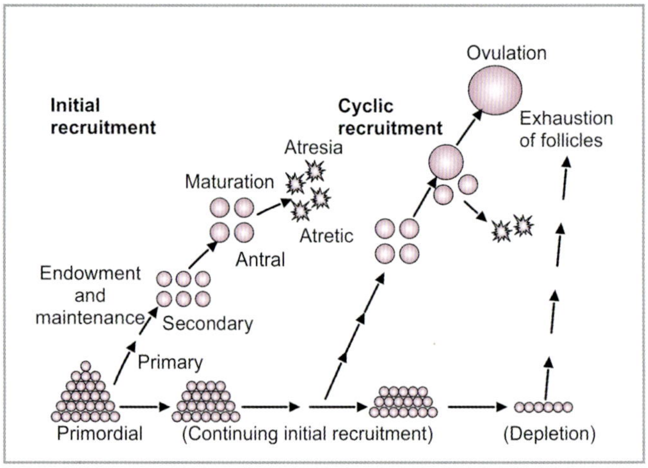

FIGURE 1 Life history of ovarian follicles. Initial recruitment occurs from primordial follicle pool. Follicles develop through different stages, whether primordial, primary and secondary stages. Then, they acquire an antral cavity. Most follicles undergo atresia; however, few of them are rescued (cyclic recruitment) under optimal gonadotropin stimulation. [*Source:* From McGee E and Hsueh A. Initial and Cyclic Recruitment of Ovarian Follicles. Endocrine Reviews. 2000;21(2):200-214].

and fractionation schedule.[18] It was estimated that half of the PMF in the ovaries can be destroyed by less than 2 Gy.[19] Further, low-dose cranial irradiation for central nervous system tumors may adversely affect fertility by disruption of the hypothalamic–pituitary–ovarian axis.[20,21] This effect, however, may become evident many years after cancer treatment.[18]

The mechanism by which chemotherapeutic agents lead to progressive loss of PMF is not clearly understood. There are variations between the individual gonadotoxic effects of different agents. The oocyte or its surrounding granulosa cells may be the primary targets of different agents.[22] Chemotherapeutic agents can be mainly classified into alkylating agents (e.g. cyclophosphamide, mechlorethamine etc.), antitumor antibiotics (e.g. bleomycin, adriamycin, etc.), plant alkaloids (e.g. taxanes, vinblastine, etc.), antimetabolites (e.g. 5-fluorouracil, methotrexate, etc.), topoisomerase inhibitors (e.g. etoposide phosphate, etc.) and others (e.g. cisplatin).[23] The degree of gonadal dysfunction associated with different agents is illustrated in **Table 1**.[24] Notably, there is controversy regarding the effect of some agents like taxanes, with some studies reporting its gonadotoxic effect,[25,26] while others deny that effect.[27]

TABLE 1 The degree of gonadal dysfunction associated with different chemotherapeutic agents

High risk	*Intermediate risk*	*Low or no risk*
Cyclophosphamide	Cisplatin	Methotrexate
Melphalan	Adriamycin	5-Fluorouracil
Busulfan	Paclitaxel	Vincristine
Nitrogen mustard		Bleomycin
Chlorambucil		Actinomycin D
Procarbazine		

Source: From Sonmezer M and Oktay K. Fertility Preservation in Young Women Undergoing Breast Cancer Therapy. Oncologist. 2006;11: 422-434.

Alkylating agents such as cyclophosphamide and topoisomerase inhibitors, such as doxorubicin, are toxic against the non-proliferating population of PMF (**Figure 2**).[28] These agents lead to apoptotic cell death through induction of breaks in double-stranded DNA.[28] This effect has indeed major impact in reducing the OR and the reproductive life span of the survivor.

Cyclophosphamide is the most gonadotoxic, with an almost 4-fold increased risk of induced amenorrhea when compared with other agents. The higher the cumulative dose of cyclophosphamide, the higher the observed incidence of gonadal toxicity is.[29] In a mouse study, follicular damage occurred in a dose-dependent manner with cyclophosphamide, with a dose of 20–100 mg/kg. Notably, PMF destruction occurred even at the lowest dose.[30]

The proliferating nature of granulosa cells allows almost all chemotherapeutic agents to damage the developing follicles, with subsequent development of temporary amenorrhea. New follicles, however, will develop from the undamaged PMF within 3 to 6 months.

Therefore, non-DNA-damaging agents cause temporary amenorrhea and do not affect fertility thereafter. Anti-metabolites such as methotrexate have their impact only on the developing follicles with development of temporary amenorrhea without affecting the ovarian OR (**Figure 2**).[28]

Factors Affecting for the Development of Gonadal Dysfunction

Multiple studies have shown that age of the patient as well as the type and cumulative dose of chemotherapeutic agent(s) are the major determining factors for the development of gonadal failure.[3,4,30,31]

Incidence of amenorrhea, however, varies widely, from 49% to 100% in women older than the age of 40 and from 21%–71% in younger women.[3] In the study by Sukumvanich et al. (2010), chemotherapy-induced amenorrhea was reported in less than 5% of women aged 20 to 34 years, compared with 11% of women aged 35 to 39 years and 40% of women aged older than 39 years.[32] In a multivariable logistic model, age at diagnosis was significantly associated with the likelihood of ongoing menstrual bleeding ($P < 0.01$). There has been a decrease in the odds of bleeding by 24% for each additional year of age.[33] The investigators underscored that this association mostly reflects the progressively depleted follicular reserve in older women.[33]

Importantly, the extent of ovarian damage induced by chemotherapy is variable and can be presented with a variety of symptoms, such as irregular cycles, amenorrhea, or eventual development of primary ovarian insufficiency (POI).[34-38] POI, previously termed as premature ovarian failure (POF), is cessation of ovarian function before the age of 40 and usually presents with amenorrhea, hypergonadotropinism and hypoestrogenism.[39] The first sign of POI is usually missed periods; however, some women may still have irregular cycles. Admittedly, the definition of gonadal dysfunction and chemotherapy-related amenorrhea are not uniform. Therefore, wide variations in the rates of chemotherapy-related amenorrhea are reported.[3]

Furthermore, concerns of decrease in OR exist, even in young survivors with normal menstrual cycles.[40] Changes in ultrasound (ovarian volume and antral follicle counts (AFC)) as well as hormonal (follicle-stimulating hormone (FSH), luteinizing hormone (LH), estradiol (E2), inhibin B and anti-Mullerian hormone (AMH)) markers of OR are reported. Impaired OR in cancer survivors with preserved menstrual cycles was reported.[40-43] Gracia et al. (2012) reported that young menstruating cancer survivors had impaired OR measures, compared to a control group of women in of late reproductive-age.[40]

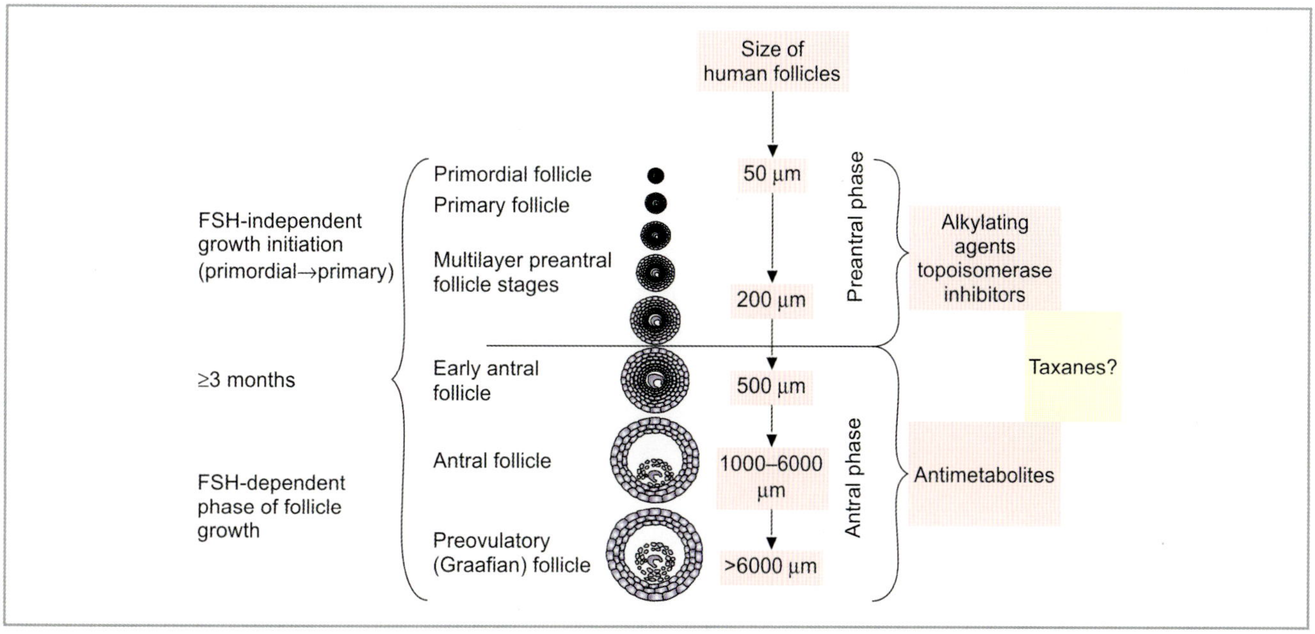

FIGURE 2 Impact of some chemotherapy agents on follicle growth. Alkylating agents and topoisomerase inhibitors affect primordial follicle reserve. Antimetabolites appear to only affect the developing follicles. The impact of taxanes is uncertain. [*Source:* From Rodriguez-Wallberg K, Oktay K. Fertility Preservation and Pregnancy in Women With and Without BRCA Mutation–Positive Breast Cancer. Oncologist. 2012;17(11):1409-17].

Therefore, restoration of menstruation post-chemotherapy does not exclude the later development of POI. On the other hand, there have been reports of cycle resumption after chemotherapy-related amenorrhea. [37,44]

Evaluation of OR appears essential in identifying the degree of gonadal dysfunction. Currently, AMH and AFC are the best markers for evaluating OR.[12,13] They can be used to quantify the degree of ovarian damage after cancer therapy. Early detection of compromised ovarian function in young survivors may allow these patients to start aggressive fertility treatments.[40] Longitudinal studies, however, are needed to determine whether the impairment in these markers truly coincides with the fertility potential and occurrence of pregnancy as well as in the later development of POI.

THE HYPOTHESIS BEHIND MEDICAL APPROACHES

The use of hormone suppression in gonadal function protection is based on the observation that non-cycling cells are more resistant to destruction than are the rapidly proliferating ones. This observation has been the basis for the antitumor action of many of the antineoplastic drugs. Therefore, it has been suggested that suppression of serum FSH concentrations could break the vicious circle of accelerated follicular recruitment and destruction during gonadotoxic treatment.[45] In preliminary studies, suppression of gonadotropins with gonadotropin releasing hormone (GnRH) analogs or oral contraceptive pills (OCPs)[46,47] has been suggested to suppress ovarian function and halt follicular development and division. This suppression has been proposed as a simple, attractive strategy for fertility preservation (**Figure 3**).[45]

Initiation and early stages of follicle growth are gonadotropin-independent;[16] however, other mechanisms have been suggested.[17]

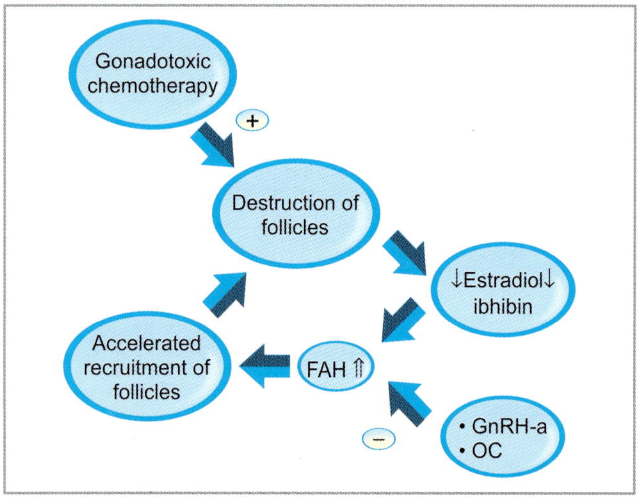

FIGURE 3 Suggested mechanisms for the protective effect of GnRH agonist and OCPs against chemotherapy induced gonadal toxicity. [*Source:* From Blumenfeld Z, von Wolff M. GnRH-analogs and oral contraceptives for fertility preservation in women during chemotherapy. Hum Reprod Update. 2008;4(6):543-52].

PRESERVATION OF OVARIAN FUNCTION WITH THE USE OF GnRH ANALOGS

GnRH and GnRH Analogs

GnRH is the principal hypothalamic regulator of reproductive function. It is a decapeptide hormone responsible for the release of gonadotropins (Gn): FSH and LH from the pituitary gland. GnRH is synthesized in the arcuate nucleus of the hypothalamus and transported via the portal circulation to the anterior pituitary in a pulsatile fashion.[48] Very low levels of GnRH exist during childhood and these levels are increased around puberty. Andrew Schally and Roger Guillemin were the first to isolate and synthesize this hormone in 1971. They were awarded the Nobel Prize in medicine and physiology for their accomplishment in December 1977.[48]

The short half-life of GnRH has evoked an intense effort to synthesize longer acting and more potent GnRH analog preparations for clinical use. GnRH analogs are synthetic peptide drugs, which interact with the GnRH receptors and modify the release of Gn. It was the amino acid substitutions that clarified the importance of specific regions for the activation and stability of pituitary gonadotrophs.[49] There are 2 types of analogs: GnRH agonists and GnRH antagonists.

For GnRH agonists, modifications accomplished mainly at positions 6 and 10 gave rise to its development with an extended half life and increased binding capacity.[50] There are different agonist preparations (Leuprolide, Buserelin, Goserelin, Histrelin, Nafarelin and Triptorelin) with either daily or depot monthly administration. GnRH agonists are not degraded nor dissociate from their receptor rapidly. Therefore, an initial increase in FSH and LH is elicited (flare-up), followed by a profound hypogonadal effect through receptor down-regulation and desensitization.[50,51] Admittedly, the introduction of GnRH agonist preparations in the 1980s and the concept of pituitary desensitization have revolutionized the field of assisted reproductive technology (ART).

After the elucidation of GnRH agonists, a considerable period of time passed before the generation of the clinically used antagonists. The third generation compounds reached the market in 2001. These compounds are more complex than the agonists with many amino acids modifications. These GnRH antagonists bind competitively to the GnRH receptors and prevent endogenous GnRH from exerting its stimulatory effects.[51,52] GnRH antagonists have no intrinsic activity and the initial flare-up, which is present with the GnRH agonists, is avoided and the secretion of gonadotropins decrease within hours.[51,52] There are 2 antagonist preparations (Cetrorelix and Ganirelix) which are administered either daily or every 4 days.

The principal proposed mechanism of GnRH analogs in gonadal protection during chemotherapy is through gonadal suppression, which will be mentioned in further detail later in this chapter. Notably, the occurrence of gonadal suppression with the agonist is achieved within 7 to 14 days, so that the initial increase in gonad activity ("flare") is followed by down-regulation. Therefore, GnRH agonists must be administered

10–14 days before starting chemotherapy to assure suppression. This regimen might not be adhered to in many oncologic illnesses due to time pressures and the need to start early chemotherapy. Indeed, this protocol might limit the use of the agonist for gonadal protection. Alternatively, there is an additional approach to avoid or suppress this flare-up.[53] The combination of GnRH antagonist with GnRH agonist, which would combine the quick onset of action of GnRH antagonist with the long-lasting effects of GnRH agonist, could be a possibility.[53,54]

Proposed Mechanisms for the Use of GnRH Analogs in Ovarian Protection and their Controversy

Induction of a Temporary, Pre-pubertal Hormonal Milieu

Induction of a temporary pre-pubertal hormonal milieu was suggested as the main rationale for the use of GnRH analogs. Chemotherapy induces follicular damage with subsequent decrease in inhibin and estrogen production (**Figure 3**).[45] An increased secretion of FSH is followed by further maturation and recruitment of pre-antral follicles. This will result in further exposure to the gonadotoxic chemotherapy and more acceleration of follicular depletion. Pituitary desensitization will prevent the increase in FSH secretion and stop the vicious circle of further follicular developments and destruction.[55,56]

The development of PMF, which constitutes the main bulk of OR, is a gonadotropin-independent process.[16] Some studies, however, have reported that maturation of PMF is triggered by some growth factors, which are secreted by more mature follicles.[57] These growth factors are induced by FSH; therefore, pituitary desensitization will prevent their release with subsequent non-stimulation of further PMF development.[56,57]

There have been reports that most long-term female survivors have preserved their ovarian function when treated pre-pubertally with gonadotoxic treatment, in contrast to similarly treated adult women.[58,59] Long-term follow-up of 240 children receiving chemotherapy for treating Hodgkin's disease (HD) showed azoospermia in 83% of the boys compared with the development of POI in only 13% of the girls.[58] Similar results were reported by other investigators[60,61] with lower susceptibility of pre-pubertal female gonads to chemotherapy than pre-pubertal male gonads.[58,62] Therefore, developing a hypogonadotropic milieu like that in the pre-pubertal period with the use of analogs appears to be an attractive strategy for preserving gonadal function in adult females.

Other studies, however, reported that pre-pubertal females (or males) are susceptible to the adverse effects of cancer therapies.[17] This finding was also documented in a series of studies emerging from the United States Childhood Cancer Survivor Study (CCSS).[63-65] Increased risks of POI and subsequent reduction of fertility in a large series of 5-year childhood cancer survivors was observed. These studies underscored the increased risk, especially following alkylating agent-based chemotherapy and abdominal pelvic irradiation. Further, the diagnosis of Hodgkin's lymphoma (HL) was associated with a specific adverse effect, which might be related to the immune-regulatory nature of this cancer.[63-65] In the last study of Green et al. (2009) upon 5149 participants, they emphasized the decreasing fertility of young survivors and the strict need for proper counseling of patients and their parents.[65] Larsen et al. (2003) also reported diminished OR in childhood cancer survivors. They suggested that cessation of fertility may occur much earlier than anticipated and focused on the need of adult survivors to plan for early childbearing.[66]

Indeed, the later studies challenge the concept of possible gonadal protection upon the inducement of pre-pubertal hormonal milieu and further clarification of this issue is required.

Decrease in Utero-ovarian Perfusion

GnRH analogs may decrease the utero-ovarian perfusion. This decrease results from the hypo-estrogenic state induced by pituitary-gonadal desensitization.[67,68] In a rat model, high estrogen concentrations were reported to significantly increase ovarian perfusion in dose dependent manner; however, this effect was inhibited by GnRH agonists.[68] Agonist administration will, thus, decrease the utero-ovarian perfusion with resultant lower delivery of the gonadotoxic chemotherapeutic agents to the ovary. The same effect was not tested with the antagonist.

Activation of GnRH Receptors and Direct Effects on Ovarian Follicles

GnRH receptors were detected in human gonads.[69,70] GnRH1 and GnRH2 receptor activation in the ovary were shown to result in decreased apoptosis.[69] There has been a suggestion that GnRH agonists may up-regulate sphingosine-1-phosphate (S1P), an intragonadal anti-apoptotic molecule.[45] Further, in vitro study has demonstrated that GnRH analogs retarded the doxorubicin-induced granulosa cell damage in a dose dependent manner.[71]

On the contrary, a pro-apoptotic effect of GnRH agonists has been suggested in many studies by different mechanisms. Agonists were shown to increase apoptosis incidence in porcine and human cultured granulosa cells and decrease proliferation of in vitro human luteinized granulosa cells.[72] Further, GnRH agonists were shown to induce granulosa-luteal cells apoptosis through activation of caspase-8, -9 and -3 and cleavage of poly-(ADP-ribose)-polymerase (PARP).[73]

Whether the GnRH agonist protects against apoptosis or induces it appears controversial and further studies are needed to answer this question.

For the antagonists, Meirow et al. (2004) demonstrated that prior exposure of mice ovaries to GnRH antagonists had significantly increased the number of surviving PMF upon exposure to cyclophosphamide.[74] Two doses of cyclophosphamide were tested (50 and 75 mg/kg). Higher numbers of PMF were destroyed in the high dose group (35% of PMF were destroyed in the antagonist group, versus 54% in animals treated without it) than the low dose group (14% of PMF were destroyed in the antagonist group, compared with 53% in animals treated without it). The investigators concluded that the antagonist had protected against the gonadotoxic effects of cyclophosphamide. This effect, however, was dose dependent and decreased with the increasing doses of cyclophosphamide. A possible protective effect in women undergoing chemotherapy was suggested.[74]

On the other hand, in a murine model, Danforth et al. (2005) showed that the antagonist did not protect PMF from chemotherapeutic destruction by cyclophosphamide with an almost 50% reduction in PMF. Both antagonists even caused a significant decrease in PMF number without the presence of cyclophosphamide.[75] In accordance, Peng et al. (2007), in a rat model, demonstrated the absence of gonadal protection in the presence of GnRH antagonist.[76]

These observations cast doubt on the possible protective effect of antagonists in minimizing the chemotherapy-associated gonadotoxicity. Further, an important question is whether the initial co-administration of the antagonist to the agonist for reducing the flare-up could adversely affect its possible protective role. These concerns, however, remain theoretical and prospective evaluation in human is warranted.

Studies Using GnRH Agonists for Ovarian Protection

GnRH agonists are accessible drugs with easy administration as well as relatively few side effects. Indeed, the use of these agents for gonadal protection appears to be a simple and attractive option, especially in comparison to the other alternative strategies, including in vitro fertilization and embryo cryopreservation before treatment.

Agonist use was tested in animals first. Glode and colleagues (1981) were the first to test this hypothesis in male mice and reported that agonists appeared to protect the gonads from cyclophosphamide.[77] In female rats, Ataya and colleagues (1985) also reported a protective effect of agonists in preventing chemotherapy-induced ovarian damage.[46] In rhesus monkeys, Ataya and colleagues (1995) demonstrated that agonists had protected the ovaries from the damaging effect of cyclophosphamide and had significantly decreased the number of lost non-primordial follicles and PMF.[35] The same group also reported an absence of protective effect of GnRH agonist co-treatment against radiation-induced ovarian damage in rhesus monkeys,[78] which was consistent with the reported results in rodents.[79] Letterie (2004), however, in a mouse study did not find evidence that suppression of the ovaries by either agonists or OCPs conferred any protection against cyclophosphamide-induced gonadal toxicity.[80]

Importantly, it appears from basic studies that some of the principles applied in animals do not necessarily apply in humans.[55,62] There are lower concentrations of human ovarian GnRH receptors[55,62] and the human ovary might not respond in the same way as experimental animal models. Many studies evaluated the efficacy of GnRH agonists in protecting the ovaries from chemotherapy. Co-administration of agonists were tested in different indications, whether hemato-oncology, breast cancer or even non-malignant diseases, requiring chemotherapy as autoimmune diseases.

There have been many non-randomized trials, some of which reported beneficial impact for agonist addition,[81-85] while other studies have failed to show any protective effect[86-89] (**Table 2**).

Limitations exist to these studies and the main drawback is non-randomization.[90] The control groups consisted of women treated with similar chemotherapy or historical controls without agonist co-treatment. Different age groups, chemotherapy regimens, and doses might have contributed to the inconsistent results. Basal characteristics and chemotherapy regimens did not even match between the study and control groups in some studies. Treatment protocols were different between the control and study groups in the study of Pereyra Pacheco et al. (2001).[81] In another study, the control group had longer disease duration than the study group.[82] Additionally, markers of OR were not highlighted in many of these studies.[90]

It appears that data from both human and animal studies is controversial. Biological plausibility of fertility preservation by GnRH agonists was questioned[24,91] and the need for urgently performing randomized controlled trials (RCTs) has been emphasized.[24]

TABLE 2 Non-randomized studies on the use of GnRH agonists for gonadal protection.

Study	*Age group*	*GnRH agonist*	*Control*
Pereyra Pacheco et al. 2001 (Lymphoma, Leukemia)	14–20	0% (0/12)	100%(4/4)
Dann et al. 2005 (Non-HL)	18–40	0% (0/7)	17% (1/6)
Somers et al. 2005 (SLE)	24–28	5.0% (1/20)	30.0%(6/20)
Elis et al. 2006 (Non-HL)	17–40	0% (0/3)	8.7% (2/24)
Castelo-Branco et al. 2007 (HL)	14–45	10.0%(3/30)	76.9%(20/26)
Blumenfeld et al. 2008 (HL, Non-HL)	14–40	3.1% (2/65)	63.0%(29/46)
Huser et al. 2008 (HL)	18–35	20.8%(15/72)	71.1%(32/45)
Azem et al. 2008 (HL)	20-40	0%(0/9)	30.7%(4/13)
Nitzschke et al. 2010 (HL)	???		

Abbreviation: SLE. Systemic lupus erythematosus.

GnRH AGONIST: HUMAN RANDOMIZED CONTROLLED TRIALS

Waxman et al. (1987) were the first to perform a RCT with 18 women, between the ages of 17 and 46, who had HL.[92] One chemotherapy regimen was used in all women. Four of the 8 women in the study group were amenorrheic, while 6 of the 8 women in the control group were amenorrheic. The investigators concluded that agonist co-treatment was ineffective in protection against chemotherapy-induced gonadal toxicity.

Gilani et al. (2007) performed a RCT with 30 women, between the ages of 12 and 40, with different ovarian tumors.[93] Different chemotherapy regimens were used. None of the 15 women in the study group were amenorrheic, while 5 women in the control group were amenorrheic. The investigators reported that the agonist could have a protective effect against gonadal damage.

Giuseppe et al. (2007) randomly allocated 29 women, between the ages of 20 and 38, with HD to chemotherapy alone or chemotherapy with an agonist.[94] Different chemotherapy regimens were used. None of the 14 women in the agonist group had amenorrhea, while 8 of the 15 women in the control group were amenorrheic. OR parameters (tested by FSH, LH, inhibin B, AMH and AFC) were comparable between both groups. They concluded that a GnRH agonist could delay ovarian failure development, but that it does not protect the OR.

Sverrisdottir et al. (2009) performed a RCT with women who had pre-menopausal breast cancer.[95] One regimen of chemotherapy was used. All patients were randomly assigned to receive 2 years of: (a) an agonist (n=63), (b) an agonist plus tamoxifen (n=74), (c) tamoxifen alone (n= 60), or (d) no endocrine treatment (n=63). One year after complete therapy, 36% of the women in the agonist group reported menses, compared to 7% in the agonist plus tamoxifen group, 13% in the tamoxifen group and 10% of the control group. There was some evidence of a protective effect of the agonist on ovarian function; meanwhile, this effect was absent in the combined tamoxifen and agonist treatment.

Badawy et al. (2009) performed a RCT with 80 women, between the ages of 18 and 40, who had breast cancer (hormone positive and negative). One regimen of chemotherapy was used.[96] In the agonist/chemotherapy group, 89.6% resumed menses while 33.3% in the control group resumed menses 8 months after the end of chemotherapy. At 6 months after the end of agonist/chemotherapy, FSH and LH levels were significantly lower in the agonist group. The investigators reported a beneficial effect for agonist co-administration for protecting gonadal function.

Gerber et al. (2011) performed a multi-center RCT with 60 patients, who had hormone-insensitive breast cancer (ZORO study, Zoladex Rescue of Ovarian Function).[97] All women were younger than age 46 and were allocated to receive anthracycline/cyclophosphamide chemotherapy with or without an agonist. Reappearance of menstruation was comparable between both groups at 6 months after chemotherapy (70.0% with an agonist versus 56.7% without an agonist). All patients except only 1 woman reported regular menses 2 years after chemotherapy. Decrease in OR, evidenced by decreasing inhibin B and AMH levels, was detected in both groups. It was concluded that agonist co-administration to chemotherapy had no protective effect against gonadal toxicity.

Del Mastro et al. (2011) also performed a multicenter RCT with 281 patients, between the ages of 18 and 45, with hormone positive and negative breast cancer.[98] Multiple regimens of chemotherapy were used and only 12 of the 281 women received cyclophosphamide-based chemotherapy. Incidence of early menopause (defined in the study as absent menstruation and postmenopausal levels of FSH and E2 1 year after the end of chemotherapy) was evaluated in both groups. Early menopause was reported in 25.9% of the control group and in 8.9% of the study group. The investigators concluded that ovarian suppression during chemotherapy reduced the occurrence of chemotherapy-induced early menopause.

Munster et al. (2012) performed a RCT with women aged ≤44 years who had early-stage breast cancer.[99] Participants were stratified by age (<35, 35 to 39, >39 years), regimen of chemotherapy and estrogen receptor status. The study attempted to target 124 patients with a planned follow-up for 5 years. The trial, however, was stopped for futility after the enrollment of 49 patients. Nineteen (90%) of 21 patients in the control group had resumed menses, compared to 23 (88%) patients of 26 patients in the study group. Menses returned after a median of 5.8 and 5 months in the study group and control group, respectively. Inhibin B and FSH were correlated with menstrual status. The investigators concluded that amenorrhea rates were comparable between those taking agonist/chemotherapy and chemotherapy only, when stratified for age, treatment regimen and estrogen receptor status.

Demeestere et al. (2012) performed a multicenter RCT with women, between the ages of 18 and 45, treated for HL and non-HL.[100] Alkylating agents containing chemotherapy was used in all groups. POF rate, defined as FSH ≥ 40 IU/L after 1 year of follow-up, was the primary outcome. Eighty-four of 129 randomly assigned patients completed the 1 year follow-up. POF was exhibited in 20% and 19% of patients in the agonist and control groups. Good FSH levels (<10IU/L) were reported in more than half of patients in each group; however, AMH levels were higher in the agonist group than in the control group. The investigators concluded that about 20% of women developed POF after 1 year of chemotherapy, irrespective of the agonist co-administration. Further, it was suggested that agonists probably had a protective effect on OR.[100]

Elgindy et al. (2013), in a multi-center RCT, evaluated the effectiveness of not only GnRH agonist co-treatment, but also GnRH antagonist/agonist co-administration in the prevention of chemotherapy-induced amenorrhea.[54] One hundred hormone-insensitive breast cancer participants, between the ages of 18 and 40, undergoing one regimen of cyclophosphamide-based chemotherapy were included. The protocol of analog co-treatment was dependent on the available time until the start of chemotherapy. Participants ready for early chemotherapy (n=50) were randomly allocated to either chemotherapy alone or chemotherapy after down-regulation (E2 <50 pg/mL) by both antagonist and agonist. For chemotherapy planned to start at least 10 days later, 50 women were randomly allocated to either chemotherapy alone or chemotherapy after down-regulation with agonist. At 12 months after the end of chemotherapy, there were no significant differences in menstruation resumption between analog co-treated patients and their respective controls. Amenorrhea ranged from 16% to 20% in the 4 studied groups. No significant differences existed in hormonal (FSH, LH, E2 and AMH) and ultrasound (AFC) markers of OR between analog users and control groups. Seventeen women in each group were followed up at 18 months after the end of chemotherapy, with no significant differences regarding cycle resumption and regularity as well as OR parameters. The investigators concluded that GnRH analog co-treatment did not offer a significant protective effect on ovarian function in patients treated by cyclophosphamide-based chemotherapy.

In all of these RCTs, inconsistent results existed regarding the efficacy of agonist co-administration in ovarian protection. Variations in age, chemotherapy regimens and the variable primary end points (whether amenorrhea or POF), might explain these differences. Additionally, different length and method of follow-up were reported.

Furthermore, the use of tamoxifen in women with hormone positive breast cancer is another confounding factor. Tamoxifen does not have a detrimental effect on fertility; but, it has an effect on menstrual resumption and was reported to cause amenorrhea.[4,95,101] The study of Badawy et al. (2009)[96] was criticized as the analysis did not control for tamoxifen use. This failure might have confounded the amenorrhea rate in the control group in addition to the short follow-up time of 8 months. Only the studies of Elgindy et al. (2013) and ZORO included hormone-insensitive breast cancer participants without the confounding use of tamoxifen.[54,97] The study of Munster et al. (2012) was acknowledged due to stratification of participants by the important predictors.[99] Nevertheless, the premature end of the study might have limitations.

OR markers, measured at baseline and serially in follow-up visits, appear to decline in all groups over time. Demeestere et al. (2012) reported that AMH, one of the best markers for OR prediction, was relatively spared upon agonist co-treatment;[100] other investigators, however, did not find evidence to support that report.[54,94,97]

GnRH AGONIST FOR GONADAL PROTECTION: CURRENT EVIDENCE

Kim et al. (2010), in a systematic review and meta-analysis of 11 published studies, showed a favorable effect for agonist co-treatment in gonadal protection.[90] The separate analysis, however, of the 3 included RCTs[92,94,96] failed to prove the statistically significant protective effects of the agonist co-treatment. The investigators emphasized that the results are influenced by non-randomized studies and they underscored the need for more RCTs.

Bedaiwy et al. (2011),[102] in a systematic review and meta-analysis of 6 RCTs,[92-96,103] reported a potential benefit of agonist co-treatment. The overall conclusion was that GnRH-a is beneficial based on the available evidence at the time of publication. Despite this conclusion, the meta-analysis is limited by the inherent weakness of 2 of the included trials. The larger of these 2 studies was by Badawy et al. (2009), [96] which was criticized for significant methodological weaknesses.[104,105] The other study was the ZORO trial that showed a benefit of GnRH analog co-treatment, only at the 6 month follow-up. However, when the 2 year follow-up became available, it did not show a difference in menstrual resumption between agonists and control groups.

In an informative letter to the editor, Balkenende et al. (2011) performed a new meta-analysis for the studies in Bedaiwy et al.'s meta-analysis, but with the exclusion of the controversial study and the inclusion of the 2 year follow-up in the ZORO study.[105] According to this new meta-analysis, the potential benefit of GnRH agonist was excluded (OR = 2.25, 95% CI, 0.65–7.78) in contrast to the original meta-analysis (OR 3.46; 95% CI 1.13–10.57).

A Cochrane review by Chen et al. (2011) reported that GnRH agonists could be effective in protecting ovaries during chemotherapy.[23] This review included 4 RCTs. [92-94,96] However, the largest one of these studies, with 80 women from the study of Badawy et al. (2009),[96] was the one with some inherent weaknesses.[104,105] Furthermore, the sum of women in the 3 remaining studies was.[77]

Many of the RCTs in recent years are not yet included in meta-analyses. Additionally, there are other ongoing trials such as the OPTION (Ovarian Protection Trial In Estrogen Negative) trial[106] and the SWOG (Southwest Oncology Group) study[107] on women with hormone receptor-negative breast cancer. Preliminary data from the OPTION trial were presented at the 46th Annual Meeting of the ASCO. The data of 87 women, younger than 40 years old, were presented. There was an absence of menstruation in 34.7% of participants in the agonist co-treatment group compared to 15.8% in the chemotherapy-only group. The conclusion was an absence of clear benefit regarding menstrual resumption in women having ovarian suppression during chemotherapy.[106] The results of the SWOG study have not yet been reported and will undoubtedly, with the completed OPTION trial, provide additional complementary information for our evolving understanding of the potential role of ovarian suppression during gonadotoxic treatment.

STUDIES USING GnRH ANTAGONISTS FOR OVARIAN PROTECTION

Use of Antagonist in Combination with the Agonist for Gonadal Protection

Initially, GnRH antagonists were used in combination with agonists to achieve faster down-regulation and avoid the 10–14 day delay before the start of chemotherapy. Then, the antagonist is stopped with continuation of the agonist co-treatment with chemotherapy.

Mardesic et al. (2004) have evaluated this combination, in 6 postmenarchal young participants (aged 15.4 ± 0.7 years) with hematological malignancies.[108] Down-regulation of LH was reported in all 6 patients within 96 hours. The investigators concluded that this combination had induced a rapid, reliable, and cost-effective gonadal suppression. They emphasized the need to monitor gonadal function of treated patients. Notably, a historical group of healthy patients was used and both groups were compared regarding LH concentration.

Nahari et al. (2007) tried to test this combination in 9 young patients (aged ≤35 years) receiving different chemotherapy regimens for different malignant diseases and medical conditions.[108] GnRH agonist and antagonist were administered with chemotherapy. A GnRH antagonist was given for the first 2 weeks and then stopped with continuation of ovarian suppression using a GnRH agonist. Menstruation was resumed in 8 patients (88.9%), within 3–11 months after the end of chemotherapy. Normal levels of FSH, LH and E2 were also regained in 8 patients (88.9%) within this time. The investigators underscored the beneficial impact of using combined GnRH agonists and antagonists in preserving ovarian function during chemotherapy. Notably, there are 2 limitations in this study. First, there was no control group. Second, patients received simultaneous GnRH agonist, GnRH antagonist and chemotherapy. Importantly, the classic flare-up effect associated with GnRH agonists cannot be suppressed with the first dose of GnRH antagonist and it could be of concern to give chemotherapy at that time.

Von Wolff et al. (2010) tried to study in detail the occurrence of ovarian suppression with GnRH analoges in 24 patients treated with different chemotherapy regimens due to different indications.[53] Patients planned to start chemotherapy within 4 to 7 days after GnRH agonist administration were given daily GnRH antagonists (cetrorelix 0.25 mg/day) for 6 days (group I, n=13). For patients where chemotherapy was planned to start later than 7 days after the agonist administration, GnRH antagonists were not added (group II, n=11). Levels of FSH, LH and E2 were measured on the day of the GnRH-agonist administration (day 0) and on days 2, 4, 6 and 8. Two main results were reported. First, there was a significant reduction in FSH increase on day 2 after the antagonist/agonist combination compared with the agonist only. Second, the reduction did not occur in all patients and it took about 6 days for down-regulation to occur.[54] This study did not evaluate the impact of analoge co-treatment on ovarian function. However, its findings highlight the variable time for achieving down-regulation even after antagonist co-administration.

The only RCT testing the possible value of antagonist/agonist co-treatment was the study by Elgindy and colleagues (2013),[54] mentioned earlier in this chapter. The antagonist/agonist combination neither increased the rate of menstrual resumption, nor preserved the OR parameters at one year after the end of chemotherapy. Notably, the addition of antagonists to agonists neither improved nor averted the resumption of menses in comparison with the control group. The concern that the antagonist might have suppressive effects on the ovary[75] appears hypothetical. Indeed, such an effect would question all ART therapies, which are increasingly using antagonists nowadays.

Use of Antagonist Only for Gonadal Protection

There are only 2 preliminary non-RCTs. The first pilot study by Whitehead et al. (2011) included 18 women, aged 18 to 35 years, treated with chemotherapy due to cancer or an autoimmune disease.[110] Three doses of 250 ug GnRH antagonist were used, every 4 days, over 12 days, starting 1 to 4 days, prior to starting each chemotherapy cycle (where possible) and for the duration of their chemotherapy. Resumption of spontaneous menses occurred in 94% (14/15) of women within 12 months after the end of chemotherapy, although 3 women did not complete this pilot study. The investigators suggested that antagonist co-administration may have protected ovarian function during chemotherapy.

The second study by Digeni et al. (2012) evaluated the use of antagonist co-treatment in patients with a hematologic malignancy.[111] Twenty-four women with a mean age of 23.3± 6.4 years were included. Various cytotoxic agents, including cyclophosphamide, were administered to participants with 3 mg of cetrorelix, every second day. Data were compared with a historical group. Six months after cessation of treatment, 4.3% of the antagonist co-treatment group had absent menstruation versus 27.3% in the historical control. No significant differences were observed between the 2 groups in the levels of FSH, E2, and AMH after completion of chemotherapy. The investigators concluded that the GnRH antagonist appeared to decrease the incidence of secondary amenorrhea post-chemotherapy; however, it did not give full protection of ovarian function.

Notably, the 2 studies appear to have limitations. The first study is preliminary upon a small number of patients without a control group.[110] Meanwhile, the second study had historical controls and only 6 months of follow-up were reported after the end of chemotherapy.[111] The cetrorelix protocol of administration varied between the 2 studies with insufficient data about its optimal use. Admittedly, the investigators in the second study had emphasized the need for adjustment of cetrorelix administration. They also underscored the need for future large RCTs for proper evaluation.[111]

THE USE OF ORAL CONTRACEPTIVES FOR OVARIAN PROTECTION

Chapman and Sutcliffe (1981) were the first to study whether ovarian function suppression by OCPs would protect the ovary from gonadotoxic chemotherapy.[47] Six young women, aged 18 to 31-years-old, with HD were included and had taken OCPs at the start of chemotherapy. Three women underwent ovarian biopsy, 6 to 12 weeks, after the last cycle and menstrual history was followed up to 20–29 months after the end of chemotherapy. Resumption of menses was reported in all women and PMF as well as primary follicles were comparable in the 3 women having ovarian biopsies before and after therapy.

In contrast, Whitehead et al. (1983) did not find evidence to support that result in a larger study of 44 adult females treated for HD.[112] Median age at treatment was 23 years old and the time of follow-up ranged from 6 months to 10 years (median, 30 months) after the end of chemotherapy. Nine women took the OCPs throughout chemotherapy; however, amenorrhea and oligo-menorrhea occurred in 4 and 3 women respectively. The investigators emphasized the absence of an apparent protective role for OCPs in chemotherapy-induced ovarian damage.

In accordance, Longhi et al. (2003) tried to study the concomitant use of OCPs in a larger group of osteosarcoma patients receiving chemotherapy.[113] Early chemotherapy-induced menopause occurred in 3 out of 19 post-pubertal patients who received the OCPs and in 3 out of 71 post-pubertal patients in the control group. Furthermore, 2 patients had thrombophlebitis in the OCP group, which might be attributed to the increased thrombophilic tendency caused by both OCPs and chemotherapy. No delay in menarche was seen in pre-pubertal patients in both groups. The investigators underscored that age and chemotherapy doses are the most important predictors for early menopause, whereas OCPs did not appear to have a protective role for the ovary.[113]

Elis et al. (2006) also tried to evaluate the fertility status of 36 women, aged ≤ 40 years, treated for non-HL with cyclophosphamide-based chemotherapy.[87] Three patients received GnRH agonists, while 9 patients received OCPs with chemotherapy. Menses was resumed in all participants except in two 40-year-old women. Resumption of menstruation, cycle regularity and pregnancy were comparable between all groups. The investigators emphasized the low incidence of gonadal dysfunction among young women, so that fertility-preserving modalities are not needed.

Behringer et al. (2005) studied the menstrual status of 405 patients younger than 40 years treated for advanced-stage HL.[114] One hundred forty-nine participants underwent OCP co-treatment with chemotherapy. A statistical association was reported between the use of OCPs and menstrual resumption. The investigators, however, emphasized the need for a properly conducted RCT for further investigation.

The German Hodgkin Study Group (GHSG) investigated the use of GnRH agonists and OCPs in young women, aged 18 to 40 years, with advanced HL.[115] Participants were randomly assigned to receive either daily OCPs or monthly agonist during cyclophosphamide-based chemotherapy. Premature closure of the study was done after an interim analysis of 12 and 11 patients in the OCP and agonist co-treatment groups, respectively. The median age was 25 years in both groups and AMH was reduced in all participants at ≥ 12 months after the end of chemotherapy. The ovarian follicle preservation rate was 0% (95% CI, 0% to 12%) in the entire study cohort. The investigators concluded that hormonal co-treatment during chemotherapy did not offer protection of the OR. They emphasized the need for alternative strategies for protecting fertility in these women.

ETHICAL ISSUES CONCERNING FERTILITY PRESERVATION IN CANCER PATIENTS

The ASCO 2006 has emphasized that the 2 methods of fertility preservation with the highest likelihood of success among cancer survivors are sperm cryopreservation for males and embryos freezing for females.[11] Other approaches, however, should be considered investigational and need further evaluation. Patrizio and Caplan (2010) also underscored that all of the available approaches for fertility preservation are considered experimental, except for embryo and semen freezing.[1] More recently, the ASRM reconsidered its opinion that oocyte cryopreservation was experimental and now considers it a viable option for fertility preservation.[116] Depending on investigational fertility preservation strategies, including medical approaches raises ethical issues.

CONCLUSION

Currently, the role of ovarian suppression for fertility preservation during chemotherapy remains uncertain. The value of this strategy is not established, with an absence of rigorous data demonstrating the actual improvement in gonadal function upon its suppression with various treatments. Given the current level of evidence, medical approaches for fertility preservation should be considered experimental. Results from ongoing RCTs and firm evidence are awaited to have a better understanding on the role of ovarian suppression during chemotherapy as a viable fertility preservation option.

REFERENCES

1. Patrizio P, Caplan AL. Ethical issues surrounding fertility preservation in cancer patients. Clin Obstet Gynecol. 2010;53(4):717-26.
2. Jemal A, Siegel R, Xu J, Ward E. Cancer Statistics, 2010. CA Cancer J Clin. 2010;60:277-300.
3. Bines J, Oleske DM, Cobleigh MA. Ovarian function in premenopausal women treated with adjuvant chemotherapy for breast cancer. J Clin Oncol. 1996;14:1718-29.
4. Goodwin PJ, Ennis M, Pritchard KI, et al. Risk of menopause during the first year after breast cancer diagnosis. J Clin Oncol. 1999;17: 2365-70.
5. Donnez J, Martinez-Madrid B, Jadoul P, et al. Ovarian tissue cryopreservation and transplantation: a review. Hum Reprod Update. 2006;12:519-35.
6. Schover LR. Patient attitudes toward fertility preservation. Pediatr Blood Cancer. 2009;53:281-4.
7. Brydoy M, Fossa SD, Dahl O, Bjoro T. Gonadal dysfunction and fertility problems in cancer survivors. Acta Oncol. 2007;46:480-9.
8. Partridge AH, Gelber S, Peppercorn J, et al. Web-based survey of fertility issues in young women with breast cancer. J Clin Oncol. 2004;22:4174-83.

9. Avis NE, Crawford S, Manuel J. Psychosocial problems among younger women with breast cancer. Psychooncology. 2004;13:295-308.
10. Degner LF, Kristjanson LJ, Bowman D, et al. Information needs and decisional preferences in women with breast cancer. J Am Med Assoc. 1997;277:1485-92.
11. Lee SJ, Schover LR, Partridge AH, et al.; American Society of Clinical Oncology. American Society of Clinical Oncology recommendations on fertility preservation in cancer patients. J Clin Oncol. 2006;24(18):2917-31.
12. Broekmans FJ, Kwee J, Hendriks DJ, et al. A systematic review of tests predicting ovarian reserve and IVF outcome. Hum Reprod Update. 2006;12:685-718.
13. Broer SL, Mol BW, Hendriks D, Broekmans FJ. The role of antimullerian hormone in prediction of outcome after IVF: comparison with the antral follicle count. Fertil Steril. 2009;91:705-14.
14. Lass A, Silye R, Abrams DC, et al. Follicular density in ovarian biopsy of infertile women: a novel method to assess ovarian reserve. Hum Reprod. 1997;12:1028-31.
15. Oktay K, Nugent D, Newton H, et al. Isolation and characterization of primordial follicles from fresh and cryopreserved human ovarian tissue. Fertil Steril. 1997;67:481-6.
16. McGee E, Hsueh A. Initial and Cyclic Recruitment of Ovarian Follicles. Endocr Reviews. 2000;21(2):200-14.
17. Anderson R, Wallace W. Fertility preservation in girls and young women. Clin Endocrinol. 2011;75(4):409-19.
18. Wallace WH, Anderson RA, Irvine DS. Fertility preservation for young patients with cancer: who is at risk and what can be offered? Lancet Oncol. 2005;6:209-18.
19. Wallace WH, Thomson AB, Kelsey TW. The radiosensitivity of the human oocyte. Hum Reprod. 2003;18:117-21.
20. Bath LE, Critchley HO, Chambers SE, et al. Ovarian and uterine characteristics after total body irradiation in childhood and adolescence: response to sex steroid replacement. Br J Obstet Gynaecol. 1999;106:1265-72.
21. Hall JE, Martin KA, Whitney HA, et al. Potential for fertility with replacement of hypothalamic gonadotropin-releasing hormone in long term female survivors of cranial tumors. J Clin Endocrinol Metab. 1994;79:1166-72.
22. Meirow D, Biederman H, Anderson RA, Wallace WH. Toxicity of chemotherapy and radiation on female reproduction. Clin Obstet Gynecol. 2010;53: 727-39.
23. Chen H, Li J, Cui T, Hu L. Adjuvant gonadotropin-releasing hormone analoges for the prevention of chemotherapy induced premature ovarian failure in premenopausal women (Review). Cochrane Database Systematic Reviews. 2011, Issue 11. Art. No.: CD008018.
24. Sonmezer M, Oktay K. Fertility Preservation in Young Women Undergoing Breast Cancer Therapy. Oncologist. 2006;11(5):422-34.
25. Fornier MN, Modi S, Panageas KS, et al. Incidence of chemotherapy-induced, long-term amenorrhea in patients with breast carcinoma age 40 years and younger after adjuvant anthracycline and taxanes. Cancer. 2005;104:1575-79.
26. Davis AL, Klitus M, Mintzer DM. Chemotherapy-induced amenorrhea from adjuvant breast cancer treatment: the effect of addition of taxanes. Clin Breast Cancer. 2005;6:421-4.
27. Martin M, Pienkowski T, Mackey J, et al. Adjuvant docetaxel for node-positive breast cancer. N Engl J Med. 2005;352:2302-13.
28. Rodriguez-Wallberg K, Oktay K. Fertility Preservation and Pregnancy in Women With and Without BRCA Mutation–Positive Breast Cancer. Oncologist. 2012;17(11):1409-17.
29. Oktem O, Oktay K. A novel ovarian xenografting model to characterize the impact of chemotherapy agents on human primordial follicle reserve. Cancer Res. 2007;67:10159-62.
30. Meirow D, Lewis H, Nugent D, Epstein M. Subclinical depletion of primordial follicular reserve in mice treated with cyclophosphamide: clinical importance and proposed accurate investigative tool. Hum Reprod. 1999;14:1903-7.
31. Sonmezer M, Oktay K. Fertility preservation in female patients. HumReprod Update. 2004;10:251-66.
32. Sukumvanich P, Case LD, Van Zee K, et al. Incidence and time course of bleeding after longterm amenorrhea after breast cancer treatment: A prospective study. Cancer. 2010;116:3102-11.
33. Petrek JA, Naughton MJ, Case LD, et al. Incidence, time course, and determinants of menstrual bleeding after breast cancer treatment: a prospective study. J Clin Oncol. 2006;24:1045-51.
34. Ataya K, Moghissi K. Chemotherapy-induced premature ovarian failure: mechanisms and prevention. Steroids. 1989;54:607-26.
35. Ataya K, Rao LV, Lawrence E, Kimmel R. Luteinizing hormone-releasing hormone agonist inhibits cyclophosphamide-induced ovarian follicular depletion in rhesus monkeys. Biol Reprod. 1995;52:365-72.
36. Blumenfeld Z, Avivi I, Linn S, et al. Prevention of irreversible chemotherapy induced ovarian damage in young women with lymphoma by a gonadotropin-releasing hormone agonist in parallel to chemotherapy. Hum Reprod. 1996;11(8):1620-26.
37. Lutchman Singh K, Davies M, Chatterjee R. Fertility in female cancer survivors: pathophysiology, preservation and the role of ovarian reserve testing. Hum Reprod Update. 2005;11:69-89.
38. Meirow D, Nugent D. The effects of radiotherapy and chemotherapy on female reproduction. Hum Reprod Update. 2001;7:535-43.
39. Robert R. Premature ovarian failure. Obstet Gynecol. 2009;113(6): 1355-63.
40. Gracia C, Sammel M, Freeman E, et al. Impact of cancer therapies on ovarian reserve. Fertil Steril. 2012;97:134-40.
41. Larsen EC, Muller J, Schmiegelow K, et al. Reduced ovarian function in long-term survivors of radiation- and chemotherapy-treated childhood cancer. J Clin Endocrinol Metab. 2003;88:5307-14.
42. Lie Fong S, Lugtenburg PJ, Schipper I, et al. Anti-Mullerian hormone as a marker of ovarian function in women after chemotherapy and radiotherapy for haematological malignancies. Hum Reprod. 2008;23:674-78.
43. Lie Fong S, Laven JS, Hakvoort-Cammel FG, et al. Assessment of ovarian reserve in adult childhood cancer survivors using anti-Mullerian hormone. Hum Reprod. 2009;24:982-90.
44. Byrne J, Fears TR, Gail MH, et al. Early menopause in long-term survivors of cancer during adolescence. Am J Obstet Gynecol. 1992;166:788-93.
45. Blumenfeld Z, von Wolff M. GnRH-analoges and oral contraceptives for fertility preservation in women during chemotherapy. Hum Reprod Update. 2008;14 (6): 543-52.
46. Ataya M, McKanna JA, Weintraub AM, et al. A luteinizing hormone-releasing hormone agonist for the prevention of chemotherapy-induced ovarian follicular loss in rats. Cancer Research. 1985;45: 3651-56.
47. Chapman RM, Sutcliffe SB. Protection of ovarian function by oral contraceptives in women receiving chemotherapy for Hodgkin's disease. Blood. 1981;58:849-51.
48. Weissman A, Shoham Z. GnRH and its agonistic analoges: basic knowledge. In: Shoham Z, Howles CM, and Jacobs HS (Eds.) Female Infertility Therapy Current Practice. Martin Dunitz Ltd. Press. 1999: 157-66.
49. Schally AV. Luteinizing hormone-releasing hormone analogs: their impact on the control of tumorigenesis. Peptides. 1999;20: 1247-62.
50. Conn PM, Crowley WF Jr. Gonadotropin-releasing hormone andits analogs. Ann Review Med. 1994;45:391-405.
51. Couzinet B, Lahlou N, Thomas G, et al. Effects of gonadotrophin releasing hormone antagonist and agonist on the pulsatile release of gonadotropins and alpha-subunit in postmenopausal women. Clin Endocrinol. 1991;34:477-83.

52. Matikainen T, Ding YQ, Vergara M, et al. Differing responses of plasma bioactive and immunoreactive follicle-stimulating hormone antagonist and agonist treatments in postmenopausal women. J Clin Endocrinol Metabol. 1992;75:820-5.
53. Von Wolff M, Kämmerer U, Kollmann Z, et al. Combination of gonadotropin-releasing hormone (GnRH) agonists with GnRH antagonists before chemotherapy reduce but does not completely prevent a follicle-stimulating hormone flare-up. Fertil Steril. 2011;95:452-4.
54. Elgindy E, El-Haieg D, Khorshid O, et al. Gonadatropin Suppression to Prevent Chemotherapy-Induced Ovarian Damage. A Randomized Controlled Trial. Obstet Gynecol. 2013;121(1):78-86.
55. Lobo RA. Potential options for preservation of fertility in women. N Engl J Med. 2005;353:64-73.
56. Blumenfeld Z. How to preserve fertility in young women exposed to chemotherapy? The role of GnRH agonist cotreatment in addition to cryopreservation of embrya, oocytes, or ovaries. Oncologist. 2007;12:1044-54.
57. Knight PG, Glister C. TGF-beta superfamily members and ovarian follicle development. Reprod. 2006;132:191-206.
58. Ortin TT, Shostak CA, Donaldson SS. Gonadal status and reproductive function following treatment for Hodgkin's disease in childhood: The Stanford experience. Int J Radiol Oncol Biol Phys. 1990;19:873-80.
59. Blumenfeld Z. Gender difference: fertility preservation in young women but not in men exposed to gonadotoxic chemotherapy. Minerva Endocrinol. 2007;32:23-34.
60. Blumenfeld Z, Avivi I, Ritter M, Rowe JM. Preservation of fertility and ovarian function and minimizing chemotherapy-induced gonadotoxicity in young women. J Soc Gynecol Investig. 1999;6: 229-39.
61. Chiarelli AM, Marrett LD, Darlington G. Early menopause and infertility in females after treatment for childhood cancer diagnosed in 1964-1988 in Ontario, Canada. Am J Epidemiology. 1999;150: 245-54.
62. Blumenfeld Z. Gynecologic concerns for young women exposed to gonadotoxic chemotherapy. Curr Opin Obstet Gynecol. 2003;15: 359-70.
63. Chemaitilly W, Mertens AC, Mitby P, et al. Acute ovarian failure in the childhood cancer survivor study. J Clin Endocrinol Metabol. 2006; 91:1723-28.
64. Sklar CA, Mertens AC, Mitby P, et al. Premature menopause in survivors of childhood cancer: a report from the childhood cancer survivor study. J Nat Cancer Instit. 2006;98:890-6.
65. Green DM, Kawashima T, Stovall M, et al. Fertility of female survivors of childhood cancer: a report from the childhood cancer survivor study. J Clin Oncol. 2009;27(16):2677-85.
66. Larsen EC, Müller J, Rechnitzer C, et al. Diminished ovarian reserve in female childhood cancer survivors with regular menstrual cycles and basal FSH <10 IU/l. Hum Reprod. 2003;18(2):417-22.
67. Saitta A, Altavilla D, Cucinotta D, et al. Randomized, double-blind, placebo-controlled study on effects of raloxifene and hormone replacement therapy on plasma NO concentrations, endothelin-1 levels, and endotheliumdependent vasodilation in postmenopausal women. Arterioscler Thromb Vasc Biol. 2001;21:1512-19.
68. Kitajima Y, Endo T, Nagasawa K, et al. Hyperstimulation and a gonadotropin-releasing hormone agonist modulate ovarian vascular permeability by altering expression of the tight junction protein claudin-5. Endocrinol. 2006;147:694-9.
69. Grundker C, Emons G. Role of gonadotropin-releasing hormone (GnRH) in ovarian cancer. Reprod Biol Endocrinol. 2003;1:65-71.
70. Harrison GS, Wierman ME, Nett TM, Glode LM. Gonadotropin-releasing hormone and its receptor in normal and malignant cells. Endocr Relat Cancer. 2004;11:725-48
71. Imai A, Sugiyama M, Furui T, et al. Direct protection by a gonadotropin releasing hormone analog from doxorubicin-induced granulosa cell damage. Gynecol Obstet Invest. 2007;63:102-6.
72. Zhao S, Saito H, Wang X, et al. Effects of gonadotropin-releasing hormone agonist on the incidence of apoptosis in porcine and human granulosa cells. Gynecol Obstet Invest. 2000;49:52-6.
73. Park EJ, Shin JW, Seo YS, et al. Gonadotropin-releasing hormone-agonist induces apoptosis of human granulosa-luteal cells via caspase-8, -9 and -3, and poly-(ADP-ribose)-polymerase cleavage. Biosci Trends. 2011;5(3):120-8.
74. Meirow D, Assad G, Dor J, Rabinovici J. The GnRH antagonist cetrorelix reduces cyclophosphamide-induced ovarian follicular destruction in mice. Hum Reprod. 2004;19:1294-99.
75. Danforth DR, Arbogast LK, Friedman CI. Acute depletion of murine primordial follicle reserve by gonadotropin-releasing hormone antagonists. Fertil Steril. 2005;83:1333-38.
76. Peng P, Yang DZ, Zheng CY, et al. Effects of gonadotropin releasing hormone analoges on chemotherapy-induced ovarian function damage in rats. Zhonghua Fu Chan Ke Za Zhi. 2007;42:546-50.
77. Glode LM, Robinson J, Gould SF. Protection from cyclophosphamide induced testicular damage with an analoge of gonadotropin-releasing hormone. Lancet. 1981;1:1132-34.
78. Ataya K, Pydyn E, Ramahi-Ataya A, et al. Is radiation-induced ovarian failure in rhesus monkeys preventable by luteinizing hormone-releasing hormone agonists? Preliminary observations. J Clin Endocrinol Metab. 1995;80:790-5.
79. Gosden RG, Wade JC, Fraser HM, et al. Impact of congenital or experimental hypogonadotrophism on the radiation sensitivityof the mouse ovary. Hum Reprod. 1997;12:2483-88.
80. Letterie GS. Anovulation in the prevention of cytotoxic-induced follicular attrition and ovarian failure. Hum Reprod 2004;19:831–7.
81. Pereyra Pacheco B, Méndez Ribas JM, Milone G, et al. Use of GnRH analogs for functional protection of the ovary and preservation of fertility during cancer treatment in adolescents: a preliminary report. Gynecol Oncol. 2001;81:391-7.
82. Somers EC, Marder W, Christman GM, et al. Use of a gonadotropin-releasing hormone analog for protection against premature ovarian failure during cyclophosphamide therapy in women with severe lupus. Arthritis Rheum. 2005;52: 2761-67.
83. Castelo-Branco C, Nomdedeu B, Camus A, et al. Use of gonadotropin-releasing hormone agonists in patients with Hodgkin's disease for preservation of ovarian function and reduction of gonadotoxicity related to chemotherapy. Fertil Steril. 2007;87:702-5.
84. Blumenfeld Z, Avivi I, Eckman A, et al. Gonadotropin-releasing hormone agonist decreases chemotherapy-induced gonadotoxicity and premature ovarian failure in young female patients with Hodgkin lymphoma. Fertil Steril. 2008;89:166-73.
85. Huser M, Crha I, Ventruba P, et al. Prevention of ovarian function damage by a GnRH analoge during chemotherapy in Hodgkin lymphoma patients. Hum Reprod. 2008;23:863-8.
86. Dann EJ, Epelbaum R, Avivi I, et al. Fertility and ovarian function are preserved in women treated with an intensified regimen of cyclophosphamide, adriamycin, vincristine and prednisone (Mega- CHOP) for non-Hodgkin lymphoma. Hum Reprod. 2005;20: 2247-49.
87. Elis A, Tevet A, Yerushalmi R, et al. Fertility status among women treated for aggressive non-Hodgkin's lymphoma. Leuk Lymphoma. 2006;47:623-7.
88. Azem F, Samara N, Cohen T, et al. Assessment of ovarian reserve following ovarian tissue banking and/or GnRH-a co-treatment prior to chemotherapy in patients with Hodgkin's disease. J Assist Reprod Genet. 2008;25:535-8.

89. Nitzschke M, Raddatz J, Bohlmann MK, et al. GnRH analogs do not protect ovaries from chemotherapy-induced ultrastructural injury in Hodgkin's lymphoma patients. Arch Gynecol Obstet. 2010;282:83-8.
90. Kim SS, Lee JR, Jee BC, et al. Use of hormonal protection for chemotherapy-induced gonadotoxicity. Clin Obstet Gynecol. 2010;53:740-52.
91. Oktay K, Briggs D, Gosden RG. Ontogeny of follicle-stimulating hormone receptor gene expression in isolated human ovarianfollicles. J Clin Endocrinol Metab. 1997;82:3748-51.
92. Waxman JH, Ahmed R, Smith D, et al. Failure to preserve fertility in patients with Hodgkin's disease. Cancer Chemother Pharmacol. 1987;19:159-62.
93. Gilani MM, Hasanzadeh M, Ghaemmaghami F, Ramazanzadeh F. Ovarian preservation with gonadotropin-releasing hormone analog during chemotherapy. Asia-Pac J Clin Oncol. 2007;3:79-83.
94. Giuseppe L, Attilio G, Edoardo DN, et al. Ovarian function after cancer treatment in young women affected by Hodgkin disease (HD). Hematology. 2007;12:141-7.
95. Sverrisdottir A, Nystedt M, Johansson H, Fornander T. Adjuvant goserelin and ovarian preservation in chemotherapy treated patients with early breast cancer: results from a randomized trial. Breast Cancer Res Treat. 2009;117:561-7.
96. Badawy A, Elnashar A, El-Ashry M, Shahat M. Gonadotropin-releasing hormone agonists for prevention of chemotherapy-induced ovarian damage: prospective randomized study. Fertil Steril. 2009;91:694-7.
97. Gerber B, von Minckwitz G, Stehle H, et al. Effect of luteinizing hormone-releasing hormone agonist on ovarian function after modern adjuvant breast cancer chemotherapy: the GBG 37 ZORO study. J Clin Oncol. 2011;29:2334-41.
98. Del Mastro L, Boni L, Michelotti A, et al. Effect of the Gonadotropin-Releasing Hormone Analoge Triptorelin on the Occurrence of Chemotherapy-Induced Early Menopause in Premenopausal Women With Breast Cancer. A Randomized Trial. J Am Med Assn. 2011;306(3): 269-76.
99. Munster P, Moore A, Ismail-Khan R, et al. Randomized Trial Using Gonadotropin-Releasing Hormone Agonist Triptorelin for the Preservation of Ovarian Function During (Neo) Adjuvant Chemotherapy for Breast Cancer. J Clin Oncol. 2012;30(5):533-8.
100. Demeestere I, Brice P, Peccatori F, et al. Gonadotropin-Releasing Hormone Agonist for the Prevention of Chemotherapy-Induced Ovarian Failure in Patients With Lymphoma: 1-Year Follow-Up of a Prospective Randomized Trial. J Clin Oncol 2012; Published Ahead of Print on November 5, 2012 as 10.1200/JCO.2012.42.8185.
101. Partridge A. Ovarian Suppression for Prevention of Premature Menopause and Infertility: Empty Promise or Effective Therapy? J Clin Oncol. 2012;30:479-81.
102. Bedaiwy M, Abou-Setta A, Desai N, et al: Gonadotropin-releasing hormone analog cotreatment for preservation of ovarian function during gonadotoxic chemotherapy: a systematic review and meta-analysis. Fertil Steril. 2011;95(3):906-14.
103. Gerber B, Stehle H, Ricardo F, et al. ZORO: a prospective randomized multicenter study to prevent chemotherapy-induced ovarian failure with the GnRH-agonist goserelin in young hormone-insensitive breast cancer patients receiving anthracycline containing (neo) adjuvant chemotherapy (GBG 37). Abstract ID 34455. American Society of Clinical Oncology (ASCO) Annual Meeting. J Clin Oncol, 2009:15s. Available at: http://www.asco.org/ascov2/Meetings/Abstracts.
104. Oktay K, Sonmezer M. Questioning GnRH analogs for gonadal protection in cancer patients. Fertil Steril. 2009;92:e32.
105. Balkenende E, Dahhan T, Van der Veen F, Goddijn M. Comment on GnRH analoge cotreatment with chemotherapy for preservation of ovarian function. Fertil Steril. 2011 Oct;96(4):e155-e156.
106. Leonard RC, Adamson D, Anderson R, et al. The OPTION trial of adjuvant ovarian protection by goserelin in adjuvant chemotherapy for early breast cancer. J Clin Oncol. 28:89s, 2010 (suppl; abstr 590)
107. Southwest Oncology Group Protocol Fast Fact Sheet: SWOG S0230: Phase III Trial of LHRH Analog Administration During Chemotherapy to Reduce Ovarian Failure Following Standard in Early Stage, Hormone-Receptor Negative Breast Cancer. http://swog.org/intergroup/GetSecuredFile.asp?ProtocolNumber=S0230&AccessCode=p5guFuf&Document=MISC1-0230.pdf.
108. Mardesic T, Snajderova M, Sramkova L, et al. Protocol combining GnRH agonists and GnRH antagonists for rapid suppression and prevention of gonadal damage during cytotoxic therapy. Eur J Gynaecol Oncol. 2004;25:90-2.
109. Nahari ab C, Fishman A, Cohen I. Protection of ovarian function and fertility using a combination of gonadotropin-releasing hormone (GnRH) agonist and GnRH antagonist during cancer treatment in young females. Gynecol Endocrinol. 2007;23(5):290-4.
110. Whitehead J, Toledo MG, Stern CJ. A pilot study to assess the use of the gonadotropin antagonist cetrorelix in preserving ovarian function during chemotherapy. Aust N Z J Obstet Gynaecol. 2011 Oct;51(5):452-4.
111. Digeni A, Symeonidis A, Georgopoulos NA. Effect of the gonadotropin-releasing hormone antagonist cetrorelix on the prevention of chemotherapy-induced ovarian damage in women with hematological malignancy. Int J Gynaecol Obstet. 2012;118(1):73-4.
112. Whitehead E, Shalet SM, Blackledge G, et al. The effect of combination chemotherapy on ovarian function in women treated for Hodgkin's disease. Cancer 1983;52:988-93.
113. Longhi A, Pignotti E, Versari M, et al. Effect of oral contraceptive on ovarian function in young females undergoing neoadjuvant chemotherapy treatment for osteosarcoma. Oncol Rep. 2003;10: 151-5.
114. Behringer K, Breuer K, Reineke T, et al. German Hodgkin's Lymphoma Study Group. Secondary amenorrhea after Hodgkin's lymphoma is influenced by age at treatment, stage of disease, chemotherapy regimen, and the use of oral contraceptives during therapy: a report from the German Hodgkin's Lymphoma Study Group. J Clin Oncol. 2005;23:7555-64.
115. Behringer K, Wildt L, Mueller H, et al. German Hodgkin Study Group. No protection of the ovarian follicle pool with the use of GnRH-analoges or oral contraceptives in young women treated with escalated BEACOPP for advanced-stage Hodgkin lymphoma. Final results of a phase II trial from the German Hodgkin Study Group. Ann Oncol 2010;21(10): 2052-60.
116. Practice Committee of The American Society of Reproductive Medicine; Practice Committee of the Society for Assisted Reproductive Technology. Mature oocyte cryopreservation: a guideline. Fertil Steril. 2013;99(1):37-43.

6

Ovarian Transposition as a Fertility Preservation Strategy

Ayman Al-Talib, Togas Tulandi

CHAPTER OUTLINE

OVARIAN AND REPRODUCTIVE PHYSIOLOGY

The ovary has two functions, it produces oocytes for the purpose of procreation and ovarian hormones for maintaining ovarian function. As the number of oocytes declines with increasing age, fertility decreases. Al-Sunaidi et al. found that the antral follicle count number significantly decreased at the age of 35 years.[1]

RADIATION-INDUCED OVARIAN FAILURE

Depending on the site and stage of the disease, pelvic or abdominal irradiation is often indicated in women with hematological, neurologic, genitourinary, or low intestinal malignancies. Ionizing radiation affects gonadal function adversely by damaging the germ cells, depleting the number of follicles and eventually causing ovarian atrophy. As a result, sterility and premature ovarian failure occur.

The estimated dose at which half of the follicles are lost (LD50) is 4 Gy.[2] Compared to an adult ovary, the ovary of prepubertal children and adolescents are relatively resistant to chemotherapy and radiotherapy. Ovarian failure in this age group occurs with an estimated dose of 20 Gy.[3]

TERMINOLOGY AND HISTORIC OVERVIEW

Advances in cancer therapy, including radiation therapy, have resulted in improved long-term survival of young patients with malignancies. In order to decrease radiation exposure to the ovaries, they can be repositioned outside the radiation field; a procedure named ovarian transposition, oophoropexy, or ovariopexy. McCall et al. first described this technique in 1958 for patients with cervical cancer.[4] However, scattered radiation could still affect the ovaries. Today, intensity modulated radiotherapy (IMRT), which concentrates radiotherapy towards the target tumor in three dimensions, minimizes radiation exposure to the surrounding tissue.[5, 6]

INDICATIONS AND SURGICAL TECHNIQUES

Traditionally, ovarian transposition is performed by laparotomy during the staging procedure for the primary disease. The ovaries could be transpositioned behind the uterus away from the radiation field and protected with a lead block (*medial transposition*).[7] Today, surgery staging and ovarian transposition could be performed by laparoscopy.[8] Surgical exteriorization of the ovaries under the skin through an opening in the flank has also been described, but is not commonly used.[9]

The ovaries have been transposed laterally to a variety of sites and levels, from the base of the round ligament[10] to the level of low kidney pole[11] and to low and high paracolic gutters (*lateral ovarian transposition*).[12-14] To be effective, the ovaries should be transposed to the level above the pelvic brim and as lateral as possible. Transposition to this level can be achieved easily without separating the fallopian tubes from their uterine origin, allowing the possibility of spontaneous conception.[15] With the increasing popularity of robotic surgery, robotic-assisted ovarian transposition has also been described.[16, 17]

Before surgery, the radiation field should be outlined on the abdominal wall. This process assists the surgeon in determining the best location of transposition. Age and type of radiation are important factors to be considered when planning ovarian transposition. Patients older than 40 years generally have reduced fertilization potential as well as a high risk for ovarian failure, despite ovarian transposition.[14,18]

LAPAROTOMY VERSUS LAPAROSCOPY

As with any laparotomy, ovarian transposition by this approach is associated with a large abdominal incision, a long hospital stay and an increased risk of adhesion formation and intestinal obstruction. In addition, the healing process is longer than that by laparoscopy, delaying radiation treatment. The transposed ovaries might also fall back into the pelvis.[8] Both laparotomy and laparoscopic procedures are equally effective in preserving ovarian function. Ovarian transposition by laparotomy is associated with preservation of ovarian function in 83% of women after pelvic radiation,[19] while ovarian transposition by laparoscopy preserves ovarian function in 88.6% of women.[15]

Despite ovarian transposition, ovarian failure could still occur. This has been attributed to the surgical techniques, radiation injury to the vascular pedicles, or scattered radiation.[20,21]

SURGICAL PROCEDURE

The operation is performed under general anesthesia; the patient is placed in lithotomy position. We use three trocars, a primary trocar is inserted 2 cm above the umbilicus to facilitate relocation of the ovaries above the pelvic brim and two secondary trocars at the same level or slightly lower. A thorough examination of the abdominal cavity, including the liver and diaphragm and peritoneal lavage for cytologic examination are done first. To maximize future fertility options for women undergoing pelvic irradiation, we perform a unilateral ovarian wedge resection for ovarian cryopreservation. Hemostasis is achieved by a few interrupted sutures of 4-0 polydioxanone (PDS) to approximate the ovarian incision. Dissection of the mesosalpinx with the laparoscopic scissors is done, the ovaries are then mobilized along with the infundibulopelvic ligaments. Both fallopian tubes are kept intact and the transposed ovaries securely sutured to the peritoneum of the anterior abdominal wall using non-absorbable suture. A surgical hemoclip is applied to the ovaries to indicate the site of transposed ovary by future imaging.

COMPLICATIONS

Complications of the procedure are rare. Injury and torsion of the ovarian blood vessels have been described.[19] Ovarian functional cyst formation is commonly reported and usually is unilateral. In a study of 54 women with early stage cervical cancer who underwent ovarian transposition, 3 of 54 patients (5.5%) developed symptomatic ovarian cysts. Subsequently, 2 women required surgical intervention due to pain symptoms.[21]

In another study including 84 premenopausal women with cervical cancer who underwent radical hysterectomy, the incidence of symptomatic ovarian cyst formation in women with ovarian transposition was 24% and in those without this procedure was 7%.[22] Adjuvant pelvic radiation appears to decrease ovarian cyst formation, perhaps due to additional damage to the ovaries.[23] Whether ovarian cyst formation is related to the procedure remains unclear.[23] Feeney et al., however, reported that among 132 women who underwent ovarian transposition, the incidence of adnexal disease that required analgesia and surgical intervention was only 3%.[20]

The mechanism of ovarian cyst formation is unknown. Extensive mobilization of the ovaries, previous endometriosis or pelvic adhesions has been proposed.[21] Although rare, metastasis of the primary cancer to the ovaries has been reported.[18,24] Other rare complications include metastasis on the trocar site[25] and adhesion formation leading to bowel obstruction.[18]

OVARIAN FUNCTION AFTER TRANSPOSITION

Several factors have been proposed as determinant of the ovarian function after transposition. The two most important factors are the dose absorbed by the ovaries during radiotherapy[26] and the age of the patient.[3,27] The type of radiation also plays an important role in maintaining ovarian function. It has been reported that a dose of more than 300 cGy leads to menopause-induced ovarian failure in 60% of cases.[19,23]

Morice et al. found that the rates of ovarian preservation were 100% in patients treated exclusively by surgery, 90% in patients treated by postoperative vaginal brachytherapy and 60% in patients treated by postoperative external radiation therapy and vaginal brachytherapy, suggesting that the occurrence of ovarian failure is mainly due to external radiation.[18] Ovarian function following ovarian transposition is shown in **Table 1**.

FERTILITY OUTCOME

If many studies evaluated ovarian function after ovarian transposition, there were few studies describing the reproductive outcome. Due to the increase in spontaneous abortion and low birth weight in women who conceive shortly after treatment, Fenig et al. recommended delaying pregnancy one year after radiation exposure.[28]

In the largest series in the literature, the authors evaluated 37 cases of ovarian transposition. They divided the patients into two groups. Group 1 consisted of 27 women with clear cell adenocarcinoma of the vagina and/or the cervix and who were treated with surgery and brachytherapy (60 Gy) or external irradiation (15 Gy). Group 2 consisted of 9 women with ovarian dysgerminoma and another with uterine sarcoma treated with surgery followed by postoperative external irradiation of iliac and para-aortic lymph nodes (25 to 35 Gy). A total of 18 pregnancies were achieved in 12 patients (12/37; 32%). The pregnancy rate in group 1 was 15% (4/27) and in group 2 it was 80% (8/10). Of 18 pregnancies, 5 ended in a miscarriage and 13 pregnancies produced 15 live births (one was premature at 28 weeks gestation). The low pregnancy rate in group 1 may be related to diethylstilbestrol-related anomalies of the reproductive tract as an etiologic factor of the cancer type in this group in addition to brachytherapy.[29]

Another report included 11 girls with Hodgkin's lymphoma who underwent bilateral ovarian transposition at a median age of 13 years. Fourteen pregnancies were recorded with 12 live births (1 twin) and 3 miscarriages.[30] The literature also contains several case reports as well as spontaneous pregnancy following ovarian transposition.[15,31-35]

Successful surrogate pregnancies after radical hysterectomy, lymphadenectomy and ovarian transposition for cervical cancer, followed by radiation therapy have also been reported. The oocytes were retrieved transabdominally.[36-40]

EFFECT OF RADIATION ON ENDOMETRIUM AND FERTILITY OUTCOME

It is well-documented that estrogen deficiency after radiation-induced ovarian failure leads to uterine atrophy. However, in

TABLE 1 Ovarian function following ovarian transposition

Author (year)	*No. of patients*	*Type of Malignancy*	*Mean age of patients (years)*	*Follow up period (years)*	*Menses or continued ovarian function No. (%)*	*Ovarian failure No. (%)*
Olejek et al. (2001)[47]	25	Cervical cancer	34.5	5	13 (52)	12(48)
Morice et al. (2000)[18]	84	Cervical cancer	33.5	2.6	68 (81)	16 (19)
Williams et al. (1999)[8]	10	Hodgkin's disease	27.9	6	5 (50)	5 (50)
Classe et al. (1998)[48]	4	Hodgkin's disease,	31	2.9	4 (100)	0
Clough et al. (1996)[14]	14	Cervical cancer, Hodgkin's disease, and ependymoma of the cauda equina.	32.8	2	12 (85.7)	2 (14.3)
Coven et al. (1996)[12]	3	Cervical cancer	26.5	2.7	2 (66.7)	1 (33.3)
Feeny et al. (1995)[20]	28	Cervical cancer	33.5	2	14 (50)	14 (50)
Anderson et al. (1993)[24]	24	Cervical cancer	31.5	6.4	4 (16.7)	20 (83.3)
Thibaud et al. (1992)[33]	18	Hodgkin's disease , Ewing sarcoma , medulloblastoma, ovarian seminoma and vaginal or uterine tumor	9.4	8.9	13 (72.2)	3 (16.7)
Husseinzadeh et al. (1984)[19]	18	Cervical and vaginal cancer	29	6	12 (66.7)	6 (33.3)
Total	228				147(64.5)	79(34.6)

TABLE 2 Reproductive outcome following ovarian transposition

Author (year)	No. of patients	Indication for ovarian transposition	Pregnancy no (%)	Abortion no (%)	Live birth	Premature birth
Terenziani et al. (2009)[30]	11	Hodgkin's disease	14 (100)*	3 (27.3)	12	-
Williams et al. (1999)[8]	10	Hodgkin's disease	4 (40)	0	4	-
Morice et al. (1998)[27]	37	Ovarian dysgeminoma and parauterine sarcoma	18 (48.6)	5 (13.5)	15	1
Thibaud et al. (1992)[33]	18	Hodgkin's disease	2 (11.2)	0	2	-
Gabriel el al. (1986)[7]	17	Hodgkin's disease	8 (47.1)	2 (11.8)	5	1
Thomas et al. (1976)[49]	22	Hodgkin's disease	4 (18.2)	0	4	-
Le Floch et al. (1976)[50]	9	Hodgkin's disease	5 (55.6)	2 (22.2)	8	-
Baker et al. (1972)[51]	65	Hodgkin's disease	3 (4.6)	0	3	-
Total	189		58(30.7)	12(6.3)	53(28)	2(1.1)

*More than one pregnancy per patient

those with normal ovarian function, direct damage to the endometrium could also occur, leading to an increased risk of miscarriage, mid-trimester pregnancy loss, preterm birth and low birth weight. In any event, an irradiated uterus can carry a pregnancy.[41-44] There have been no reports of increased risks of either congenital abnormalities or childhood malignancy in children born to long-term survivors of childhood cancer.[42,45,46] Reproductive outcome after pelvic irradiation is shown in **Table 2**.

CONCLUSION

Ovarian transposition should be considered in young women undergoing pelvic irradiation. This procedure could be performed by laparoscopy and is associated with preservation of ovarian function in most patients. Due to the high rate of ovarian failure in women over 40 years old, ovarian transposition is not recommended. During surgery, ovarian tissue could be excised for ovarian cryopreservation and possible transplantation in the future.

REFERENCES

1. Al-Sunaidi M, Al-Mahrizi S, Tan S, Tulandi T. Age-related changes in antral follicle count among women with and without polycystic ovaries. Gynecol Obstet Invest. 2007;64:199-203.
2. Wallace W, Kelsey T. Ovarian reserve and reproductive age may be determined from measurement of ovarian volume by transvaginal sonography. Hum Reprod. 2004;19:1612-7.
3. Lushbaugh C, Casarett G. The effects of gonadal irradiation in clinical radiation therapy: a review. Cancer. 1976;37:1111-25.
4. McCall M, Keaty E, Thompson J. Conservation of ovarian tissue in the treatment of carcinoma of the cervix with radical surgery. Am J Obstet Gynecol. 1958;75:590-600.
5. Wo J, Viswanathan A. Impact of radiotherapy on fertility, pregnancy, and neonatal outcomes in female cancer patients. Int J Rad Oncol Biol Phys. 2009;73:1304-12.
6. Kochanski J, Mell L, Roeske J, Mundt A. Intensity-modulated radiation therapy in gynecologic malignancies: Current status and future directions. Clin Adv Hematol Oncol. 2006;4:379-86.
7. Gabriel DA, Bernard SA, Lambert J, Croom RD 3rd. Oophoropexy and the Management of Hodgkin's Disease: A Reevaluation of the Risks and Benefits. Arch Surg. 1986;121:1083-5.
8. Williams R, Littell R, Mendenhall N. Laparoscopic oophoropexy and ovarian function in the treatment of Hodgkin disease. Cancer. 2000;86:2138-42.
9. Kovacev M. Exteriorization of ovaries under the skin of young women operated upon for cancer of the cervix. Am J Obstet Gynecol. 1968;101:756-9.
10. Lee C, Lai Y, Soong Y, Lin T, Tang S. Laparoscopic ovariopexy before irradiation for medulloblastoma. Hum Reprod. 1995;10:372-4.
11. Schulz-Lobmeyr I, Schratter-Sehn A, Huber J, Wenzl R. Laparoscopic lateral ovarian transposition before pelvic irradiation for a Non Hodgkin lymphoma. Acta Obstet Gynecol Scand. 1999;78:350-2.
12. Covens A, Van der Putten H, Fyles A, et al. Laparoscopic ovarian transposition. Eur J Gynaecol Oncol. 1996;17:177-82.
13. Yarali H, Demirol A, Bükülmez O, Coskun F, Gürgan T. Laparoscopic high lateral transposition of both ovaries before pelvic irradiation. J Am Assoc Gynecol Laparosc. 2000;7:237-9.
14. Clough K, Goffinet F, Labib A, et al. Laparoscopic unilateral ovarian transposition prior to irradiation: prospective study of 20 cases. Cancer. 1996;77:2638-45.
15. Bisharah M, Tulandi T. Laparoscopic preservation of ovarian function: an underused procedure. Am J Obstet Gynecol. 2003;188:367-70.
16. Molpus K, Wedergren J, Carlson M. Robotically assisted endoscopic ovarian transposition. JSLS. 2003;7:59-62.
17. Al-Badawi I, Al-Aker M, Tulandi T. Robotic-Assisted Ovarian Transposition Before radiation. Sur Technol Int. 2010;19:141-3.

18. Morice P, Juncker L, Rey A, El-Hassan J, Haie-Meder C, Castaigne D. Ovarian transposition for patients with cervical carcinoma treated by radiosurgical combination. Fertil Steril. 2000;74:743-8.
19. Husseinzadeh N, Nahhas W, Velkley D, Whitney C, Mortel R. The preservation of ovarian function in young women undergoing pelvic radiation therapy. Gynecol Oncol. 1984;18:373-9.
20. Feeney D, Moore D, Look K, Stehman F, Sutton G. The fate of the ovaries after radical hysterectomy and ovarian transposition. Gynecol Oncol. 1995;56:3-7.
21. Van Eijkeren M, Van Der Wijk I, El Sharouni S, Heintz A. Benefits and side effects of lateral ovarian transposition (LOT) performed during radical hysterectomy and pelvic lymphadenectomy for early stage cervical cancer. Int J Gynecol Cancer. 2001;9:396-400.
22. Chambers S, Chambers J, Holm C, Peschel R, Schwartz P. Sequelae of lateral ovarian transposition in unirradiated cervical cancer patients. Gynecol Oncol. 1990;39:155-9.
23. Chambers S, Chambers J, Kier R, Peschel R. Sequelae of lateral ovarian transposition in irradiated cervical cancer patients. Int J Rad Oncol Biol Phys. 1991;20:1305-8.
24. Anderson B, LaPolla J, Turner D, Chapman G, Buller R. Ovarian transposition in cervical cancer. Gynecol Oncol. 1993;49:206-14.
25. Picone O, Aucouturier J, Louboutin A, Coscas Y, Camus E. Abdominal wall metastasis of a cervical adenocarcinoma at the laparoscopic trocar insertion site after ovarian transposition: case report and review of the literature. Gynecol Oncol. 2003;90:446-9.
26. Haie-Meder C, Mlika-Cabanne N, Michel G, et al. Radiotherapy after ovarian transposition: ovarian function and fertility preservation. Int J Rad Oncol Biol Phys. 1993;25:419-24.
27. Morice P, Castaigne D, Haie-Meder C, et al. Laparoscopic ovarian transposition for pelvic malignancies: indications and functional outcomes. Fertil Steril. 1998;70:956-60.
28. Fenig E, Mishaeli M, Kalish Y, Lishner M. Pregnancy and radiation. Cancer Treat Rev. 2001;27:1-7.
29. Morice P, Haie-Meder C, Pautier P, Lhomme C, Castaigne D. Ovarian metastasis on transposed ovary in patients treated for squamous cell carcinoma of the uterine cervix: report of two cases and surgical implications. Gynecol Oncol. 2001;83:605-7.
30. Terenziani M, Piva L, Meazza C, Gandola L, Cefalo G, Merola M. Oophoropexy: a relevant role in preservation of ovarian function after pelvic irradiation. Fertil Steril. 2009;91:935-e15-6.Epub.
31. Kurt M, Uncu G, Cetintas S, Kucuk N, Guler S, Ozkan L. Successful spontaneous pregnancy in a patient with rectal carcinoma treated with pelvic radiotherapy and concurrent chemotherapy: the unique role of laparoscopic lateral ovary transposition. Eur J Gynaecol Oncol. 2007;28:408-10.
32. Kim S. Fertility preservation in female cancer patients: current developments and future directions. Fertility and sterility. 2006;85:1-11.
33. Thibaud E, Ramirez M, Brauner R, et al. Preservation of ovarian function by ovarian transposition performed before pelvic irradiation during childhood. J Pediatrics. 1992;121:880-4.
34. Nakamura G, Sumii Y, Kato K, Yoshimitu K, Hamada M, Nakano H. Vascular pedicle transposition of an ovary with subsequent intrauterine pregnancy. Fertil Steril. 1989;52:688-90.
35. Ferrari S, Persico P, Di Puppo F, Giardina P, Ferrari A. Laparoscopic lateral ovarian transposition: a fertility sparing procedure. Minerva Ginecol. 2009;61:465-8.
36. Agorastos T, Zafrakas M, Mastrominas M. Case Report: Long-term follow-up after cervical cancer treatment and subsequent successful surrogate pregnancy. Reprod Biomed Online. 2009;19:250-1.
37. Steigrad S, Hacker N, Kolb B. In vitro fertilization surrogate pregnancy in a patient who underwent radical hysterectomy followed by ovarian transposition, lower abdominal wall radiotherapy, and chemotherapy. Fertil Steril. 2005;83:1547-9.
38. Zinger M, Liu J, Husseinzadeh N, Thomas M. Successful surrogate pregnancy after ovarian transposition, pelvic irradiation and hysterectomy. J Reprod Med. 2004;49:573-4.
39. Azem F, Yovel I, Wagman I, Kapostiansky R, Lessing J, Amit A. Surrogate pregnancy in a patient who underwent radical hysterectomy and bilateral transposition of ovaries. Fertil Steril. 2003;79:1229-30.
40. Giacalone P, Laffargue F, Bénos P, Dechaud H, Hédon B. Successful in vitro fertilization-surrogate pregnancy in a patient with ovarian transposition who had undergone chemotherapy and pelvic irradiation. Fertil Steril. 2001;76:388-9.
41. Green D, Whitton J, Stovall M, et al. Pregnancy outcome of female survivors of childhood cancer: A report from the childhood cancer survivor study. Am J Obstet Gynecol. 2002;187:1070-80.
42. Hawkins M, Smith R. Pregnancy outcomes in childhood cancer survivors: probable effects of abdominal irradiation. Int J Cancer. 1989;43:399-402.
43. Signorello L, Cohen S, Bosetti C, et al. Female survivors of childhood cancer: preterm birth and low birth weight among their children. J Natil Cancer Inst. 2006;98:1453-61.
44. Urbano M, Tait D. Can the irradiated uterus sustain a pregnancy? A literature review. Clin Oncol. 2004;16:24-8.
45. Blatt J. Pregnancy outcome in long-term survivors of childhood cancer. Med Pediatr Oncol. 1999; 33:29-33.
46. Li F, Fine W, Jaffe N, Holmes G, Holmes F. Offspring of patients treated for cancer in childhood. J Natl Cancer Inst. 1979;62:1193-7.
47. Olejek A, Wala D, Chimiczewski P, Rzempoluch J. Hormonal activity of transposed ovaries in young women treated for cervical cancer. Gynecol Endocrinol. 2001;15:5-13.
48. Classe J, Mahé M, Moreau P, et al. Ovarian transposition by laparoscopy before radiotherapy in the treatment of Hodgkin's disease. Cancer. 1998;83:1420-4.
49. Thomas P, Winstanly D, Peckham M, Austin D, Murray M, Jacobs H. Reproductive and endocrine function in patients with Hodgkin's disease: effects of oophoropexy and irradiation. Br J Cancer. 1976;33:226-31.
50. Le Floch O, Donaldson S, Kaplan H. Pregnancy following oophoropexy and total nodal irradiation in women with Hodgkin's disease. Cancer. 1976;38:2263-8.
51. Baker J, Peckham M, Morgan R, Smithers D. Preservation of ovarian function in patients requiring radiotherapy for para-aortic and pelvic Hodgkin's disease. Lancet. 1972;299:1307-8.

7

Surgical Strategies for Fertility Preservation in Women with Cancer

Mohamed A Bedaiwy, William W Hurd, Kristine Zanotti

CHAPTER OUTLINE

INTRODUCTION

For women of reproductive age who are diagnosed with cancer, their survival rates have significantly improved primarily due to remarkable advancements in cancer treatment.[1] Specifically, as a result of recent diagnostic and treatment developments in the fields of breast and colorectal cancer, the overall death rates due to cancer for women fell by 11.4% from 1991 to 2005. Moreover, between 1991 and 2005, over 160,000 cancer deaths were prevented in women in the United States.[1]

Roughly 70% of reproductive-aged women, who are diagnosed with cancer, want children after they complete their cancer therapy.[2,3] Notwithstanding the fact that modern cancer therapy significantly improves survival, it frequently negatively impacts a woman's fertility because of chemotherapy and radiotherapy effects on reproductive organs. Additionally, for gynecologic cancers specifically, the surgical removal of reproductive organs can also harm or completely prevent future fertility.

The growing need to deal with fertility preservation in female cancer patients is well-acknowledged. The American Society of Clinical Oncology advises that, for cancer patients in their reproductive years, fertility preservation be raised as an issue and addressed.[4] The President's Cancer Panel also published a strong recommendation focusing on the necessity for further research in the field of fertility preservation.[5]

For women of reproductive age diagnosed with cancer, the following strategies for fertility preservation were developed: (a) changing the surgical treatment of gynecologic cancer, (b) protection of reproductive organs during radiation or chemotherapy treatment and (c) removal and cryopreservation of ovarian tissue before cancer treatment in anticipation of subsequent transplantation back into the patient after remission is achieved. This chapter will consider the surgical approaches for these enumerated strategies, which currently are being used for reproductive-age women with cancer.

GYNECOLOGIC CANCERS: SURGICAL TREATMENTS THAT PRESERVE FERTILITY

For most gynecologic cancers, treatment involves procedures that often render the patient sterile, like removal of the uterus, ovaries and Fallopian tubes. That said, in the case of reproductive-age women with early disease, occasionally fertility-sparing surgery can be undertaken. In this section, we will outline fertility-preserving surgical approaches to cervical, ovarian and endometrial cancer (**Table 1**).

Cervical Cancer

Cervical cancer is the most frequent gynecologic cancer diagnosed during a woman's reproductive years. Even though cervical cancer only encompasses 16% of all cancers in women, 40% of women are diagnosed before the age of 45.[6] In the United States specifically, the age-adjusted incidence rate is roughly 8 per 100,000 women per year.[6] Moreover, approximately 1/3 of these American women will die from their disease.[6] The 5-year survival rate is currently measured at 70%.

Standard Treatment Approach

Depending on the stage of the cancer at diagnosis, the therapy for cervical cancer can differ. About 50% of cervical cancers are between Stages II-IV, where the cancer has spread beyond the cervix (either to adjacent structures, to regional lymph nodes, or to more distance sites).[6] The standard therapy for the majority of these women combines chemotherapy and radiotherapy.

The other 50% of women with cervical cancer are Stage I, where the disease is only in the cervix.[6] For women with this condition who do not wish for future fertility, the surgical therapy is radical hysterectomy with pelvic lymphadenectomy.[3] In some case reports regarding women who have undergone this procedure, they have had children using in vitro fertilization (IVF) and a surrogate to carry the pregnancy.[7,8] Adjuvant pelvic radiotherapy may also be administered after radical hysterectomy depending on recurrence risk factors. Nonetheless, the ovary's tolerance for radiation is low, and thus, the standard pelvic radiotherapy doses of 45 to 50 Gy will consistently induce premature ovarian failure. Some case reports note successful surrogate pregnancies when, at the time of radical hysterectomy, oocytes were removed from the ovaries or the ovaries were surgically transposed out of the pelvic radiation field.[7,8]

Fertility-Sparing Approach

Cone Biopsy

It is suggested by observational data that lesions that meet the criteria for microinvasive cervical carcinoma (designated as "Stage Ia1") have an insignificant risk for lymphatic metastasis and they can be excised using less drastic procedures, such as cold knife conization.[9] The impact of cone biopsy on obstetric outcomes is controversial. Although some studies note no increase in adverse outcome,[10,11] other studies, including a recent large meta-analysis, suggest that such an approach does increase the risk of not only pre-term delivery but also low birth weight infants.[12,13]

Radical Trachelectomy

Radical trachelectomy is another fertility-sparing method for patients who have very early, invasive cervical cancer.[14-17] In radical trachelectomy, the cervix is removed as is the surrounding vaginal and parametrial tissue, while the uterine fundus is preserved.[14-17] This approach may be used for smaller, cervix-confined lesions such as lesions otherwise meeting criteria for microinvasion, but which are also accompanied by lymphovascular invasion, Stage IA2 lesions and Stage IB1 lesions, and visible lesions < 4 cm that are confined to the cervix with superficial invasion and no vascular space invasion.[9]

Radical trachelectomy via an abdominal approach can be used with pelvic lymphadenectomy in order to exclude lymphatic spread.[18] On the other hand, radical trachelectomy can also be performed vaginally in conjunction with laparoscopic lymphadenectomy.[19] After the cervix and parametria are excised, a permanent cerclage is usually placed and the vaginal mucosa is then re-approximated to the uterine stump.

TABLE 1 Fertility-sparing surgery for reproductive-age women with gynecologic cancers.

Cancer type	*Standard therapy*	*Fertility-sparing approach*	*Requirements*
Cervical	Total abdominal hysterectomy, bilateral salpingo-oophorectomy	1. Cone biopsy 2. Radical trachelectomy	1. Stage IA1 2. Stage IA2- IB1
Ovarian	Total abdominal hysterectomy, bilateral salpingo-oophorectomy	Unilateral oophorectomy	1. Borderline tumors 2. Stage IA-C Grade I or II
Endometrial	Total abdominal hysterectomy, bilateral salpingo-oophorectomy	Surgical staging without hysterectomy or oophorectomy; Progestin therapy	Stage I, Grade I endometriod cancer

Reproduced with permission from: Bedaiwy MA, Zanotti K, Shahin A, Abdel Rahman M, Hurd WW. Surgical strategies for fertility preservation in women with cancer. Current Women Health Reviews. 2010; 6: 167.

The survival and recurrence rates for radical hysterectomy appear to be comparable to traditional radical hysterectomy in appropriate early-stage cervical cancer patients. Three studies involving 151 patients who were followed for 23-60 months reported satisfactory recurrence rates of 2.8% to 5%.[15,20,21] For women with larger cervical lesions, the oncologic outcome data is more limited.

As far as preserving fertility, radical trachelectomy is usually effective, but obstetric complications are increased. Rates of miscarriage in the first trimester are comparable to those in the general population. Second trimester miscarriage rates and preterm delivery, however, are appreciably increased in patients who have previously undergone radical trachelectomy. Ramirez et al. conducted a review of 520 radical vaginal trachelectomy patients and found that, of the 43% who attempted to conceive after surgery, 70% of those women actually achieved pregnancy.[22] Of the 70%, or 227 pregnancies, 21% ended in first trimester miscarriage, 8% ended in second trimester miscarriage, 21% were born prematurely and 50% were delivered at < 36 weeks. Because many women have a permanent cerclage placed at the time of their radical trachelectomy, delivery by elective cesarean section is usually warranted.

Ovarian Cancer

In the United States in 2009, the fifth leading cause of cancer death was ovarian cancer.[1] Notwithstanding the fact that the peak age of occurrence of ovarian cancer is after menopause, up to 17% of all ovarian cancers happen in women <40 years of age.[23] Many women in this age group of <40 years of age desire preserved reproductive potential and ovarian endocrine function.

By examining the stage and histological grade of ovarian cancer at the time of diagnosis, clinicians can predict survival rates. Generally, women with ovarian cancer that is confined to the ovary (stage I) experience a >90% 5-year survival rate. Women with ovarian cancer that have stages III-IV tumors experience <40% 5-year survival rates. Due to the fact that >75% of ovarian cancers at diagnosis are stages III-IV, the overall 5-year survival rate for ovarian cancer is <45%.[6, 24]

Ovarian Cancer Subtypes

Ovarian cancer can be separated into three major histologic classes: (a) epithelial ovarian tumors, (b) germ cell tumors and (c) stromal tumors. Each histologic subtype is related to specific clinical features that are pertinent to the determination process of advising a fertility-sparing procedure. Those specific clinical features include the following: age at presentation, typical stage at presentation and incidence of bilateral ovarian involvement. Auspiciously, many of the more commonly seen histologic subtypes that occur during a woman's reproductive years are amenable to less drastic surgical approaches.

Epithelial ovarian malignancies typically arise from either the ovarian surface epithelium or within epithelial inclusion cysts. These malignancies comprise no less than 80% of all ovarian malignancies.[25] At the time of presentation, an estimated 75% of invasive epithelial cancers are at Stages III or IV; yet, most of these epithelial cancers are diagnosed in post-reproductive-age women.[24] It is imperative to distinguish low malignant potential tumors (borderline epithelial tumors). These comparatively indolent lesions are often found in women of reproductive age. Furthermore, these lesions have a tendency to remain confined to the ovary for long periods of time, often reaching an impressive size before diagnosis. An estimated 90% of women present with stage I disease (confined to one or both ovaries), which is bilateral in 25% of patients.[26,27]

Germ cell tumors comprise an estimated 10–15% of all ovarian tumors, although malignant germ cell tumors are uncommon. Even though germ cell malignancies account for less than 5% of all ovarian cancers, they comprise two-thirds of the ovarian malignancies that are seen in the first two decades of life.[28] Comprising 40% of germ cell cancers, ovarian dysgerminoma is the most frequently seen malignant germ cell tumor. At diagnosis, an estimated 75% of ovarian dysgerminomas are stage I and at least 15% present with bilateral ovarian involvement. Immature teratoma, endodermal sinus tumor and choriocarcinoma are other germ cell malignancies, which are seldom bilateral.

Ovarian stromal tumors, which include granulosa-theca and Sertoli-Leydig cell tumors, are rarely seen and usually are low-grade, with approximately 70% presenting at stage I. Ovarian stromal tumors are also seldom bilateral.[24,29]

Standard Treatment Approach

For women with ovarian cancer who do not desire future fertility, their surgical therapy includes hysterectomy and bilateral salpingo-oophorectomy. Many patients also undergo lymphadenectomy and partial omentectomy for staging purposes. For women who have a sufficient risk for recurrence, postoperative adjuvant combination chemotherapy may be appropriate.[25]

Fertility-Sparing Approach

For women with ovarian malignancies, fertility-sparing surgery includes unilateral oophorectomy, often with removal of the neighboring Fallopian tube. Usually, staging lymphadenectomy and appropriate biopsies are also undertaken. Nonetheless, the contralateral ovary and uterus are left in place. A multitude of circumstances exist where removal of the contralateral ovary and uterus do not affect the overall oncologic outcomes or prognosis. In such instances, fertility-sparing surgery is a very practical option.

The majority of sex cord stromal and unilateral germ cell malignancies are amenable to fertility-sparing surgery. Luckily, aggressive histologic subtypes and/or advanced surgical stages are rare in women of reproductive age. In those women, adjuvant multi-agent chemotherapy frequently is recommended in order to decrease the risk of recurrence.[30] Thomas et al. reported a 90%10-year overall survival rate after fertility-sparing surgery for germ cell malignancies.[31] Additionally, they reported successful subsequent pregnancies—even among women who had received chemotherapy.[31]

Not only is fertility-sparing surgery frequently appropriate for unilateral borderline tumors, but also there is little data that oncologic outcomes are compromised, even with metastatic disease.[32] Park et al. reported that the recurrence rate was an estimated 5%, regardless of whether patients had radical or fertility-sparing surgery. That said, bilateral ovarian involvement is frequent in borderline malignancies. The residual ovarian tissue was the most frequent location of tumor recurrence in those women choosing fertility-sparing procedures, which indicates the necessity for close surveillance of the remaining ovary.[32] In Park et al.'s study, 18% of 184 patients had successful subsequent pregnancies after the fertility-sparing surgery.

Conservative fertility-sparing surgery for specific unilateral stage I cases of invasive epithelial ovarian cancer can be appropriate.[33] In such cases, full staging is nonetheless recommended. In 15% of women who present with apparent ovary-confined disease, pelvic washings, lymph node sampling, and omentectomy will disclose occult metastases.[25,34] Some specialists advise doing a wedge biopsy on the contralateral normal-appearing ovary with intraoperative frozen section in order to rule out occult malignancy.[35] With the exception of cases of low-grade histology, the majority of women who are diagnosed with invasive epithelial ovarian carcinoma of any stage will undergo postoperative adjuvant chemotherapy.

Despite undergoing unilateral oophorectomy and chemotherapy, the majority of women who have malignant epithelial ovarian tumors will be able to get pregnant. Many of these women will resume menstrual function and in one study over 70% of women had a subsequent, successful pregnancy.[25, 36]

Endometrial Cancer

The most common gynecologic cancer is endometrial cancer, which accounts for an estimated 6% of all cancers in women.[37,38] That said, many of the women who are diagnosed with endometrial cancer are past reproductive age. No more than 5% of endometrial cancers occur in women who are less than 40 years of age.[6] In this cohort of women, these neoplasms tended to be well-differentiated with not only an indolent biology but also confinement to the uterus at diagnosis.[6] A surfeit of estrogen, such the levels seen in obesity and anovulation, is the chief risk factor for the occurrence of low-grade endometrial neoplasms. Moreover, an estimated 25% of young women who do develop endometrial cancer will also have polycystic ovary syndrome (PCOS).[37] This alleged "low risk" cancer has an overall 5-year survival rate of over 90%.

Standard Treatment Approach

For endometrial cancer, the standard treatment approach is hysterectomy and bilateral salpingo-oophorectomy.[39] For women with high-risk histology or advanced disease, adjuvant postoperative radiation therapy or chemotherapy may be appropriate. Because most women with endometrial cancer are past their reproductive years, fertility-sparing surgery is not commonly considered.

Fertility-Sparing Approach

In certain younger women who not only have low-grade endometrial carcinoma but also desire fertility preservation, fertility-sparing approaches may be appropriate. These treatment approaches usually use medical treatment with progestin therapy. Such an approach is recommended only for young women who have non-invasive (stage IA), hormone-sensitive lesions (typically Grade I histology) with a desire for future fertility and an otherwise reasonable likelihood for conception after therapy.[40-42]

Pre-Treatment Studies

Essential, prior to beginning a medical management strategy for endometrial carcinoma, is a meticulous endometrial sampling through D&C and an accurate pathology review.[40] Immunohistochemistry studies looking at progesterone receptor content are also valuable in predicting the patient's reaction to progestin therapy. That said, in a study by Thigpen et al. of metastatic endometrial carcinoma, 37% of patients who had tumors indicating progesterone receptor content responded to progestin therapy, while only 8% of patients with tumors without established progesterone receptor content responded.[43] To varying degrees, the majority of FIGO Grade I endometrial neoplasms will express progesterone receptors. The worth of further quantifying progesterone content in patients who are considering medical management has yet to be evaluated.

An important element of pre-treatment assessment for endometrial carcinoma is the determination of depth of myometrial invasion because non-invasive or minimally invasive lesions are regarded as the only candidates possibly amenable to medical management. The most appropriate imaging method available for this assessment is the contrast-enhanced MRI.[44,45] Additionally, pelvic MRI is very sensitive for the discovery of neoplastic lymph node involvement, although lymphatic metastasis is otherwise a very rare occurrence for non-invasive and early-invasive FIGO Grade I endometrial lesions.[46]

Progestin Therapy

In order to avoid the necessity of hysterectomy, progestin therapy can be used in an effort to eliminate early-stage, well-differentiated endometrial cancer.[11,47,48] Even though there is no set treatment regimen, the two most commonly used progestin regimens are: (a) megestrol acetate, 80 mg/day, or (b) medroxyprogesterone, 200 mg/day. Doses of medroxyprogesterone as high as 1000 mg/day have been recommended by some, but this higher dose has yet to be found more effective than 200 mg/day for patients with advanced disease and thromboembolic complications were distinctly elevated.[43]

Follow-Up

In order to have a definitive assessment of treatment response, endometrial sampling, either by D&C or biopsy every 1 to 3 months, is required.[41] As soon as D&C confirms that the endometrium has returned to normal histology, the patient can attempt pregnancy.[40] Useful early indicators of disease progression include monthly transvaginal ultrasonography and serum CA-125 levels.[41,49]

Outcomes

An estimated 50% of well-differentiated tumors demonstrate a full response to hormonal treatment. Because of continuing risk factors, about 25% of responders will have a relapse after the initial successful therapy.[50] Therefore, patients should be advised about the possibility of failure with this approach.

Subsequent Fertility

A few studies have described successful pregnancies following progestin therapy for endometrial carcinoma.[40] Even though the studies are limited to some extent, it does appear that at least one-third of women conceive after progestin therapy. Regrettably, as mentioned previously, recurrence is frequent and requires continued close follow-up so long as the patient retains her uterus.[40] Moreover, the reported rates of conception are low, which reflects both the poor regression of endometrial pathology and the inherent fertility issues that occur in these classically subfertile patients. Because these patients frequently have PCOS and anovulation, it is usually necessary to use ovulation induction in this population.

PROTECTING OVARIES AND OOCYTES DURING CANCER TREATMENT

Cancer therapy frequently has destructive consequences for ovarian function and future fertility. For several cancers frequent in young women, including gynecologic cancers and lymphomas, pelvic irradiation can be restorative. That said, when the ovaries are inside the treatment field, then commonly premature ovarian failure occurs. Similarly, systemic chemotherapy is a successful therapy for these types of cancers, as well as for cancers that occur outside of the pelvis, such as leukemia and breast cancer. Multi-agent chemotherapy produces ovarian failure in an estimated 40% of women who are less than 40-years-old and in more than 75% in women who are more than 40-years-old, and it is expected to harm the fertility in an even greater number of women who are more than 40-years-old.[51]

Protecting oocytes from damage is the most essential concern for fertility preservation in women who need pelvic irradiation or systemic chemotherapy. Thus, for fertility preservation, women undergoing these cancer therapies have the option of both non-surgical and surgical methods.

Non-Surgical Approaches

Even though the subject of this chapter is surgical approaches to preserve fertility, it would be remise not to mention existing non-surgical approaches. These non-surgical approaches can be divided into two classes: (a) oocyte retrieval for in vitro manipulation and cryopreservation and (b) pituitary down-regulation during chemotherapy.

Controlled Ovarian Stimulation and Cryotechnology

The most effective fertility preservation approach that is non-surgical is oocyte removal for in vitro manipulation.[52] By combining hormonal stimulation followed by timed transvaginal recovery of mature oocytes, in vitro fertilization (IVF) and then embryo cryopreservation, the highest pregnancy rates have been achieved. For this approach, the cumulative rate of pregnancy (after thawing and intrauterine transfer) is presently > 60% per embryo.[53] If the patient does not desire immediate fertilization of her oocytes, oocyte cryopreservation can be done, in which the present rate of pregnancy after thawing, IVF and intrauterine transfer is 57% per embryo.[54] Several disadvantages of these techniques exist and include: (a) delayed plan for cancer therapy for two or more weeks after the commencement of the next menstrual period and (b) exposure of the women to higher than average estrogen levels during ovarian stimulation.

In order to diminish the time until retrieval and to circumvent high estrogen levels in women who have estrogen dependent cancers (e.g. breast, endometrial), different approaches have been used to retrieve immature oocytes.[55,56] In a process called in vitro maturation (IVM), the immature oocytes are hormonally treated. The mature oocytes that result can be fertilized and then the embryos are frozen. In a slightly different approach, the mature oocytes can be frozen without first being fertilized. Even though some reports of pregnancy rates are comparable to those achieved with the traditional IVF method with embryo transfer, these IVM approaches have yet to become universally applied.[57]

Gonadotropin Releasing Hormone Agonists During Chemotherapy

Down-regulation of the pituitary gland with the use of a gonadotropin-releasing hormone agonist (GnRH-a) is a pharmacologic treatment to decrease ovarian damage that results from chemotherapy.[58] There are several hypotheses regarding why this method may reduce chemotherapy's gonadotoxic effects. The first hypothesis addresses the inhibition of follicle-stimulating hormone (FSH) secretion, which may prevent recruitment of pre-antral follicles. A second hypothesis identifies the decrease of FSH and luteinizing hormone (LH) stimulation as factors that would reduce ovarian perfusion. Lastly, another hypothesis describes decreased FSH stimulation of the ovary as an up-regulator of sphingosine-1-phosphate, which may be used as an ovarian cytoprotectant.[52,58,59]

The ability of pituitary down-regulation to hinder pre-antral follicle recruitment is currently in question. In a patient with Hodgkin's disease who was treated with GnRH-a, continued growth of primordial follicles was observed.[60] It has been suggested by in vitro studies of human ovarian tissue that pre-antral follicles display growth that is FSH independent and that this observation might give an explanation of why antral follicle development is not completely inhibited by pituitary down-regulation.[52] Other studies have observed that, during GnRH-a therapy and the hypogonadal state preceding puberty, primordial follicles continue to begin growth.[61]

In a review of GnRH-a use during chemotherapy in clinical studies it was concluded that, even though some evidence exists that GnRH-a therapy does diminish chemotherapy-related gonadotoxicity, such a concept has yet to be statistically proven.[62] In the nine studies analyzed, the frequency of ovarian failure following chemotherapy was 11% in women who received GnRH-a, as compared with 56% in women who had not received GnRH-a. That said, because the majority of these studies were small, retrospective and non-randomized, uncertainty remains regarding the benefit of GnRH-a.

Surgical Approaches for Preserving Ovarian Function

Commonly used approaches for gynecologic cancers and other cancers in a woman's reproductive years (specifically lymphomas and breast cancer) include radiation therapy and chemotherapy. Because both pelvic irradiation and systemic chemotherapy can cause harm to the ovaries, several surgical approaches have been devised to attempt preservation of ovarian function. Two of such surgical techniques are: (a) ovarian transposition and (b) ovarian tissue cryopreservation and re-implantation (**Table 2**).

Ovarian Transposition

Oophoropexy, or ovarian transposition, surgically mobilizes the ovary, with its vascular pedicle and then relocates the ovary outside of the planned field of radiation therapy. Minimization of ovarian radiation exposure is the goal in order to safeguard ovarian function and hopefully fertility.[63] For women undergoing radiotherapy, both local pelvic and abdominal, for a number of cancers, including cervical, vaginal, dysgerminona and Hodgkin's disease, the techniques and results of ovarian transposition have been described.[64-67]

The traditional external beam radiation and brachytherapy are devised to send a radiation dose of >4000 cGy to the pelvis.[68] A dose of >1200 cGy to the ovary will produce premature ovarian failure in >50% of patients. After ovarian transposition from the pelvis, the ovaries get an estimated 5–10% of the total pelvic dose because of scatter.[69] Due to both radiation scatter and the circulation changes from surgery, surgical transposition does not consistently save ovarian function.

Technique

Originally, ovarian transposition was undertaken via laparotomy.[70,71] Recently, however, a laparoscopic approach has been used.[67] Typically, ovarian transposition starts with occlusion and division of the utero-ovarian ligament, which is then followed by separation of the ovary from the Fallopian tube.[66] By incising the peritoneum along the length of the infundibulopelvic ligament, the ovaries are then mobilized. Lastly, the ovaries are laterally moved and affixed to the peritoneum high in paracolic gutters.

As an alternative transposition location, the ovaries can be placed behind the uterus should lateral pelvic radiation therapy be needed, as is usually the circumstance with lymphomas.[67] In theory, a potential disadvantage of midline oophoropexy is a larger radiation exposure to the ovaries because of internal scatter.

Ovarian Function Preservation

In 50–79% of women, ovarian transposition before pelvic irradiation has preserved ovarian function.[66,70] However, these comparatively short-term studies have yet to have determined just how many of these patients will subsequently have premature ovarian failure.

Fertility Preservation

In terms of efficacy, ovarian transposition is worse at fertility preservation than at ovarian hormonal function preservation. Likely, this significant decrease in fertility is due to the severing of the ovaries from the Fallopian tubes and the subsequent lateral displacement. In a study by Morice et al. of 37 patients, 16 pregnancies spontaneously occurred; however in 12 of these patients, the ovaries were not severed from the Fallopian tubes.[66]

In the event that spontaneous pregnancy does not occur after the ovaries were separated from the Fallopian tubes, retrieval of oocytes followed by IVF has had some success. That said, transvaginal oocyte retrieval is usually difficult after lateral transposition and may necessitate a transabdominal or laparoscopic approach for oocyte retrieval.

OVARIAN TISSUE TRANSPLANTATION

Transplantation of ovarian tissue is an experimental treatment with significant promise for many cancer patients, particularly adolescent girls and children. For ovarian tissue transplantation,

TABLE 2 Surgical methods for preserving ovarian function for reproductive-age women with cancer undergoing pelvic irradiation or systemic chemotherapy.

Method	*Indication*	*Approaches*	*Effectiveness*
Ovarian transposition	Cancer requiring pelvic radiation therapy	• Lateral transposition • Medial transposition	• Often preserves ovarian function • Might require IVF to restore fertility
Ovarian transplantation	Cancer requiring pelvic irradiation or systemic chemotherapy	1. Laparoscopic removal of ovarian tissue 2. Cryopreservation 3. Transplantation of ovarian tissue	• Remains experimental • Preservation of ovarian function and fertility is possible

Reproduced with permission from: Bedaiwy MA, Zanotti K, Shahin A, AbdelRahman M, Hurd WW. Surgical strategies for fertility preservation in women with cancer. Current Women Health Reviews. 2010; 6: 167.

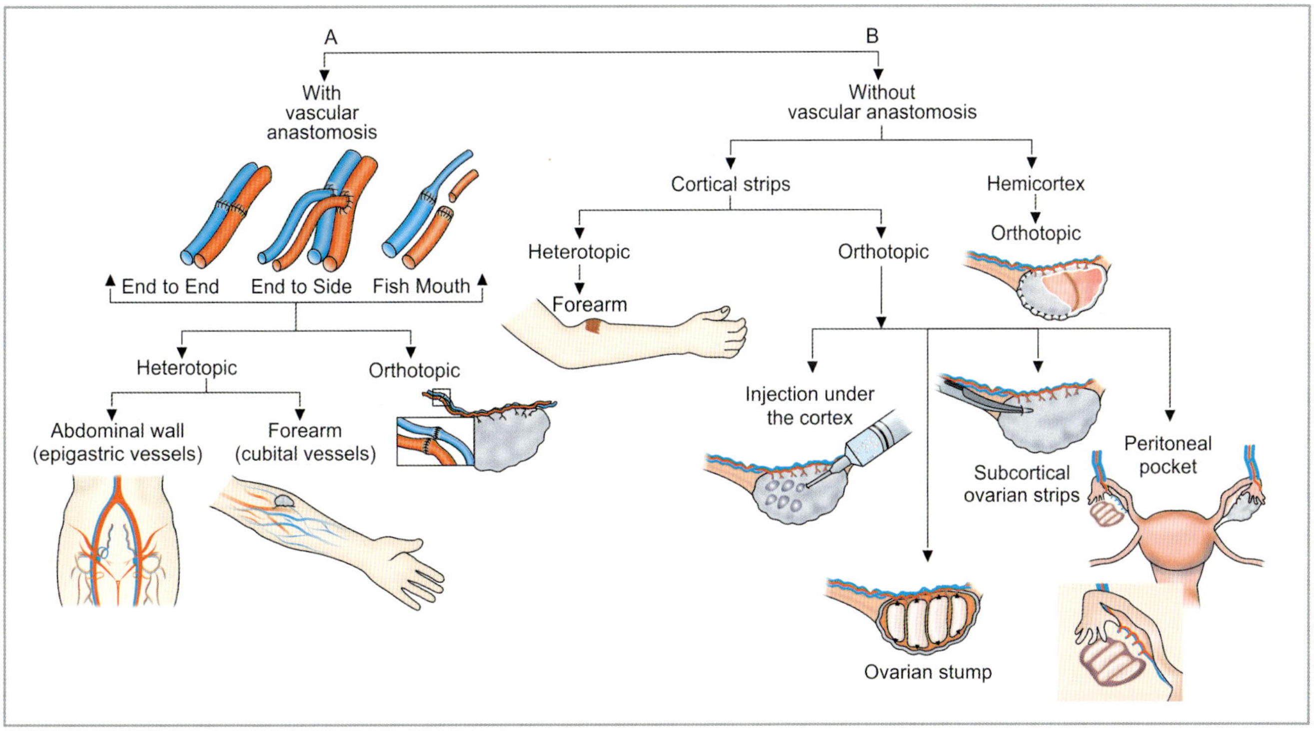

FIGURE 1 Various proposed sites of ovarian transplantation with and without vascular anastomosis. Reproduced with permission from: Bedaiwy MA, Shahin AY, Falcone T. Reproductive organ transplantation: advances and controversies. Fertil Steril. 2008 Dec;90(6):2031-55.

ovarian tissue is surgically removed before radiation or chemotherapy and then cryopreserved. Following completion of cancer therapy and when the patient is in remission, autologous transplantation is undertaken (e.g. the ovarian tissue is transplanted back into the patient). This approach is experimental but has been used in order to protect both ovarian function and fertility.

There are two approaches that have been used for the first stage of ovarian tissue transplantation: (a) removal of the whole ovary, or large sections of the ovary with a vascular pedicle and (b) removal of ovarian cortex tissue. In "orthotopic" transplants, ovarian cortex tissue is transplanted back onto the ovary. In "heterotopic" transplants, the ovarian cortex tissue is transplanted onto subcutaneous locations distant from the pelvis. **Figure 1** illustrates the varying locations and methods for ovarian transplantation.

Ovarian Tissue Transplant with Vascular Pedicles

In order to restart ovarian function in women who have premature ovarian failure, surgical removal of ovarian tissue with a vascular pedicle followed by orthotopic transplantation back into the adnexal region has been performed with transplantation of the patient's identical twin's ovary into the patient's adnexa as well.[72] Presently, microvascular anastomoses are undertaken via laparotomy, though laparoscopic methods are also being explored.[73]

Ovarian tissue transplantation is still experimental. In animal models where ovaries were removed with their vascular pedicles and then auto-transplanted, it has shown success. The vessels of the ovaries were anastomosed to the deep inferior epigastric vessels by means of end-to-end (**Figure 2**), end-to-side (**Figure 3**), or fish mouth modification (**Figure 4**). Of these three techniques, the end-to-end anastomosis provided the highest patency rate of the vascularized grafts.[73]

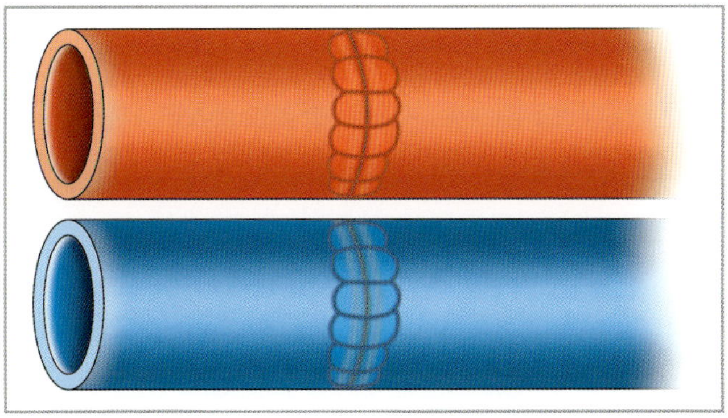

FIGURE 2 Microvascular anastomosis technique using end-to-end anastomosis. Reproduced with permission from: Bedaiwy MA, Falcone T. Harvesting and autotransplantation of vascularized ovarian grafts: approaches and techniques. Reprod BioMedicine Online. 2007; 14(3): 360-371.

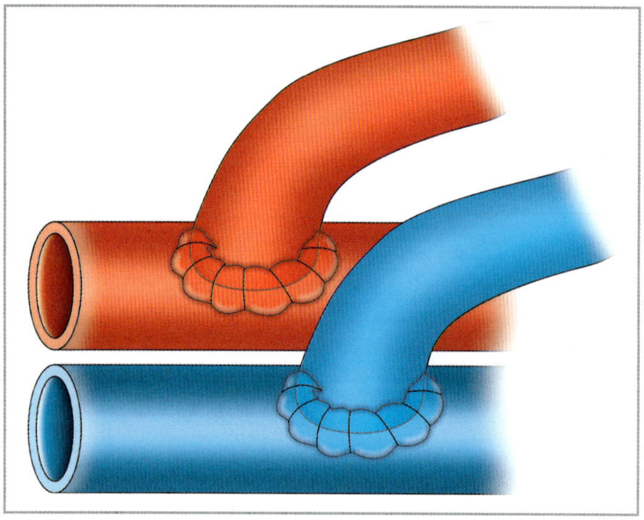

FIGURE 3 Microvascular anastomosis technique using end-to-side anastomosis. Reproduced with permission from: Bedaiwy MA, Falcone T. Harvesting and autotransplantation of vascularized ovarian grafts: approaches and techniques. Reprod BioMedicine Online. 2007; 14(3): 360-371.

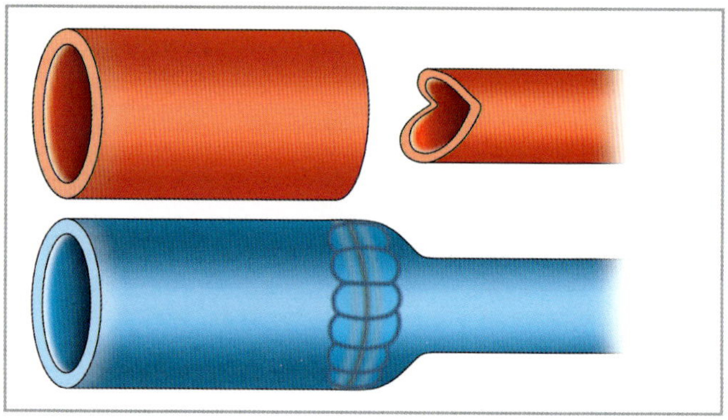

FIGURE 4 Microvascular anastomosis technique using fish mouth modification anastomosis. Reproduced with permission from: Bedaiwy MA, Falcone T. Harvesting and autotransplantation of vascularized ovarian grafts: approaches and techniques. Reprod BioMedicine Online. 2007; 14(3): 360-371.

Ovarian Cortex Transplant

In humans, surgically removing the ovarian cortex with subsequent cryopreservation followed by orthotopic transplantation back into the patient's adnexal region has had some success.[74] Additionally, heterotopic transplantation of the ovarian cortex in humans to a subcutaneous site away from the adnexal region has been reported.[75-77]

Orthotopic Transplantation

Several investigators have reported re-implantation of human ovarian cortex back onto the surface of the ovary.[78-80] After transplantation, re-establishment of ovarian function often takes longer than four months.[81] The duration of time that the grafts stay viable after the transplantation varies and reports range from a few months to over five years.[81] Even though, through this technique, menstrual function is returned, in patients who have previous ovarian failure, their basal FSH levels stay elevated, which indicates a diminished ovarian reserve.[82] **Table 3** sums up ovarian functions after orthotopic ovarian transplantation.

TABLE 3 Ovarian functions following orthotopic ovarian transplantation.

Reference	*Aproach of transplantation*	*Number and size of the graft*	*Chemo before freezing*	*Recovery time*	*Follicular development after transplantation*	*Laboratory findings*
Oktay and Karlikaya, 2000[50]	O: Pelvic peritoneum	eight pieces each 5–10 × 2 mm	No	16 weeks	folliculogenesis	↑ E_2, ovulation, menses
Radford et al., 2001[51]	O: Ovarian	2 pieces each 10 × 5 × 1	Yes	8 weeks	folliculogenesis	↓ FSH, ↓ LH, ↑ E_2 ovulation, menses (one cycle)
Donnez et al., 2004[1]	O: ovarian fossa	67 pieces each 2 × 2 × 1	No	18 weeks	folliculogenesis	
Meirow et al.l 2005[2]	O: Ovarian	3 + 8 pieces, sized 15 × 2 × 2	Yes	32 weeks	folliculogenesis	
Schmidt et al., 2005[52]	O: ovarian + peritoneum H: abdominal wall	12 pieces in three different undetemined sizes (4 + 4 + 4)	No	19/22 weeks	folliculogenesis	
Donnez et al., 2006[53]	Orthotopic: ovarian (a) + ovarian fossa peritoneum (b)	69 pieces (2 × 2 × 1 mm): 45 (a) + 24 (b)	No	16 weeks	A follicle of 20 mm in diameter	↓ FSH, ↑ AMH and inhibin B modified natural cycle IVF, oocyte retrieval, one MII oocytes, IVF-ICSI, four-cell embryo, pregnancy, live birth

Note: ICSI = intracytoplasmic sperm injection

Reproduced with permission from: Bedaiwy MA, Shahin AY, Falcone T. Reproductive organ transplantation: advances and controversies. Fertil Steril. 2008 Dec;90(6):2031-55.

TABLE 4 Ovarian functions following heterotopic ovarian transplantation

Reference	*Aproach of transplantation*	*Number and size of the graft*	*Chemo before freezing*	*Recovery time*	*Follicular development after transplantation*	*Laboratory findings*
Oktay et al., 2001[41,42]	H: fore arm	16 strips of 1 × 50	No	10–26 weeks	Folliculogenesis, menstruation, documented ovulation and egg retrieval	↓ FSH, ↑ E_2, ovulation retrieval of MII oocyte
Callejo et al., 2001[58]	H: rectus abdomins	40–45 pieces each 2–3 mm	No	12–16 weeks	Folliculogenesis (20 mm)	↑ E_2
Kim et al., 2004 [57,59]	H: breast H: rectus	40 pieces each 5 × 5 × 5	No	14 weeks	Folliculogenesis	↓ FSH, ↑ E_2, ovulation
Oktay et al., 2004[44]	H: SC abdominal wall	15 pieces each 15 × 2 × 2	No	12 weeks	Folliculoenesis	Retrieval, 20 oocytes, eight IVF-ICSI, four-cell embryos and one aneuploid embryo
Wolner-Hanseen et al. (2005)	Heterotopic: SC forearm	10 pieces (1–2 × 1–2 × 0.5–1 mm)	No	18 weeks	Folliculogenesis of two follicles: 12.6 and 6.7 mm in diameter after local gonadotrophin stimulation	↓ FSH, ↓ LH, ↑ E_2, ovulation, regular cycles, pregnancy, live birth
Hilders et al., 2004[61]	Heterotopic: arm	whole fresh ovary	No	No comment	–	Doppler indicating normal blood flow in anastomosed artery and vein, local vault reccurence
Oktay et al., 2006[54]	Heterotopic: SC abdominal wall	Left ovary in pieces	Yes	8 weeks	Folliculogenesis, documented ovulation	↓ FSH, ↑ E_2, menses, no stimulation, empty follicle (20 mm)

Note: ICSI = intracytoplasmic sperm injection

Reproduced with permission from: Bedaiwy MA, Shahin AY, Falcone T. Reproductive organ transplantation: advances and controversies. Fertil Steril. 2008 Dec;90(6):2031-55.

Fertility Preservation

Successful pregnancies have occurred after frozen-thawed cortical tissue is autologously transplanted to orthotopic sites.[78-80] Most of these reported pregnancies occurred spontaneously after menstrual function returned and FSH levels normalized. These spontaneous pregnancies often occurred at some point in the first year after the transplantation. Oocytes that were harvested from ovarian cortex that was transplanted have the tendency to be immature and of poor quality when IVF is later attempted.[83]

Heterotopic Transplantation

Also reported in humans is the re-implantation of ovarian cortex to subcutaneous locations distant to the pelvis.[84,85] This technique avoids the risks associated with a second surgery to re-transplant the ovarian cortex tissue back onto the ovary. That said, the ischemia that the tissue experiences before spontaneous neovascularization likely is harmful to the tissue transplant's subsequent functionality. Moreover, future fertility requires oocyte retrieval and IVF. So far, there have been no reported pregnancies using this technique. **Table 4** sums up ovarian functions after heterotopic ovarian transplantation.

CONCLUSION

Some women of reproductive-age who have gynecologic cancers can benefit from fertility-sparing surgery. Proper selection of patients can not only yield survival rates similar to traditional radical surgery but also spare a woman's fertility. Appropriate women who have borderline or grade I, stage I ovarian cancer can have unilateral oophorectomy. Stage I cervical cancer patients can undergo radical trachelectomy. Lastly, young women who have stage I endometrial cancer can have progestin therapy in order to avoid the necessity of a hysterectomy.

Surgical approaches that take into account fertility preservation additionally can be used for women of reproductive-age who are diagnosed with cancer and require pelvic irradiation or systemic chemotherapy. Subsequent ovarian function can be preserved if the ovaries are translocated before pelvic irradiation. Should systemic chemotherapy be planned, developing experimental methods include the surgical removal and cryopreservation of ovarian tissue. Following remission by the patient, ovarian tissue is transplanted back into the patient. This technique has restored not only ovarian function but also resulted in successful pregnancies in some women.

Continuing efforts are being made to develop methods to conserve ovarian function and fertility in cancer patients who are of reproductive-age. For the best chance at continued ovarian function and fertility, these techniques must be put into practice as part of the preliminary approach to cancer therapy and before definitive radiation or chemotherapy. Looking forward, fertility preservation for women of reproductive-age who have cancer will likely involve ovarian tissue removal, followed by in vitro follicle culture of the tissue and then oocyte removal.[86] This technique will provide immature eggs, which will then be the subject of in vitro maturation. Currently, more effective cryopreservation techniques are being developed for not only oocytes, but also embryos.

REFERENCES

1. Jemal A, Siegel R, Ward E, et al. Cancer statistics 2009. CA Cancer J Clin. 2009;59(4):225-49.
2. Schover LR, Holmes D, Makin G. Knowledge and experience regarding cancer, infertility, and sperm banking in younger male survivors. J Clin Oncol. 2002;20(7):1880-9.
3. Schover LR, Rybicki LA, Martin BA, Bringelsen KA. Having children after cancer. A pilot survey of survivors' attitudes and experiences. Cancer. 1999;86(4):697-709.
4. Lee SJ, Schover LR, Partridge AH, et al. American Society of Clinical Oncology recommendations on fertility preservation in cancer patients. J Clin Oncol. 2006;24(18):2917-31.
5. Panel, A.R.o.P.s.C., Annual Report of President's Cancer Panel 2005-2006. Available at: http:// deainfo.nci.nih.gov/advisory/pcp/pcp06rpt/pcp06rpt.pdf. 2005-2006.
6. SEERS, National Cancer Institute. Cancer Surveillance Epidemiology and End Results (SEER). <http://seer.cancer.gov/statfacts/html/corp.html>.
7. Azem F, Yovel I, Wagman I, et al. Surrogate pregnancy in a patient who underwent radical hysterectomy and bilateral transposition of ovaries. Fertil Steril. 2003;79(5):1229-30.
8. Giacalone PL, Laffargue F, Bénos P, et al. Successful in vitro fertilization-surrogate pregnancy in a patient with ovarian transposition who had undergone chemotherapy and pelvic irradiation. Fertil Steril. 2001;76(2):388-9.
9. Ramirez PT. Fertility-Sparing Options for Treatment of Women with gynecologic Cancers, in Gynecologic Cancer, Springer. 2006; p. 44-60.
10. Mathevet P, Chemali E, Roy M, Dargent D. Long-term outcome of a randomized study comparing three techniques of conization: cold knife, laser, and LEEP. Eur J Obstet Gynecol Reprod Biol. 2003; 106(2):214-8.
11. Paraskevaidis E, Koliopoulos G, Lolis E, et al. Delivery outcomes following loop electrosurgical excision procedure for microinvasive (FIGO stage IA1) cervical cancer. Gynecol Oncol. 2002;86(1):10-3.
12. Kyrgiou M, Koliopoulos G, Martin-Hirsch P, et al. Obstetric outcomes after conservative treatment for intraepithelial or early invasive cervical lesions: systematic review and meta-analysis. Lancet. 2006;367(9509): 489-98.
13. Samson SL, Bentley JR, Fahey TJ, et al. The effect of loop electrosurgical excision procedure on future pregnancy outcome. Obstet Gynecol. 2005;105(2):325-32.
14. Burnett AF, Roman LD, O'Meara AT, Morrow CP. Radical vaginal trachelectomy and pelvic lymphadenectomy for preservation of fertility in early cervical carcinoma. Gynecol Oncol. 2003;88(3):419-23.
15. Covens A, Shaw P, Murphy J, et al. Is radical trachelectomy a safe alternative to radical hysterectomy for patients with stage IA-B carcinoma of the cervix? Cancer. 1999;86(11):2273-9.
16. Rodriguez M, Guimares O, Rose PG. Radical abdominal trachelectomy and pelvic lymphadenectomy with uterine conservation and subsequent pregnancy in the treatment of early invasive cervical cancer. Am J Obstet Gynecol. 2001;185(2):370-4.
17. Shepherd JH, Mould T, Oram DH. Radical trachelectomy in early stage carcinoma of the cervix: outcome as judged by recurrence and fertility rates. Br J Obstet Gynaecol. 2001;108(8):882-5.
18. Smith JR, Boyle DC, Corless DJ, et al. Abdominal radical trachelectomy: a new surgical technique for the conservative management of cervical carcinoma. Br J Obstet Gynaecol. 1997;104(10):1196-200.
19. Cibula D, Ungar L, Palfalvi L, et al. Laparoscopic abdominal radical trachelectomy. Gynecol Oncol. 2005;97(2):707-9.
20. Dargent D, Martin X, Sacchetoni A, Mathevet P. Laparoscopic vaginal radical trachelectomy: a treatment to preserve the fertility of cervical carcinoma patients. Cancer. 2000;88(8):1877-82.
21. Plante M, Renaud MC, François H, Roy M. Vaginal radical trachelectomy: an oncologically safe fertility-preserving surgery. An updated series of 72 cases and review of the literature. Gynecol Oncol. 2004;94(3):614-23.
22. Ramirez PT, Schmeler KM, Soliman PT, Frumovitz M. Fertility preservation in patients with early cervical cancer: radical trachelectomy. Gynecol Oncol. 2008;110(3 Suppl 2):S25-8.
23. Duska LR, Chang YC, Flynn CE, et al. Epithelial ovarian carcinoma in the reproductive age group. Cancer. 1999; 85(12):2623-9.
24. Gonzalez-Lira G, Escudero-De Los Rios P, Salazar- Martinez E, et al. Conservative surgery for ovarian cancer and effect on fertility. Int J Gynaecol Obstet. 1997;56(2):155-62.
25. Schilder JM, Thompson AM, DePriest DP, et al.Outcome of reproductive age women with stage IA or IC invasive epithelial ovarian cancer treated with fertility-sparing therapy. Gynecol Oncol. 2002;87(1):1-7.
26. Barnhill DR, Kurman RJ, Brady MF, et al. Preliminary analysis of the behavior of stage I ovarian serous tumors of low malignant potential: a Gynecologic Oncology Group study. J Clin Oncol. 1995;13(11): 2752-6.
27. Seidman JD, Kurman RJ. Subclassification of serous borderline tumors of the ovary into benign and malignant types. A clinicopathologic study of 65 advanced stage cases. Am J Surg Pathol. 1996;20(11): 1331-45.
28. Imai A, Furui T, Tamaya T. Gynecologic tumors and symptoms in childhood and adolescence; 10-years' experience. Int J Gynaecol Obstet. 1994;45(3):227-34.
29. Berman ML. Future directions in the surgical management of ovarian cancer. Gynecol Oncol. 2003;90(2 Pt 2):S33-9.
30. Gershenson D. Fertility-sparing surgery for malignancies in women. J Natl Cancer Inst Monogr. 2005;34:43-7.
31. Thomas GM, Dembo AJ, Hacker NF, et al. Current therapy for dysgerminoma of the ovary. Obstet Gynecol. 1987;70(2):268-75.
32. Park JY, Kim DY, Kim JH, et al. Surgical management of borderline ovarian tumors: The role of fertility-sparing surgery. Gynecol Oncol. 2009;113(1):75-82.
33. Wright JD, Shah M, Mathew L, et al. Fertility preservation in young women with epithelial ovarian cancer. Cancer. 2009; 115(18):4118-26.
34. Cass I, Li AJ, Runowicz CD, et al. Pattern of lymph node metastases in clinically unilateral stage I invasive epithelial ovarian carcinomas. Gynecol Oncol. 2001;80(1):56-61.

35. Benjamin I, Morgan MA, Rubin SC. Occult bilateral involvement in stage I epithelial ovarian cancer. Gynecol Oncol. 1999;72(3):288-91.
36. Morice P, Camatte S, Wicart-Poque F, et al. Results of conservative treatment in epithelial ovarian carcinoma. Cancer. 2001;92(9): 2412-8.
37. DiSaia PJ,, Adenocarcinoma of the uterus. In: DiSaia PJ, Creasman WT (Eds). Clinical gynecologic oncology. 5th edition. St. Louis: Mosby. 1997;134-68.
38. American Cancer Society, Cancer facts and figures. 2002. Available at: http://www.cancer.org: p. (Last accessed: May, 13, 2007).
39. Scholten AN, van Putten WL, Beerman H, et al. Postoperative radiotherapy for Stage 1 endometrial carcinoma: long-term outcome of the randomized PORTEC trial with central pathology review. Int J Radiat Oncol Biol Phys. 2005;63(3):834-8.
40. Benshushan A. Endometrial adenocarcinoma in young patients: evaluation and fertility-preserving treatment. Eur J Obstet Gynecol Reprod Biol. 2004;117(2):132-7.
41. Kaku T, Yoshikawa H, Tsuda H, et al. Conservative therapy for adenocarcinoma and atypical endometrial hyperplasia of the endometrium in young women: central pathologic review and treatment outcome. Cancer Lett. 2001;167(1):39-48.
42. Pinto AB, Gopal M, Herzog TJ, et al. Successful in vitro fertilization pregnancy after conservative management of endometrial cancer. Fertil Steril. 2001;76(4):826-9.
43. Thigpen JT, Brady MF, Alvarez RD, et al. Oral medroxyprogesterone acetate in the treatment of advanced or recurrent endometrial carcinoma: a dose-response study by the Gynecologic Oncology Group. J Clin Oncol. 1999;17(6):1736-44.
44. Kinkel K, Kaji Y, Yu KK, et al. Radiologic staging in patients with endometrial cancer: a meta-analysis. Radiology. 1999; 212(3):711-8.
45. Zarbo G, Caruso G, Caruso S, et al. Endometrial cancer: preoperative evaluation of myometrial infiltration magnetic resonance imaging versus transvaginal ultrasonography. Eur J Gynaecol Oncol. 2000;21(1):95-7.
46. Creasman WT, Morrow CP, Bundy BN, et al. Surgical pathologic spread patterns of endometrial cancer. A Gynecologic Oncology Group Study. Cancer. 1987;60(8 Suppl):2035-41.
47. Evans-Metcalf ER, Brooks SE, Reale FR, et al. Profile of women 45 years of age and younger with endometrial cancer. Obstet Gynecol. 1998; 91(3):349-54.
48. Zanetta G, Chiari S, Rota S, et al. Conservative surgery for stage I ovarian carcinoma in women of childbearing age. Br J Obstet Gynaecol. 1997;104(9):1030-5.
49. Gotlieb WH, Beiner ME, Shalmon B, et al. Outcome of fertility-sparing treatment with progestins in young patients with endometrial cancer. Obstet Gynecol. 2003;102(4):718-25.
50. Chiva L, Lapuente F, González-Cortijo L, et al. Sparing fertility in young patients with endometrial cancer. Gynecol Oncol. 2008;111(2 Suppl):S101-4.
51. Bines J, Oleske DM, Cobleigh MA, Ovarian function in premenopausal women treated with adjuvant chemotherapy for breast cancer. J Clin Oncol. 1996;14(5):1718-29.
52. Oktay K, Sonmezer M. Fertility preservation in gynecologic cancers. Curr Opin Oncol. 2007;19(5):506-11.
53. Sonmezer M, Oktay K. Fertility preservation in female patients. Hum Reprod Update. 2004;10(3):251-66.
54. Grifo JA, Noyes N. Delivery rate using cryopreserved oocytes is comparable to conventional in vitro fertilization using fresh oocytes: potential fertility preservation for female cancer patients. Fertil Steril. 2010;93(2):391-6.
55. Huang JYJ, Tulandi T, Holzer H, et al. Combining ovarian tissue cryobanking with retrieval of immature oocytes followed by in vitro maturation and vitrification: an additional strategy of fertility preservation. Fertil Steril. 2008;89(3):567-72.
56. Huang, JYJ, Buckett WM, Gilbert L, et al. Retrieval of immature oocytes followed by in vitro maturation and vitrification: a case report on a new strategy of fertility preservation in women with borderline ovarian malignancy. Gynecol Oncol. 2007;105(2): 542-4.
57. Son WY, Chung JT, Herrero B, et al. A 38 h interval between hCG priming and oocyte retrieval increases in vivo and in vitro oocyte maturation rate in programmed IVM cycles. Hum Reprod 2008;23(9): 2010-6.
58. Blumenfeld Z, von Wolff M. GnRH-analogues and oral contraceptives for fertility preservation in women during chemotherapy. Hum Reprod Update. 2008;14(6):543-52.
59. Oktay K, Sonmezer M. Gonadotropin-releasing hormone analogs in fertility preservation-lack of biological basis? Nat Clin Pract Endocrinol Metab. 2008;4(9):488-9.
60. Azem F, Hasson J, Cohen T, et al. Retrieval of immature oocytes after chemotherapy for Hodgkin's disease and prolonged ovarian down-regulation with gonadotropin-releasing hormone agonist. Fertil Steril. 2009;92(2):828e1-2.
61. Zeleznik AJ. The physiology of follicle selection. Reprod Biol Endocrinol. 2004;2:31.
62. Blumenfeld Z. GnRH-agonists in fertility preservation. Curr Opin Endocrinol Diabetes Obes. 2008;15(6):523-8.
63. Owens, S., Roberts, W. S., Fiorica, J. V. et al. Ovarian management at the time of radical hysterectomy for cancer of the cervix. Gynecol Oncol. 1989;35(3):349-51.
64. Dursun P, Ayhan A, Yanik FB, Kuşçu E. Ovarian transposition for the preservation of ovarian function in young patients with cervical carcinoma. Eur J Gynaecol Oncol. 2009;30(1):13-5.
65. Howard FM. Laparoscopic lateral ovarian transposition before radiation treatment of Hodgkin disease. J Am Assoc Gynecol Laparosc. 1997;4(5):601-4.
66. Morice P, Castaigne D, Haie-Meder C, et al. Laparoscopic ovarian transposition for pelvic malignancies: indications and functional outcomes. Fertil Steril. 1998;70(5):956-60.
67. Terenziani M, Piva L, Meazza C, et al. Oophoropexy: a relevant role in preservation of ovarian function after pelvic irradiation. Fertil Steril. 2009;91(3):935 e15-6.
68. Covens AL, van der Putten HW, Fyles AW. Laparoscopic ovarian transposition. Eur J Gynaecol Oncol. 1996;17(3):177-82.
69. Wallace WH, Shalet SM, Crowne EC, et al. Gonadal dysfunction due to cis-platinum. Med Pediatr Oncol. 1989;17(5):409-13.
70. Feeney DD, Moore DH, Look KY, et al. The fate of the ovaries after radical hysterectomy and ovarian transposition. Gynecol Oncol. 1995;56(1):3-7.
71. Morice P, Thiam-Ba R, Castaine D. Fertility results after ovarian transposition for pelvic malignancies treated by external irradiation or brachytherapy. Hum Reprod. 1998;13(3):660-3.
72. Mhatre P, Mhatre J, Magotra R. Ovarian transplant: a new frontier. Transplant Proc. 2005;37(2):1396-8.
73. Bedaiwy MA, Falcone T. Harvesting and autotransplantation of vascularized ovarian grafts: approaches and techniques. Reprod Biomed Online. 2007;14:360-71.
74. Sánchez M, Alamá P, Gadea B, et al. Fresh human orthotopic ovarian cortex transplantation: long-term results. Hum Reprod. 2007;22(3): 786-91.
75. Donnez J, Dolmans MM, Demylle D, et al. Restoration of ovarian function after orthotopic (intraovarian and periovarian) transplantation of cryopreserved ovarian tissue in a woman treated by bone marrow transplantation for sickle cell anaemia: case report. Hum Reprod. 2006;21(1):183-8.
76. Donnez J, Squifflet J, Van Eyck AS, et al. Restoration of ovarian function in orthotopically transplanted cryopreserved ovarian tissue: a pilot experience. Reprod Biomed Online. 2008;16(5):694-704.

77. Radford JA, Lieberman BA, Brison DR, et al Orthotopic reimplantation of cryopreserved ovarian cortical strips after high-dose chemotherapy for Hodgkin's lymphoma. Lancet. 2001;357(9263):1172-5.
78. Donnez J, Dolmans MM, Demylle D, et al. Livebirth after orthotopic transplantation of cryopreserved ovarian tissue. Lancet. 2004; 364(9443):1405-10.
79. Meirow D, Levron J, Eldar-Geva T, et al. Pregnancy after transplantation of cryopreserved ovarian tissue in a patient with ovarian failure after chemotherapy. N Engl J Med. 2005;353(3):318-21.
80. Demeestere I, Simon P, Emiliani S, et al. Fertility Preservation: Successful Transplantation of Cryopreserved Ovarian Tissue in a Young Patient Previously Treated for Hodgkin's Disease. Oncologist. 2007;12(12):1437-42.
81. Bedaiwy MA, Shahin AY, Falcone T. Reproductive organ transplantation: advances and controversies. Fertil Steril. 2008;90(6): 2031-55.
82. Donnez J, Squifflet J, Dolmans MM, et al. Orthotopic transplantation of fresh ovarian cortex: a report of two cases. Fertil Steril. 2005;84: 1018.
83. Tryde Schmidt KL, Yding Andersen C, Starup J, et al. Orthotopic autotransplantation of cryopreserved ovarian tissue to a woman cured of cancer - follicular growth, steroid production and oocyte retrieval. Reprod Biomed Online. 2004;8(4):448-53.
84. Grazul-Bilska AT, Banerjee J, Yazici I, et al. Morphology and function of cryopreserved whole ovine ovaries after heterotopic autotransplantation. Reprod Biol Endocrinol. 2008;6:16.
85. Sonmezer M, Oktay K. Orthotopic and heterotopic ovarian tissue transplantation. Best Pract Res Clin Obstet Gynaecol. 2010 Feb;24(1):113-26.
86. Picton HM, Harris SE, Muruvi W, Chambers EL.The in vitro growth and maturation of follicles. Reprod. 2008;136(6):703-15.

8

Basics of Cryobiology

Amjad Hossain, Shaikat Hossain, John Phelps III

CHAPTER OUTLINE

INTRODUCTION

Assisted Reproductive Technologies (ART) revolutionized the field of reproductive medicine by introducing new clinical innovations over the last 15 years. The medical and social impact of ART has been so profound that the 2010 Nobel Prize in Medicine and Physiology was awarded to Professor R.G. Edward of England, recognizing the impact ART has had on the field of medicine. Fertility preservation created opportunities for widening the application of ART in modern medicine. About 20% of all children born worldwide are from cryopreservation cycles. Thus, it is not an exaggeration to say that cryopreservation has become an increasingly important therapeutic strategy in assisted reproduction.[1-6]

Couples with impaired reproductive abilities can now fulfill their dreams of having children and forming a family. Cancer patients have the opportunity to preserve their fertility prior to undergoing radiation or chemotherapy. People opting for sterilization have similar opportunities too. Posthumous reproduction is now a reality due to the availability of fertility preservation technologies. Fertility treatment often requires storage of reproductive materials for extended periods of time to deal with the problem of uncertain supply and demand and also in order to provide patients with the flexibility of choosing an appropriate time for conception. Extended storage also gives sufficient time to perform the requisite screening to prevent the transmission of infectious pathogens. Cryopreservation has another profound advantage that makes it highly attractive. Virtually no chemical reaction occurs in biological systems at cryogenic temperature and the biological clock comes to a halt. Thus, reproductive cells and tissues stored in cryogenic temperature (–196°C) can endure storage for infinite time, with almost no biochemical change. This is probably the most effective and perhaps the only way currently known to stop and reinitiate the reproductive clock in the preferred time.[1-6]

Cryopreservation, however, is not benign because both the freezing and thawing process puts the cells under severe stresses, often causing cell death. As the materials are exposed to subzero temperature they are subjected to profound changes in the thermal, chemical and physical properties of their surrounding environment. During freezing, as the temperature drops from + 37° C to -196° C, the cells lose up to 95% of their water. Solutes concentrate inside and outside the cells, causing intracellular and extracellular ice formation to occur. These events have a harmful impact on the cells. Further, rewarming the cells to physiological temperature from the cryogenic condition may cause osmotic shock and unnatural swelling. Thus, a basic understanding of the factors that induce stresses to live cells is necessary in order to take the appropriate preventive measures against the harmful events that may occur during freezing and thawing.[1,3,5-8]

The branch of biology that deals with the principles and procedures of preserving biological materials is called Cryobiology. Understanding the basic principles of cryobiology is vital to learning how cryopreservation protocols work. There is some essential information regarding cryopreservation that one needs to know in order to achieve successful cryopreservation outcomes. This chapter attempts to familiarize the readers with the basics of cryobiology so that they acquire a background in understanding the principles and mechanisms involved in preservation of human reproductive materials. Our aim was to focus on the fundamentals of cryobiology, in order to give the readers a conceptual understanding of what goes on behind cryopreservation.[1-3,5-9]

HISTORICAL OVERVIEW OF CRYOBIOLOGY IN PARTICULAR REFERENCE TO REPRODUCTIVE MEDICINE

The word 'cryobiology' is derived from three Greek words 'cryo (cold)', 'bios (life)' and 'logos (science)'. Accordingly, Cryobiology is the study of biological materials at cold condition. In other words, Cryobiology is the branch of biology which studies the effect of low temperature on living things. The history of Cryobiology can be traced back to 2500 BC. Low temperatures were used in Egyptian practices of ancient medicine. Additionally, the use of cold was recommended to stop bleeding and swelling by the famed Greek philosopher Hippocrates. With the emergence of modern science, Robert Boyle may have made the first attempt to study the effects of low temperatures on animals. With the progress of the diverse applications of cryopreservation, the applied Cryobiology became a distinct discipline, the history of which is relatively short, less than hundred years. The review of the cryobiological literatures indicates that the potential for obtaining an ice-free state, a crucial aspect of successful cryopreservation, was achieved as early as 1937. Discovery of the cryoprotectant occurred in 1949 while performing a cryo experiment with fowl sperm. Some subsequent breakthroughs in the application of cryopreservation in the field of mammalian reproduction that had occurred are shown below in chronological order.[10-12]

1. Success was achieved in freezing sperm of farm animals in 1950s.
2. First mammalian birth was reported from cryopreserved mouse embryos in 1972.
3. Human pregnancy from frozen-thawed embryos was first reported in 1983.
4. Successful vitrification of mouse embryos was achieved in 1985.
5. First pregnancy using cryopreserved human oocytes was reported in 1986.
6. Success in freezing ovarian tissue and subsequent transplantation in sheep gave pregnancy of this kind first reported in 1994.
7. First report on follicular development in cryopreserved marmoset ovarian tissue after transplantation was reported in 1995.
8. Full development of blastocyst formation from vitrified bovine oocytes was reported first in 1996.
9. First report of a birth from cryopreservation of immature oocytes with subsequent in vitro maturation was reported in 1998.
10. Live birth after orthotropic transplantation of cryopreserved ovarian tissue was reported in 2004.

RELEVANT CRYOBIOLOGICAL FACTS IMPORTANT TO REPRODUCTIVE BIOLOGISTS

Performing cryopreservation is a routine task for a reproductive biologist. As mentioned, the success of this task depends on his understanding of the basics of cryobiology. Some of the most relevant basics of Cryobiology are discussed below.

Phenomena Behind Ice Formation

The formation of ice requires a nucleating event. It has been proposed that the nucleation of ice is initiated by an array of hydrophilic sites. The event is referred to as heterogeneous nucleation. The temperature at which ice is nucleated varies as well as the size of the nucleating site. The smaller the nucleus, the lower the temperature of nucleation is. As the temperature progressively drops, a condition called 'super cooled' arises. Ice formation in super cooled solutions is initiated by a nucleation process, which is the stochastic aggregation of water molecules into thermodynamically stable clusters from which ice crystals can grow. Thus, the rate of crystallization depends on the kinetics of both nucleation and the subsequent crystal growth. The increased solution viscosity as well as the decline in temperature can contribute to slowing down the rate of crystallization. As expected, increased concentrations of solutes in the solution will increase the solution viscosity, thus reducing the rates of nucleation and crystal growth.[7,13-19]

Around -40° C, the radius of an ice nucleus is about 1 nm and ice starts forming spontaneously, an event called homogenous nucleation. Once an ice crystal forms, the rate of growth becomes a function of temperature. Rapid cooling will result in more crystals simply because those crystals that are nucleated first will have insufficient time to grow, leaving liquid water available to be nucleated. Therefore, the slower the cooling, the larger the crystals are. Ripening of ice (recrystallization) can occur. Smaller crystals, with a smaller surface to volume ratio, have a higher vapor pressure and thus, the larger crystals grow at the expense of the smaller. With the help of concentrated solutes (CPAs), ice crystals can remain separated from each other by viscous solution, inhibiting recrystallization. Crystallization can be avoided completely by lowering the freezing point through the addition of solutes (CPAs) at high concentration. Thus, at a low enough temperature and high enough solute, the solution becomes a glassy solid usually termed as 'vitrified.'[7,15-17,19]

Theoretically the water-ice phase transition in an aqueous solution is thermodynamically possible only at temperatures below the equilibrium melting point. When ice forms in such a super cooled solution, solutes are rejected from the growing ice lattice and the unfrozen fraction of the solution becomes increasingly concentrated. On the other hand, solutes depress the equilibrium melting temperature of the unfrozen solution. The degree of super cooling will decrease concomitantly. The final equilibrium concentration of the unfrozen fraction is a function of temperature only and can be determined by mathematical models. Essentially, the thermodynamic equilibrium between ice and water serves as a regulatory mechanism for both volume and chemical composition of the solution.[7,13-17,19,20]

Mathematical Models Explaining Biophysics of Extracellular and Intracellular Water Movement, Cell Dehydration, Ice Nucleation and Crystal Growth

As temperature dips below its equilibrium melting point, ice forms in the extracellular liquid either spontaneously (breakdown of metastable state of the super cooled solution) or by deliberate 'seeding' of ice (typically by touching the sample with a chilled object). This extracellular ice phase plays a major role in the biophysical response of the cells to the cryopreservation process. It alters the chemical environment of the cells, mechanically constrains the cells and finally can induce ice formation inside the cells. By the formation of ice in the external media, a chemical imbalance between the cell (cytosol) and the unfrozen external solution occurs, giving rise to a driving force for diffusion of solution into the cell. In other words, the unfrozen external solution creates a force for diffusion of solutes into the cell and a water flux out of the cell. Since the permeability of the cell membrane to water is typically significantly higher than the corresponding solute permeability, the plasma membrane realistically behaves as a semi-permeable membrane. Thus, the cells respond to the increased tonicity of the external milieu by expressing water via osmosis.[3,8,20-22]

The kinetics of cell dehydration during freezing is now better known than before. Several mathematical models have been proposed to explain how cell dehydration occurs during freezing. By the use of these mathematical models, it has been revealed that the rate of water efflux is proportional to the osmotic pressure across the membrane and the permeability of the membrane to water. The membrane permeability is dependent on temperature and is commonly described by an 'Arrhenius' relationship as illustrated below.[3]

$$L_p\,(T) = L_{pg} \exp\,[-\,Et_p/R\,(1/T - 1/T_{ref})]$$

Where L_p, membrane water permeability; T, temperature; L_{pg}, permeability at the reference temperature (T_{ref}); Et_p, activation energy for water transport; R, gas constant.

The cell dehydration kinetics during freezing is sensitive to the values of L_{pg} and Et_p. It is important to note that these parameters vary considerably between different cell types. Variability in the response of different cells to the same freezing protocol is thus expected. As the increasing proportion of the extracellular medium solidifies, the ice matrix surrounding the cells can cause deformation to the cells.[3,8,20-22]

The exact mechanism of intracellular ice formation is not known. However, several hypotheses have been advanced to explain ice formation in the cell. These serve as the framework for the mathematical models to predict intracellular ice formation. Some of these models are phenomenological and others are mechanistic models. According to the mechanistic model, ice formation inside cells occurs by nucleation on intracellular catalytic sites. The model uses classical nucleation theory to obtain an expression for the rate of formation of intracellular ice nuclei from which ice crystals grow. The rate of nucleation is influenced by the degree of cytoplasmic super cooling as explained by the following equation.[3]

$$J\{T\} = \Omega \exp\,[-\,kT^{3}\,\Delta T^{2}]$$

Where J, nucleation rate; ΔT, super cooling; Ω, kinetic coefficient; k, thermodynamic coefficient.

Nucleation is a stochastic process; the above equation is used to calculate the probability of ice formation in a given cell undergoing cryopreservation. It should be pointed out that nucleation theory is not sufficient to fully explain the extent of intracellular crystallization since it predicts only the onset of ice formation. Recently, mathematical models of the growth of intracellular ice nuclei into microscopic crystals have been reported. According to these models, the radius of an intracellular ice crystal is a function of time as illustrated by the equation below.[3]

$$R_c\,(t) = [\,\textstyle\int^{1}_{0} x(t)^2\, D(t)\, dt]^{1/2}$$

Where t, time after appearance of the ice nucleus; x, non-dimensional crystal growth parameter; D, effective diffusivity of intracellular water.

The dynamics of ice formation inside cells are highly modulated by the concurrent dehydration process since the cytoplasmic super cooling and the diffusion constant for intracellular water depend on the instantaneous properties of the intracellular solution. One has to remember that due to water transport during freezing, both composition and volume of the cytosol are continually changing, affecting the nucleation rates and crystal growth. Cellular water which becomes super cooled (during freezing) attains thermodynamic equilibrium by leaving the cell and forming extracellular ice, or by forming a new ice phase inside the cell. Thus, the fate of the cellular water depends on the relative magnitudes of the rate of water transport and the rate of nucleation. During slow cooling, the rate of water efflux is sufficiently high to prevent super cooling and cell dehydration dominates over intracellular ice formation. Conversely, with rapid cooling, intracellular ice formation is favored. Using the above indicated mathematical models (of water transport, intracellular nucleation and crystal growth), it became possible for cryobiologists to predict what proportion of a cell population will form intracellular ice during freezing and what fraction of the intracellular liquid will crystallize. [3,8,18,23-26]

Cryoprotection involves treating biological materials with cryoprotectants, often in high concentration. This treatment produces a driving force for the movement of water by osmosis and solutes by diffusion through cell membrane. The driving force behind this flow is pressure. The flux across unit area of membrane is proportional to the solute permeability and the difference in concentration of the solute across the membrane. The direction of flux by convention is from outside to inside. Based on these assumptions, the following two equations have been developed for the determination of flow of water pressure and solute flux.[8]

A. Flow of Water Pressure

$$J_v = L_p\ A.R.T\ (C_i - C_e)$$

B. Solute Flux

$$J_s = w_s\ A.R.T\ (S_e - S_i)$$

Where J_v, water flow (volumetric flux); L_p, hydraulic conductivity (cm/atm/s); A, area of membrane; R, universal gas constant; T, absolute temperature; C_i, internal osmolalities; C_e, external osmolalities; w_s, solute permeability; S_e, external solute concentration; S_i, internal solute concentration.

The above narrated theoretical models can predict the freezing responses of cells. Accordingly, it has been possible to develop successful cryopreservation protocols for different cell and tissue types based on the models like these. [3,8,18,23-29]

Cryoprotective Agents (CPAs)/ Cryoprotectants

Cryoprotective agents (CPAs), also known as cryoprotectants, are chemicals (**Figure 1**) that are added to freezing media to prevent freezing injury to the cells. Since the accidental discovery of cryoprotectant in 1949 (see below), its use has since become an integral part of all cryopreservation protocols. Cryoprotectants fall under two categories: penetrating and non-penetrating, depending on their ability to pass through the cell membrane. Glycerol, dimethyl sulfoxide (DMSO), methanol and ethylene glycol are some examples of penetrating CPAs. Non-penetrating CPAs include polyethylene glycols, sucrose, dextrans and albumin (**Figure 1**). Penetrating CPAs are thought to protect cell injury by creating solution effects that reduce harmful concentrations of electrolytes within the cells through their colligative properties. Stabilization of intracellular and membrane bound proteins by direct interactions has also been proposed. The protective function of non-penetrating CPAs is believed to result from their ability to reduce the concentration of intracellular water, thus limiting the rate and extent of intracellular crystallization. In vitrification, cryoprotectants increase the viscosity of the cell suspension and aid in vitrification at higher cooling rates.[7,12,30-32]

Transmembrane diffusion of cryoprotectants is a temperature-dependent phenomenon. The penetration of different cryoprotectants into different cells can vary. This variation of cryoprotectant action can be estimated by suspending the cells in an isotonic solution of cryoprotectant and visually observing the time required for the cells to swell or lyse as the cryoprotectant approaches equilibrium and osmotic support is lost. Some membrane-based functions of the cells may also get lost due to the action of cryoprotectant. Osmotic tolerance should therefore be assessed. During the removal of cryoprotectant (unloading cryoprotectants), it can create hypoosmotic stresses by causing excessive cell swelling. This can be tested by exposing cells to a hyperosmotic solution first for several minutes and then abruptly transferring the cells to a slightly hypoosmotic solution. The bottom line is that a reliable estimate of osmotic limits of cells is essential to optimizing a cryoprotective regimen for any specific cell type. [7,12,30-32]

Discovery of Cryoprotective Agents (CPAs)

It was not until 1948 that a general cryopreservation method was discovered. This discovery demonstrated that restoration of cellular structure and function in cryopreserved cells is possible using an additive in the freezing protocol. The story of the discovery was published in 1949, in which Polge, Smith and Parkes disclosed that inclusion of glycerol enabled the cryopreserved material to survive freeze-thaw. Later, it was revealed that the effectiveness of a cryoprotectant depends on a number of properties, namely 1) small size, 2) highly soluble in water and remains so at low temperatures, 3) able to penetrate into cells and 4) low toxicity. High solubility creates a profound depression of the freezing temperature. Low toxicity allows usage of cryoprotectant in high concentration, which may be required to produce protective effects. The cryoprotectants discovered so far can be placed under the following two broad categories based on their ability to penetrate into cells.[7,10,12,21,33,34]

i. **Permeating:** Glycerol, DMSO, 1, 2-Propanediol (PROH), Ethylene glycol (EG), Propylene Glycol (PG).
ii. **Non-permeating:** Sucrose, Trehalose, Glucose, Lactose, Albumin.

The chemical structures of some of the selected CPAs that are commonly used in cryopreservation of human reproductive materials are shown in **Figure 1**. As evident in the Figure, all penetrating CPAs are small in size and of similar chemical structures.

Beneficial and Harmful Effects of Cryoprotectants

Cryoprotectants are obviously used in cryopreservation protocols to gain some benefit from them. They reduce the extent of crystallization (block the ability of water to freeze), replace intracellular water (at least some) and help to maintain cell volume. In sum, they are able to decrease cryoinjuries. On the other hand, cryoprotectants can have detrimental effects, such

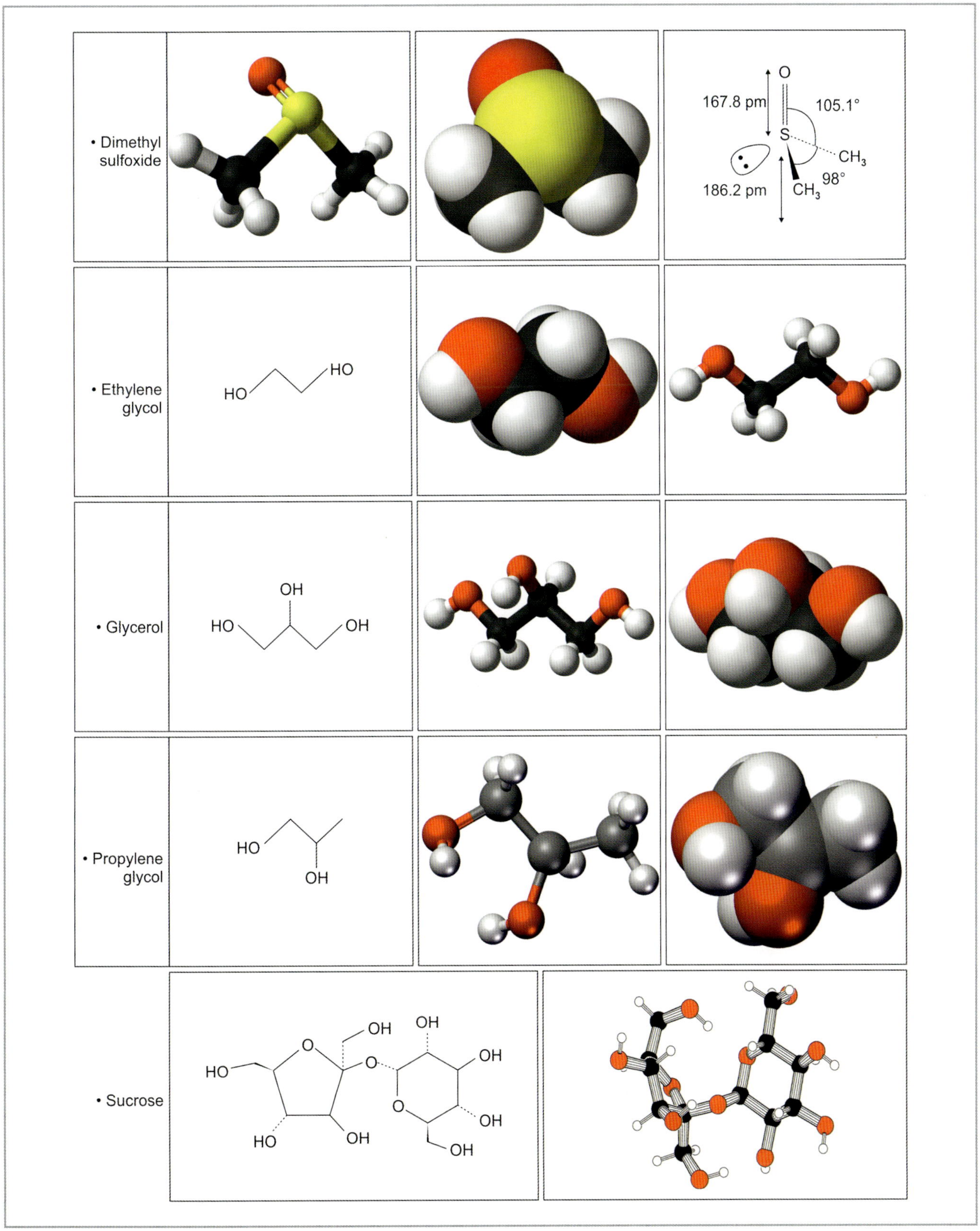

FIGURE 1 Chemical structures of some common cryoprotectants (Adapted from Wikipedia.org).

as osmotic damage and damage due to toxicity, if not properly used. In other words, improper use of cryoprotectants can lead to more harm than benefit. To minimize the harmful effects of cryoprotectants, they should be added and removed gradually in a stepwise fashion. If the exposure time is long, the toxic effects on the cells can predominate. Cryoprotectants may be toxic depending on the type, concentration, duration of exposure and temperature during exposure. [9,31,35,36]

All cryoprotectants are capable of producing some damaging effects at the concentrations used in the laboratory procedures. At the same time, they are tolerated reasonably well if properly administered and removed. The maximum concentration that can be utilized without impairment of viability is dependent on the temperature and rate of addition and removal. In slow cooling, the concentration of cryoprotectant slowly increases as ice separates. In vitrification, a much higher initial concentration is needed, but no further increase in concentration occurs during cooling simply because ice crystallizations do not occur. The concentrations of cryoprotectant needed to vitrify are usually high and carry the threat of severe toxicity. The crucial point is that there is always a toxic effect from the concentration of cryoprotectant used and that the apparent toxic effect is strongly influenced by the conditions under which the cryoprotectant is added and removed.[9,31,35,36]

Osmotic Limits of Cells and Osmotic Effects of Cryoprotectants

Although cells perform well physiologically in isotonic media, they still have limits to their stability in isotonic media. Cell shrinkage and swelling are the result of hyper- and hypoosmotic exposures, respectively. Hyperosmotic exposure of cells can cause changes in membrane permeability, integrity and function. Extreme cases can result in the extrusion of membrane components. The most common form of hyperosmotic damage results from the diffusion of non-penetrating solutes across the cell membrane. An increase in intracellular solute can severely limit the cell's tolerance to subsequent resuspension. The mechanisms of freeze related injuries to osmotic properties of cells have long been debated. It appears that different cells respond in different ways to different cryopreservation protocols. Thus, it is not possible to generalize. All living cells have a limited tolerance to hyperosmotic exposure and similarly cells have a limit to swelling if exposed to hypoosmotic condition. The cellular limitations are manifested by physical rupture.[9,29,34,35]

The osmotic effects of CPAs on living cells require special attention. Cryoprotectants penetrate cell membranes, but they do so slower compared to water, which signifies that some osmotic imbalance is inevitable during their addition or removal. High osmotic shock results in cell damage and ultimately lysis. It is therefore essential to control changes in cell volume so that acceptable limits are not transgressed. Usually two methods are followed to control cell volume during addition and removal of penetrating CPAs: (1) utilizing low rates of change in concentration i.e., change concentration in several small steps and (2) incorporation of solutes that do not penetrate the cells and therefore, function as osmotic buffer.[9,29,34,35]

Phenomena Occurring During Introduction and Removal of Cryoprotectant

Exposure of cells to high concentrations of cryoprotectant produces osmotic dehydration. If the cryoprotective agent permeates, the cells increase in volume. Water enters along with cryoprotectant until cells reach their final volume. The extent to which shrinkage and volume change will occur can be determined by analyzing the permeability parameters of the cell. During the removal of the permeating cryoprotectant, the cells are exposed to lower concentrations of the compound, which causes osmotic uptake of water, leading to cells swelling above their initial volume. The cells then shrink again as the cryoprotectant moves out, accompanied by sufficient water to maintain osmotic equilibrium. The cells can return to physiological volume only if the non- permeating solute has neither been lost nor gained during the process. Since cells are more sensitive to swelling than to shrinkage, cryoprotectant removal becomes more hazardous than its addition. Therefore, both the rate of change of volume and the final volume must be considered when designing protocols for the recovery of cryopreserved cells.[7,8,33,35]

As mentioned previously, cryopreservation protocols use penetrating cryoprotectant to reduce ice formation, lower the freezing point and raise the vitrification temperature. Since the cells have limited ability to withstand swelling and shrinking, the osmotic disequilibria induced during the addition and removal of cryoprotectants can be a critical factor. It is possible that cryo damage may be the result of solute leakage during the addition and/or removal of the cryoprotectant, rather than from freezing injury. Therefore, the addition and removal of penetrating cryoprotectants without exceeding the cell's full range of osmotic tolerance is important to remember. In an ideal protocol, one should use a concentration of cryoprotectant that does not exceed the cell's hypertonic limit. Regardless of the freezing procedure used, the loading and unloading of cryoprotectant must not be allowed to jeopardize the end result, cryosurvival. Cautions therefore should be exercised during the addition of cryoprotectants in both sequential and continuous dilution methods. It should be remembered that unloading of cryoprotectants is more of a challenge than loading, because of the fact that cells have more limited ability to swell. The main point is that the loading and unloading of cryoprotectant, whether by stepwise or continuous dilution, must not exceed the osmotic tolerance of the cells.[7,8,33,35]

CRYOPRESERVATION METHODOLOGIES

Human reproductive materials are preserved by two main approaches of cryopreservation, namely freeze-thaw and vitrification. The fundamental differences between these two approaches are that in freeze-thaw, extracellular ice formation is deliberately induced so that intracellular ice formation can be prevented, while in vitrification the ice formation is altogether avoided. Instead, attempts are taken to maintain the sample in glassy state. The first approach (freeze-thaw) involves slow freeze technique. On the contrary, in vitrification, extremely high cooling rates are a must. The example of end results of slow freeze and vitrification can be seen in **Figure 2**.

It is convincingly evident in **Figure 2** that, in slow freeze, ice formation occurs while vitrification turns the material into glass. The following strategies are reported to be followed in cryopreservation of biological materials. However, the control rate freezing (slow freeze) and vitrification are the commonly used methods. [10,27,36,37]

A. Controlled-rate Freezing
B. Equilibrium Freezing
C. Ultrarapid Freezing
D. Vitrification

PHYSICS OF FREEZING BIOLOGICAL MATERIALS

Under isotonic conditions, water in biological materials has an equilibrium melting point (EMP) around -0.6°C. Below this EMP, water becomes thermodynamically unstable and tends to crystallize (ice formation). A certain degree of super cooling occurs before the first ice nucleus is formed. The temperature at which ice nucleation occurs is usually around -5°C, but can vary. Ice formation begins preferentially in the extracellular medium due to a spontaneous breakdown of the metastable state in temperatures ranging between -5°C and -15°C. To be on the safe side, the nucleation is induced by the deliberate external seeding of ice. Intracellular water remains unfrozen at this time range.[1,13,16,22]

The above mentioned extracellular ice formation greatly influences the cellular responses to freezing. With the growth of ice, solutes accumulate into the unfrozen portion of the extracellular medium. With the extracellular medium becoming increasingly concentrated by the continuous fall of temperature, an imbalance between the cellular cytosol and the extracellular medium is created, which establishes a driving force for the diffusion of solutes into the cell and a water flux out of the cell. Since the cell membrane is semi-permeable, an osmotic gradient is created. Concurrently, as intracellular super cooling intensifies, cellular water starts to freeze. At this moment, the cell attains equilibrium either by losing water or by freezing intracellularly. However, the actual route to equilibrium depends on the velocity of cooling.[1,2,16,22]

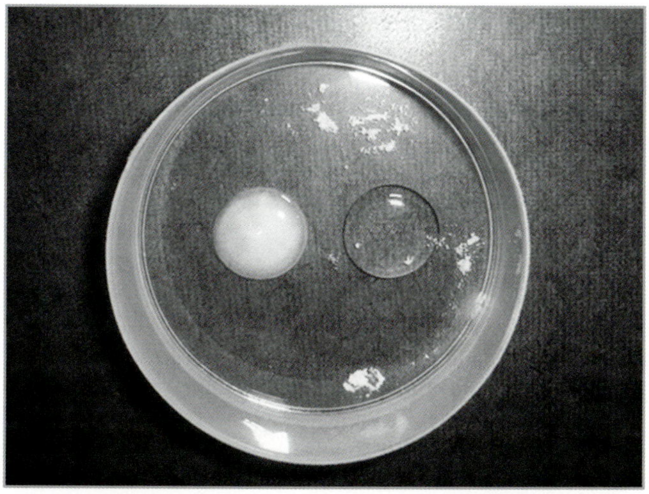

FIGURE 2 End results of slow freeze and vitrification.

In the event of slow cooling, intracellular water has sufficient time to leave the cell, leading to cell dehydration. If the cooling is faster, the cellular water does not have enough time to leave the cell. Thus, the probability of intracellular ice formation becomes higher (**Figure 2**). Several hypotheses have been proposed to explain the mechanisms behind intracellular ice formation: 1) extracellular ice catalyzes intracellular ice formation through pores in the plasma membrane (Mazur), 2) intracellular ice is seeded by extracellular ice following the rupture of the plasma membrane and subsequent exposure of the cytoplasm to extracellular ice and 3) intracellular ice formation takes place by nucleation on intracellular catalytic sites. If the cooling is extremely rapid, ice formation does not occur and instead the entire cell suspension forms glass (**Figure 2**). [1,2,13,16,26]

PHYSICOCHEMICAL AND BIOLOGICAL EVENTS OCCURRING DURING FREEZING

Cells can suffer from physical insults during freezing, which may adversely affect their biological functions. Typically, cells that survive cryopreservation respond to cooling rates in an inverted U-shaped pattern. This means cell survival is low at very slow and very fast rates of cooling and there is an intermediate rate of cooling at which survival is at a maximum. There seems to be two independent mechanisms of cell damage during cryopreservation, one occurring at slow cooling and the other at fast cooling. In the first category, the damages occur due to the result of cell dehydration and increased extracellular solute concentration. Denaturation of lipoproteins and associated lyses of the plasma membrane is suspected to happen. Some believe that there is a critical minimum cell volume that is necessary to maintain the cell in a living state, shrinkage below which is lethal. The cells that shrink osmotically during freezing can only tolerate a fixed increase in surface area (volume) during thawing.[13,24,33,35,36]

At fast (rapid) cooling, high survival rates typically demand the avoidance of intracellular ice formation. It is generally believed that cell injuries are likely caused by mechanical forces created by growing ice, which may disrupt the plasma membrane and the membranes of various sub-cellular organelles. Induction of gas bubble formation (nonmechanical mode of injury) has also been proposed. In addition to solution injuries and intracellular ice related cell injuries, there can be direct mechanical interactions between extracellular ice and the cell, which can also cause injuries. Cells can become sequestered and deformed. As a result, they can suffer possible physical damage. Ultrastructural changes in plasma membrane are supposedly caused by mechanical stresses from the extracellular ice.[13,24,33,35,36]

PHYSICOCHEMICAL AND BIOLOGICAL EVENTS OCCURRING DURING THAWING

Cells at cryogenic temperature (–196°C) must be returned to normal physiological temperature (+37°C) to be useful. There is no guarantee that a cell that has survived freezing will survive thawing, if thawing is not done properly. One has to note that the warming rate (thaw) can influence survival as much as the cooling rate. A reversed phenomenon of freezing occurs during thawing. The impact of warming will depend on the specific cryopreservation procedure used. For slowly cooled materials, response to warming rate is variable among cell types. Most slowly cooled cells have been found to be sensitive to rapid thawing since it induces a kind of osmotic shock. Also, if thawing is rapid, the cryoprotectants do not have adequate time to leave the cells. In addition, with the melting of extracellular ice, there can be rapid influx of water into the cells. All of these features, individually or collectively, can cause the cell to swell abruptly on rapid thawing, which may lead to cell injuries as extreme as lyses and death. In vitrified cells, nucleation, crystal growth, recrystallization and toxic effect of cryoprotectant can occur during warming (thaw) and the extent of these phenomena depend upon the warming rate used. If warming is slow, small crystals melt and larger crystals grow at their expense as there is sufficient time for recrystallization to occur during slow warming.[13,23,24,28,33,36]

SAFETY ISSUES IN CRYOPRESERVATION

Liquid nitrogen is utilized for cryopreservation as well as post cryopreservation storage of biological materials. It is a cryogenic liquid (–196°C). Contact of liquid nitrogen with body parts like fingers, skin, eyes, etc. may cause freezing injuries similar to frostbite. Laboratory personnel handling liquid nitrogen should be familiar with safe practices in its use. Transmission of infective agents via liquid nitrogen is of concern for both slow freezing and vitrification. Measures should be taken to minimize such risk. Direct contact between liquid nitrogen and the vitrified materials, or materials preserved by slow freeze, could be avoided as a measure to reduce such risk. A sterile secondary enclosure is reported to be an effective precaution. Procedural fault can arise from the careless handling, transport and storage of materials in liquid nitrogen, the consequences of which can be devastating. In such cases, vitrified material is more vulnerable than material preserved by slow freeze. In vitrification, conversion of a biological system from a fluid (viscous liquid) to a solid (glass) occurs solely by an increase in viscosity, without a phase-change, and without any crystallization of water (complete absence of ice). Vitrified cells and tissues are inevitably at risk of devitrification if allowed to warm some degree during handling, transport or storage. Maintaining vitrified material in a stable state (same temperature) can eliminate the risk of devitrification. The glass transition temperatures are generally in the range of –100°C to –125°C, but devitrification does not occur unless temperatures exceed that range. It is, therefore, advisable to allow a safety margin and store the materials below the glass transition temperature. Vitreous materials are brittle and liable to damage, if subjected to thermal stress.[33,38,39]

PRESERVATION OF CELLS AND TISSUES

For each type of cell there is a set of conditions that may be optimal for cryopreservation. Thus, by knowing the characteristics of a cell type, it is possible to predict a set of conditions that may produce effective preservation. The situation becomes more complicated when cryopreservation is attempted on complex multicellular systems (tissues). One has to remember that tissues contain a heterogeneous collection of cells, which may have quite different optimum requirements for preservation, which is unlike the situation in cell preservation, where one deals with a single type. It will be necessary to find a method that will secure at least adequate survival of different cells to fully reactivate the function of that tissue.[2,39,40]

CONCLUSION

As we have seen above, in cryopreservation, obtaining high viability is difficult due to the hostile environment to which cells and tissues are exposed during freezing and thawing. In freezing, temperature drops from +37°C to –196°C, with the loss of >95% water and several fold elevation of electrolyte concentration inside the cells relative to isotonic conditions. Concentrated solvents in the freezing media permeate the cells. Ice crystals intercalate the tissue and can mechanically damage the cells by disrupting intracellular structures. On the other hand, during thawing, unusual cell swelling leading to cell bursting can occur. The basic concept of Cryobiology illustrated in this chapter is expected to help to overcome these obstacles for one involved with the preservation of reproductive materials.

REFERENCES

1. Bagchi A, Woods EJ, Crister JK. Cryopreservation and Vitrification: recent advances in fertility preservation technologies. Expert Rev Med Devices. 2008;5(3):359-70.
2. Fuller B, Paynter S. Fundamentals of cryobiology in reproductive medicine. Repro BioMed Online. 2004;9(6):680-91.
3. Karlsson J, Toner M. Long-term storage of tissues by cryopreservation: critical issues. Biomaterials. 1996;17:243-56.
4. Kim SS. Fertility preservation in female cancer patients: current developments and future directions. Fertil Steril. 2006;85(1):1-11.
5. Mazur P. Freezing of living cells: mechanisms and implications. Am J Physiol. 1984;247:125-42.
6. Woods E, Benson J, Agca Y, Critser J. Fundamental cryobiology of reproductive cells and tissues. Cryobiology. 2004;48:146-56.
7. Meryman HT. Cryopreservation of living cells: principles and practice. Transfusion. 2007;47:935-45.
8. Pegg DE. Principles of Cryopreservation. Methods Molecul Biol. 2007; 368:39-57.
9. Pegg DE. The History and Principles of Cryopreservation. Seminars Reprod Med. 2002;20(1):5-13.
10. Juergen L. Cryopreservation as a tool to optimize ART outcomes. ASRM Postgraduate course. 12;2009:1-27.
11. Pegg DE. The role of vitrification techniques of cryopreservation in reproductive medicine. Human Fertil. 2005;8(4):231-9.
12. Polge C, Smith A, Parkes A. Revival of spermatozoa after vitrification and dehydration at low temperatures. Nature. 1949;164:666.
13. Franks F. Biophysics and Biochemistry at Low Temperatures. Cambridge University Press, Cambridge, UK. 1985;209 pages.
14. Karlsson JM. Effects of solution composition on the theoretical prediction of ice nucleation kinetics and thermodynamics. Cryobiology. 2010;60:43-51.
15. Luyet B. On various phase transitions occurring in aqueous solutions at low temperatures. Ann NY Acad Sci. 1960;85:549-69.
16. Mazur P. A biologist's view of the relevance of thermodynamics and physical chemistry to cryobiology. Cryobiology. 2010;60:4-10.
17. Meryman H. X-ray analysis of rapidly frozen gelatin gels. Biodynamica. 1938;8:69-72.
18. Toner M, Cravalho G, Karel M. Thermodynamics and kinetics of intracellular ice formation during freezing of biological cells. J Appl Phys. 1990;67:1582-92.
19. Turnbull D. Formation of crystal nuclei in liquid. J Appl Phys. 1950;21:1022-28.
20. Mazur P, Rall F, Leibo P. Kinetics of water loss and the likelihood of intracellular freezing in mouse ova. Cell Biophys. 1984;6:197-213.
21. Lynch M, Diller K. Analysis of the kinetics of cell freezing with cryophylactic additives. Trans ASME, 1981; 81-WA/ HT-53.
22. Pitt R. Thermodynamics and intracellular ice formation. In: Steponkus P (Ed.) Advances in Low-Temperature Biology (Vol 1), JAI Press, London, UK. 1992;63-99.
23. Karlsson J, Cravalho E, Tonner M. A model of diffusion-limited ice growth inside biological cells during freezing. J Appl Phys. 1994;75: 4442-55.
24. Muldrew K, McGann E. The osmotic rupture hypothesis of intracellular freezing injury. Biophys J. 1994;66:532-41.
25. Tonner M. Nucleation of ice crystals inside biological cells. In Steponkus P (Ed.) Advances in low-temperature Biology (Vol 2) JAI Press, London, UK. 1993;1-51.
26. Turnbull D, Fisher C. Rate of nucleation in condensed systems. J Chem Phys. 1949;17:71-3.
27. Huang Q, Pegg D, Kearney J. Banking of non-viable skin allografts using high concentrations of glycerol or propylene glycol. Cell Tissue Banking. 2004;5:3-21.
28. Kedem O, Katchalsky A. The thermodynamic analysis of the permeability of biological membranes to non-electrolytes. Biochem Biophys Acta. 1958;27:229-46.
29. Kleinhans F. Membrane permeability modeling: Kedem-Katchalsky via a two-parameter formalism. Cryobiology. 1998;37:271-289.
30. Lovelock E, Bishop M. Prevention of freezing damage to living cells by dimethyl sulfoxide. Nature. 1959;183:1394-95.
31. Meryman H. Cryoprotective agents. Cryobiology. 1971;8:172-83.
32. Renard J, Babinet C. High survival of mouse embryos after rapid freezing and thawing inside plastic straws with 1, 2-propanediol as cryoprotectant. J Exp Zool. 1984;230:443-8.
33. Chian RC, Quinn P. Fertility Cryopreservation. Cambridge University Press, Cambridge, UK. 2010; 271 pages.
34. Newton H, Pegg D, Barrass R, Gosden R. Osmotically inactive volume, hydraulic conductivity and permeability to dimethyl sulphoxide of human mature oocytes. J Reprod Fertil. 1999;117:27-33.
35. Gao D, Critser JK. Mechanisms of Cryoinjury in living cells. Instit Lab Animal R J. 1996;41(4):1-9.
36. Leibo SP. Basic Cryobiology of Embryos. Embryology certification review course compiled by AAB. 1996;14.1-14.14.
37. Leibo SP, Picton HM, Gosden RG. Cryopreservation of human spermatozoa. Gamete source, manipulation and disposition. 1994;1-9.
38. Hossain A, Nagamani M. Cryopreservation of Male Gametes. In: Rizk et al. (Eds.) Infertility and Assisted Reproduction. Cambridge University Press, Cambridge, UK. 2008: pp. 466-77.
39. Woodruff TK, Snyder KA. Oncofertility: Fertility Preservation for Cancer Survivors. Springer: New York. 2007; 262 pages.
40. Gosden RG. Gonadal tissue cryopreservation and transplantation. Reprod BioMed Online. 2001;4(1):64-7.

9

Oocyte Cryopreservation

Faten F Abdelhafez, Mohamed A Bedaiwy, Nina Desai

CHAPTER OUTLINE

INTRODUCTION

Almost fifty years ago, oocyte cryopreservation's feasibility in mice was successfully demonstrated.[1] Ever since, more and more cryopreservation protocols have been established and tried in a variety of mammalian species. Sherman et al. (1958) began the era of oocyte cryopreservation by announcing the potential for survival of cryopreserved/thawed oocytes.[1] The chief milestones along the developmental path of oocyte cryotechnology began in 1977 after the in vitro fertilization (IVF) of frozen-thawed MII mice oocytes successfully resulted in the first report of a live offspring.[2] After this milestone, there were attempts to cryopreserve the germinal vesicle (GV) oocyte,[3] which resulted in a live offspring through the use of slow freezing[4] and afterward, vitrification.[5] The accomplishments in murine cryobiology were then applied to humans. Chen et al. (1986) were the first to report a human pregnancy using slowly frozen-thawed MII oocytes.[6] Later, Kuleshova et al. (1999) used vitrified/warmed MII oocytes to achieve human pregnancy.[7] Nonetheless, low survival rates for cryopreserved/thawed mature oocytes redirected research efforts to the cryopreservation of the oocyte at an earlier developmental stage.[8,9] Before long, these efforts bore fruit and Tucker et al. (1998) reported the first pregnancy from cryopreserved GV oocytes.[10]

After the first reports of pregnancy with human frozen oocytes,[6,11-13] the following decade saw only a few reported pregnancies.[14,15] After this slowdown, interest in oocyte cryopreservation technology renewed with the report of viable pregnancies and live births from cryopreserved oocytes. In the past several years, the rates of survival for slowly frozen[16-29] and vitrified[7,30-39] MII oocytes have significantly improved.

DETERMINANTS OF OOCYTE CRYOPRESERVATION OUTCOME

Intrinsic Factors

The resulting outcomes of oocyte cryopreservation are affected by various intrinsic as well as extrinsic parameters. The intrinsic factors relate to the developmental and biological aspects of the oocyte, such as oocyte size, zona pellucida, subcellular organelles, developmental stage and the surrounding cumulus oophorus cells.

The oocyte is not just one of the biggest cells in the human body (with a diameter of 100–200 μm), but it is also likely one of the most complex as well. Although a human oocyte and a one-cell zygote have a similar shape and size, in terms of the post-thawing survival rate, the one-cell zygote has significantly better outcomes than the oocyte. This finding is partly attributed to variations between the two cell types in the lipid phase transition temperature (LPT) as well as membrane permeability. The temperature at which the cell membrane transitions from the liquid state to the gel state is what determines the LPT. It has been demonstrated that oocytes at varying developmental stages are more susceptible to thermal injury as compared to zygotes. This finding is likely due to the high LPT temperature of oocytes. It also might explain why oocytes have poor cryosurvival rates.[40]

The characteristics of an oocyte's membrane permeability change throughout its development. In the rodent model, it was shown that after maturation, the oocyte's membrane becomes less permeable to water[41] (and difficult to dehydrate), which increases the chances of intracellular ice formation. This decrease in the oocyte's water permeability can be reversed within three hours of sperm penetration.[42] Additionally, this change in water permeability may clarify why the very same freezing protocol resulted in low survival rates for frozen MII oocytes, but high survival rates for immature[43] and 2PN stage[44] oocytes. Furthermore, an oocyte's surface area to volume ratio is less than a 2PN oocyte and a cleavage stage embryo,[45] which makes adequate dehydration even more difficult.[46]

The zona pellucida, the glycoprotein layer that surrounds the plasma membrane of oocytes, can also be affected during cryopreservation by fractures[47] or hardening.[48,49] Nevertheless, whether or not oocyte cryopreservation leads to zona pellucida hardening is still controversial because some investigators did not detect a change in cortical granules.[50,51] Furthermore, the issue of zona pellucida hardening is not a real issue in current IVF protocols because of the adoption of intracytoplasmic sperm injection (ICSI) technology.

That said, Gook et al. found a comparable fertilization rate of cryopreserved oocytes for both IVF and ICSI as well as an increased cleavage rate up to the hatching blastocysts stages following ICSI.[52] Additionally, Kazem et al. (1995) found that both fertilization and cleavage rates significantly increased when ICSI was used.[53] Along the same lines, Tucker et al. (1996) reported comparable fertilization rates in fresh and cryopreserved-thawed oocytes inseminated with ICSI and also announced that the three pregnancies each resulted in early miscarriages.[14] Soon after, the first live birth from cryopreserved oocytes using propranediol (PrOH) and inseminated by ICSI was reported by Porcu et al. (1997). Consequently, all investigators then adopted ICSI to inseminate the cryopreserved-thawed oocytes.

The oocyte is structurally complex, rich in mitochondria and subcellular organelles. Such an intricate subcellular matrix is particularly vulnerable to temperature[54] and osmotic changes.[55,56] Similarly, the meiotic spindle structure can be disturbed in the process of the freeze/thaw steps. When there is a failure of spindle assembly, aneuploidy can result. Additionally, the meiotic spindle is vulnerable to cryoprotectant agents (CPAs)[57,58] and temperature changes.[59-61] In this manner, cryopreservation can induce depolymerization of the microtubules.[62] That said, clinical observations show that, after 1–3 hours of post-thaw incubation, the meiotic spindle usually reforms in most oocytes.[63,64] Human studies also show similar rates of aneuploidy between cryopreserved and fresh oocytes.[65]

Another factor that affects cryopreservation outcomes is the oocyte's developmental stage. Because of the initial low cryo-survival rates of cryopreserved-thawed MII oocytes, researchers were led to consider GV oocyte cryopreservation as a substitute. A GV oocyte is smaller in size, has a less-developed zona pellucida, and its DNA material is enclosed within a nuclear membrane (rather than organized on a meiotic spindle). Because of these criteria, the GV oocyte is a better candidate for cryopreservation than a MII oocyte. Nonetheless, human in vitro maturation (IVM) protocols are still not optimal.

Moreover, the oocyte's metabolic coupling and surrounding cumulus cells are lost in cryopreserved/thawed GV oocytes.[66] The cumulus cells' integrity and their gap junctions with the GV oocyte are vital for normal maturation and development.[66] Therefore, to date very few pregnancies have been reported using GV oocyte cryopreservation.[10,67] Furthermore, cryopreserved/thawed human GV oocytes had notably higher spindle and chromosomal abnormalities after undergoing IVM as compared to their fresh counterparts.[62,68-70] However, more clinical trials reverse order are still needed to accurately assess the effectiveness of cryopreserving GV oocytes versus MII oocytes.[71]

The significance of cumulus cells during the cryopreservation of MII oocytes is still a matter of debate. Some studies report a better cryosurvival rate after denuding the human MII oocyte of its cumulus cells,[50,72] while other studies report contradictory results.[73]

Also important the oocyte is an ephemeral cell, which should be fertilized at a specific time; otherwise, it begins to degenerate.[74] Given such a distinctive structure, oocytes are very susceptible to all kinds of insults, above all the freeze-thaw trauma.

In sum, an oocyte has many distinctive characteristics, which requires the development of an oocyte-specific cryopreservation protocol. This uniqueness in part explains the comparatively long evolutionary path for oocyte cryopreservation techniques, from the 1950s until the present, which has finally achieved a clinically meaningful outcome.

Extrinsic Factors

Oocyte cryopreservation outcomes additionally are affected by extrinsic factors that relate to the cryopreservation procedure itself, such as CPAs, cryo-device and cooling/thawing rates. Oocyte cryopreservation is usually performed with either a slow-cooling rate using the slow freeze/rapid-thaw protocol or, alternatively, by vitrification technology.

The oocyte is susceptible to chilling injury, intra- or extra-cellular ice formation and uncontrolled dehydration during the cryopreservation/thawing procedure. Using the appropriate CPAs and cooling/thawing rates can control these injuries to an extent. Nevertheless, CPAs, in and of themselves, can induce some chemical and osmotic injuries, which vary with different concentrations and types of CPAs and vary with different temperatures of exposure (reviewed in[75]).

There are many CPAs currently in use. The most commonly used slow-freezing protocols employ a combination of PrOH and sucrose,[76] while a combination of sucrose, ethylene glycol (EG) and/or dimethyl sulphoxide (DMSO) is the most popular oocyte vitrification procedure.[77] The effect of different CPAs on oocyte cryopreservation has been explained previously in detail (reviewed in[78]) and is outside the scope of the current chapter. However, presently no consensus exists regarding a universal cryopreservation procedure.

Likewise, the type of cryo-device or carrier that is used for cryopreservation can affect outcomes indirectly through the changing of cooling and warming rates. Conventional cryopreservation tools, which include the cryovial and the 0.25 mL insemination straw, have comparatively thick walls that allow restricted cooling and warming rates (around 2500°C/min)[75] and are often used for slow-freezing protocols. On the other hand, vitrification carriers often have ultra-thin walls, or no walls (open systems), which allow for the loading of micro-quantities of sample and have very high cooling and warming rates.

Numerous carriers have been proposed as vitrification vehicles, including electron microscopy grid,[79] open-pulled straw,[7] cryoloop,[39] cryotop[32,-35,37] and the McGill cryoleaf.[80] The aforementioned carriers are deemed open carrier systems because direct contact is made between the sample and liquid nitrogen (LN2). An issue that has been raised is the risk of cross-contamination during the sample's storage in LN2.[81,82] Recently, new vitrification closed systems have been developed, such as the cryotip[83,84] and high security vitrification (HSV) straw.[85] Even though the walls of these new devices are very thin, the cooling and warming rates for these closed systems are expected to be less than that of devices with open systems.

The necessity of ultra-rapid cooling devices for good embryo and oocyte vitrification outcomes has been challenged recently[86,87] Thus, in order to evaluate the efficiency of closed systems, such as conventional 0.25 mL plastic straws, cryotips and HSV straws, for embryo and oocyte vitrification, additional clinical trials are needed. Moreover, it is expected that recent FDA and European Tissue Directive regulations will greatly affect many of the techniques that customarily are used in IVF laboratories, which include cryo-devices. Therefore, the use of closed sealed systems may end up more plausible and acceptable than open system cryo-devices.

In sum, various CPAs and carriers are used in oocyte cryopreservation. The advances of open system carriers for oocyte vitrification have contributed notably to the increasingly promising outcomes obtained with oocyte vitrification.

CLINICAL APPLICATION OF FROZEN OOCYTES

Each year worldwide, the number of women of reproductive-age women diagnosed with cancer is increasing. Given the current improvements in chemo/radiotherapy protocols, these women are expected to survive their cancers. However, this expectation of survival may come at the expense of the women's reproductive potential. In order to give these women a chance at fertility preservation so that they can bear their own genetic children, oocyte cryopreservation can be a solution. Additionally, non-cancer patients, such as those with autoimmune disease, those undergoing oophorectomy for benign disease or prophylactically, or, recipients of bone marrow or stem cell transplantation, can truly benefit from oocyte cryopreservation technology.[88] Oocyte cryopreservation also can be important to women at risk of premature ovarian failure (POF) due to genetic causes, such as Turner's syndrome.[89]

The first successful use of mature oocyte cryopreservation was reported by Yang et al. as a fertility preservation tool in 2007. After embryo transfer (ET) to a surrogate, a healthy male infant was delivered from frozen-thawed oocytes that belonged to a Hodgkin's lymphoma patient.[90] Recently, Porcu et al. (2008) also reported the first pregnancy in an ovarectomized cancer patient with her own slowly frozen/rapidly thawed mature oocytes, which resulted in two healthy female infants.[91]

Nevertheless, for the majority of cancer patients, the immediate initiation of chemo/radiotherapy is compulsory, which provides no time for ovarian stimulation protocols in order to retrieve mature oocytes. However, cryopreservation of ovarian tissue and/or immature oocytes retrieval during a natural cycle are potential alternatives in such patients. Currently, more than 20 live births have been reported worldwide for autotransplanted cryopreserved/thawed ovarian tissue.[92] This systematic review of reproductive outcomes following ovarian tissue transplantation identifies the existing inefficacy of cryopreserved/thawed ovarian tissue transplantation as compared to fresh grafts.[93] This disparity is partially due to vascular insufficiency of the transplanted ovarian tissue and tissue ischemia.[94]

With the present limitations of ovarian tissue cryopreservation, it is essential to make improvements on the other available option: retrieval and cryopreservation of immature oocytes, which is then followed by IVM of frozen/thawed oocytes.[95-99] Otherwise, human GV oocytes also can be successfully cryopreserved after undergoing IVM.[100] However, the IVM technique is still in its infancy and the number of retrieved immature oocytes is often small.[101]

Moreover, for patients, an ethical dilemma arises for variety of reasons (including religion) regarding embryo freezing because of the issue of disposal of excess cryopreserved embryos. Thus, cryopreservation of unfertilized oocytes can be an appealing option for those patients who have such concerns. Freezing of oocytes is the only legal alternative for patients in some nations such as Italy, where the law absolutely prohibits embryo cryopreservation, with the exception of cases when a fresh embryo transfer is impossible.[102] In the cases of ovarian hyper-stimulation syndrome or when there is an inability to find sperm (particularly in instances of surgically retrieved spermatozoa), this technology may also be used to rescue oocytes.

A further application for oocyte cryopreservation relates to women who wish to delay childbearing for their education, career, or another reason. At a young age, cryopreservation ensures the possibility of a future pregnancy. This idea also can be applied to women who have a family history of early menopause due to these women's elevated risk of decreased ovarian reserve at a young age. The data is insufficient as of yet to recommend oocyte cryopreservation solely to evade reproductive aging in otherwise healthy women.[88] Additionally, oocyte cryopreservation potentially overcomes the existing limitations of oocyte donation, which includes cost, donor availability, travel requirements, the need to synchronize cycles of the donor and recipient and the inability to quarantine oocytes.

In sum, four main indications for oocyte cryopreservation exist. First, oocyte cryopreservation can be used as a fertility preservation strategy for women who are at risk of POF. Second, for women undergoing treatment with assisted reproductive technologies (ART) who do not consider embryo freezing an option due to ethical or other reasons, oocyte cryopreservation can be a viable option . Third, oocyte cryopreservation can be used for women who would desire preservation of their future fertility for personal, social or medical reasons (including present lack of a partner). Lastly, oocyte cryopreservation assists the oocyte donation process.

CLINICAL OUTCOME OF OOCYTE CRYOPRESERVATION

For the past two decades, more than 600 children worldwide have been born from cryopreserved-thawed oocytes.[103,104] The American Society for Reproductive Medicine (ASRM) has acknowledged that the oocyte survival, fertilization and pregnancy rates for frozen-thawed oocytes in IVF have improved.[105] ASRM also acknowledged that, presently, no increases in chromosomal abnormalities, birth defects, or developmental deficits in children born from cryopreserved oocytes have been noted. Nevertheless, until further research indicates otherwise, ASRM recommends that oocyte cryopreservation be used solely for investigational purposes and with the guidance of an Institutional Review Board.[105]

New refinements to the slow-freezing protocols have improved the reported clinical outcomes with oocyte cryopreservation. For instance, increasing the sucrose concentration from 0.1 M to 0.3 M notably increased the rate of survival of frozen-thawed oocytes from 34% to 82%.[20] This favorable effect from the use of a higher sucrose concentration also was replicated in other studies, which achieved survival rates of 74%–76%.[26,106] That said, the rates of clinical pregnancy and implantation stayed low.[26,27]

In the same way, intracellular injection of a non-permeable CPA, such as trehalose, reportedly has a positive effect on human oocytes, protecting against freeze stresses.[107] Another improvement applied to slow-freezing protocols is the replacement of sodium with choline. After being implemented in mice first,[56,108] it was later shown to increase human oocyte post-thaw survival and pregnancy rates.[22,109,110]

Recently, several studies reported improved clinical outcomes for cryopreserved-thawed oocytes (**Table 1**). Borini et al. described their 7-year cumulative experience with oocyte slow-freezing in 2006.[111] The authors reported a 43.4% survival rate and a 51.6% fertilization rate using 1.5M PROH + 0.1M sucrose on 918 slowly frozen/rapidly thawed oocytes from 67 patients. The reported rates of clinical pregnancy and implantation were 19.2% and 12.3%, respectively.

Also, Levi-Setti et al. (2006) published a large study where 2900 oocytes from 286 patients (in 303 freezing cycles) were slowly frozen with 1.5M PROH + 0.3 M sucrose.[27] In 159 of the cycles, oocytes were then rapidly thawed with a 69.9% survival rate and a 67.5% fertilization rate. Nonetheless, the reported clinical pregnancy rate (12.4%) and implantation rate (5.7%) were low.

In 2007, Bianchi et al. reported their results from a modified slow-freezing protocol on 403 slowly frozen-thawed oocytes.[112] They used a 1.5M PROH + 0.2 M sucrose solution for freezing and a decreasing concentration of PROH + 0.3 M sucrose for thawing. A 75.9% survival rate and a 76.2% fertilization rate were the result. Following ET, a 21.3% clinical pregnancy rate was reported. Of the transferred embryos, 13.5% resulted in a successful implantation.

Also in 2007, Borini et al. reported their overall experience with 5448 slowly frozen oocytes.[113] Following the thawing of 3238 oocytes from 510 patients, 68.1% of oocytes survived and 76.1% were successfully fertilized. In 590 ET cycles, the authors achieved a 14.9% clinical pregnancy rate and an 8.1% implantation rate.

Another milestone in the improvement of post-thaw survival and clinical outcomes was the application of vitrification technology to MII oocyte cryopreservation. Antinori et al. (2007) used cryotops to vitrify 463 oocytes from 120 volunteers.[34] After the 330 oocytes were warmed, 99.4% survived and 92.9% were fertilized successfully. In 120 ET cycles, the authors reported a 32.5% clinical pregnancy rate and a 13.2% implantation rate . A year later, the same group described their 3-year experience with 295 ICSI cycles and 770 vitrified/warmed oocytes.[114] Ninety-nine percent of the oocytes survived and 91.5% were fertilized. A 27.8% clinical pregnancy rate and a 12.8% implantation rate resulted. At the time of the report, 50 healthy babies had been delivered and 18 pregnancies were ongoing still.

Yoon et al. (2007) reported similar results with 364 oocytes vitrified with slush nitrogen.[35] Upon warming, 85.1% of the oocytes survived and 77.4% were fertilized. One hundred twenty embryos were transferred in 30 ET cycles. of which 14.2% were successfully implanted and a 43.3% clinical pregnancy rate resulted.

Similarly, Cobo et al. (2008) reported on their results from the vitrification of 693 oocytes from an oocyte donation program.[36] They reported a 96.1% survival rate and a 73.1% fertilization rate. Fifty-seven ETs, with 117 embryos, were transferred. The results were an implantation rate of 38.5% and a clinical pregnancy rate of 63.2%. Of note, the authors defined the clinical pregnancy rate and the implantation rate as the number of gestational sacs—not the number of fetal hearts per number of ETs and embryos transferred, respectively. Additionally, reports of successful pregnancies[115] and live births[116] after the transfer of vitrified/warmed embryos that were derived from vitrified/warmed oocytes emphasize the advancements and good performance of the vitrification cryotechnology.

TABLE 1 Summary of recent clinical studies that investigated slow freezing or vitrification of oocytes

	Borini 2006[111]	Levi-Setti 2006[27]	Bianchi 2007[112]	Borini 2007[113]	Antorini 2007[34]	Yoon 2007[35]	Antorini 2008[114]	Cobo 2008[36]	Sher 2008[39]
Technique	Slow freezing	Slow freezing	Slow freezing	Slow freezing	Vitrification	Vitrification	Vitrification	Vitrification	Vitrification
# frozen oocytes	918	2900	1083	5448	463	426	NA	693	111
#pts	67	286	141	510	120	28	NA	47	16
#thawed oocytes	705	1087	403	3238	330	364	770	693	78
#thaw cycles	101	159	90	660	120	NA	NA	NA	NA
Survival rate	43.4%	69.9%	75.9%	68.1%	99.4%	85.1%	99%	96.1%	96%
Fertilization rate	51.6%	67.5%	76.2%	76.1%	92.9%	77.4%	91.5%	73.1%	NA
Cleavage rate	86%	53.5%	93.8%	91.8%	96.7%	94.3%	NA	NA	76%
#ETs	73	145	80	590	120	30	NA	57	16
Clinical pregnancy rate /ET	19.2%	12.4%	21.3%	14.9%	32.5%	43.3%	27.8%	63.2%*	75%
Implanatation rate	12.3%	5.7%	13.5%	8.1%	13.2%	14.2%	12.8%	38.5%**	61%
Miscarriage Rate	28.6%	33.3%	11.8%	21.6%	20.5%	15.4%	NA	16.6%	6.3%
# Live births	12	13	4	60	3	5	50	28	12

*No of sacs/No of embryo transfers

** No of sacs/No of embryos transferred.

An interesting study undertook genomic hybridization on the first polar body of 323 MII human oocytes acquired from egg donors, of which only 111 oocytes were determined to be euploid.[39] On selective vitrification of those 111 euploid oocytes, 96% of them survived. Of those surviving euploid oocytes, the 46% that developed into expanded blastocysts were transferred into 16 embryo recipients. A maximum of 2 embryos were transferred per recipient. The implantation rate was 61% and the birth rate was 75%. These exciting results opened a new path for the improvement of oocyte cryopreservation outcomes. Nevertheless, additional studies regarding oocyte selection through genomic hybridization are needed in order to corroborate this promising strategy. However, it is fair and essential to acknowledge that the majority of the aforementioned vitrification studies used oocytes that were retrieved from young donors.[34,39,117]

Cil et al. (2008) conducted a systematic review and update of data that was published from January 1986 to May 2008.[103] They reported a live-birth rate per oocyte thawed of 1.7% for slow frozen oocytes and a rate of 5.0% for vitrified oocytes. The authors additionally found that the 33.4% clinical pregnancy rate and the 15% implantation rate with vitrification appeared higher than those rates for slow-freezing (15% and 8.1%, respectively). This effect could have resulted from two factors: (a) the higher number of embryos that were transferred in the vitrification group as compared to the slow-freezing group (2.7 vs. 2.2) and (b) the older mean age of women who utilized slowly-frozen/thawed oocytes (34.5 vs. 32.2). Additionally, when the authors evaluated the time trend for the accomplishments of both techniques, they found that the pre-2006 slow-freezing protocol resulted in a 22.8% clinical pregnancy rate and a 10.9% implantation rate, as compared to 42.3% and 17.6%, respectively, for the vitrification group. In the post-2006 period, the authors reported, for slow-freezing and vitrification techniques, respectively, clinical pregnancy rates of 11.1% and 31.5% and implantation rates of 6.4% and 14.3%. Even though both freezing techniques followed a downward trend, the results still favored vitrification. The authors ultimately concluded that, although oocyte vitrification was promising, larger, prospective studies were mandatory.

Which oocyte cryopreservation technique is better remains controversial. Fioravanti et al. (2007) conducted a recent prospective, randomized controlled clinical trial.[118] The authors analyzed 28 slow-freeze-thaw cycles and 35 vitrification-warming cycles. The cleavage rates, the day 3 embryo quality and the biochemical pregnancy rates were appreciably higher in the vitrification group as compared to the slow-freezing group. Even though it was statistically non-significant, the survival, fertilization and clinical pregnancy rates were also numerically higher for the vitrification group.

Recently, a randomized prospective study by Garcia et al. (2008) found no significant differences between the two techniques.[119] One hundred thirty-four oocytes were slowly frozen using 1.5M PROH + 0.2 M sucrose and 84 oocytes were vitrified on cryotops using EG, DMSO and sucrose. The resulting embryos were transferred to 30 patients. The survival rate of frozen/thawed oocytes was 88% and did not differ from the 92% survival rate of the vitrified group. Sixty-two percent of the frozen-thawed oocytes and 68% of the vitrified/warmed oocytes, were fertilized successfully. They reported a 25% clinical pregnancy rate in the slow-freezing group, which was not different from the 31% rate in the vitrification group. However, the study's participant pool was too small to come to a solid conclusion. Thus, well-designed, large randomized controlled trials are needed in order to consolidate and validate these results.

Recently, the Italian National Register collected four years worth of data between 2004–2007 on 46,517 thawed eggs, 7695 transferred embryos and 923 pregnancies after oocyte cryopreservation. This data probably constitutes the largest database on oocyte cryopreservation. More details about this database are to follow (Personal communication).

DISCUSSION

Another valuable tool used for evaluation of various oocyte cryopreservation protocols is the ultrastructure of cryopreserved thawed oocytes. For this assessment, the polarized light and transmission electron microscopes can be utilized. The polarized light microscopy (polscope) was recently used for the noninvasive spindle evaluation in live oocytes.[120] The polscope provides important information relating to the position, presence and birefringence of the meiotic spindle.

Rienzi et al. (2004) used 1.5M PROH + 0.1M sucrose to freeze the oocytes and then used the Polscope to examine them post-thaw.[63] The authors observed that, immediately following thawing, the meiotic spindle in all slowly-frozen MII oocytes totally disappeared, but then completely reformed after three hours of incubation at 37°C. The question still remained of what the functional capacity of thawed oocytes with these newly reformed spindles was. Bianchi et al. (2005) reported similar results.[24]

However, Larman et al. (2007) used vitrification and slow freezing cryopreservation methodologies in order to compare meiotic spindle stability in sibling MII oocytes.[121] When vitrification and warming were carried out at 37°C, the authors immediately observed the meiotic spindle by polscope in all oocytes (10/10) following warming. This result was the direct opposite for slowly frozen oocytes that had all steps carried out at room temperature. In that case, no spindles were exhibited in the MII oocytes (n=7) immediately after thawing. Even more interesting, the spindle retardances, as measured pre and post-vitrification, did not differ. This finding suggested that the technique did not negatively affect spindle assembly. That said, due to the small number of investigated oocytes in the study, any definitive conclusions are precluded.

Likewise, Cao et al. (2009) examined survival, fertilization, meiotic spindle configuration and embryo development, in vitrified and slowly frozen mature oocytes in humans.[122] The vitrified/warmed oocytes showed appreciably better post/warming survival, fertilization, cleavage, blastulation, spindle assembly and chromosome alignment than the slowly-frozen oocytes. Of note, though, the 54.4% cleavage rate for embryos resulting from slowly-frozen oocytes is a good deal less than the rates noted by other authors who used the same slow-freezing protocol.[25,26]

In fact, Cobo et al. (2008) recently compared immediate post-thaw survival and meiotic spindle assembly in slowly-frozen and vitrified oocytes after thawing.[84] After three hours of a 37°C incubation post-thaw, the cryopreserved-thawed oocytes were fixed. Although the vitrified oocytes had better survival, both cryopreservation methodologies showed comparable rates of normal meiotic spindle configuration, which ranged from 74–89%. Therefore, whether or not, oocyte vitrification is better at preserving meiotic spindle assembly than slow-freezing is still controversial and up for debate.

Also helpful for evaluating oocyte cryopreservation methodologies is electron microscopic examination, specifically for cellular structures and organelles of cryopreserved-thawed oocytes. With the use of transmission electron microscopy, Nottola et al. examined the efficiency of various slow-freezing[49,123] and vitrification[124] techniques in the preservation of the ultrastructure of cryopreserved MII oocytes in humans. The slowly frozen oocytes from an EG protocol demonstrated many ultrastructural changes when they were compared to fresh counterparts: (a) disorganized mitochondria-smooth endoplasmic reticulum aggregates, (b) less microvilli and cortical granules and (c) higher number of vacuoles and secondary lysosomes.[49] Even though less ultrastructural disorganizations in the frozen/thawed oocytes resulted when Nottola et al. used PROH as the CPA, there were still fewer cortical granules and abundant vacuolization as compared to the fresh control group.[123] Although, the vitrified warmed oocytes demonstrated sparse micro-vacuolization and disorganized mitochondria-smooth endoplasmic reticulum aggregates, they still showed few cortical granules and non-homogenous microvilli.[124]

An essential issue for any methodology used in humans is safety. Luckily, data relating to the safety of oocyte cryopreservation is starting to be gathered. Borini et al. (2007) followed 105 children who were born from slowly-frozen oocytes.[125] Of these children, only two have been found to have congenital anomalies: choanae atresia and Rubinstein-Taydi syndrome. It is of note that, in these two children, the fathers suffered from severe male factor infertility.

Concerns have been raised regarding the safety of the high concentrations of CPAs used in oocyte vitrification. Fortunately, recent reports have noted some reassuring data relating to the birth weights and congenital anomalies of children who were born from embryos derived from vitrified/warmed oocytes.[80,126]

The psychomotor development of 52 children who were born from vitrified/warmed oocytes with the use of the cryotop was followed up upon by Chavez-Badiola et al. (2008), with a mean follow-up of 18.4 months.[126] Of these children, only one child was found to have a congenital anomaly: an inter-ventricular septal defect. Additionally, all of the 52 children demonstrated normal psychomotor development, as measured by the Gesell's scale.

Moreover, the McGill cryoleaf and cryotop was examined by Chian et al. (2008) in 3 countries: Canada, Colombia and Mexico.[80] The authors examined the obstetric and perinatal outcome of 200 children born from vitrified oocytes. Five children had the following congenital anomalies: biliary atresia, club foot, skin hemangioma and ventricular septal defect. Still, the mean birth weight and the incidence of congenital anomalies were found to be similar to those in children born after spontaneous or assisted pregnancies.

CONCLUSION

An expanding spectrum of indications exists for oocyte cryopreservation. In contrast to the original decade-long frustration after the initial report of oocyte cryopreservation by Chen in 1986,[6] oocyte cryopreservation is presently more efficacious and reproducible. Over the past decade, the mean survival and birth rates per thawed oocyte doubled. Currently, both slow-freezing and vitrification are used worldwide. Moreover, there is no definitive evidence that one methodology is superior to the other. That said, well-designed, randomized controlled trials are necessary in order to determine whether one methodology is truly better than the other. In spite of the initial concerns about meiotic spindle integrity and aneuploidy risk, recent data supports the meiotic spindle's re-polymerization potential and the nullification of the aneuploidy risk in humans. Continuous improvements in the existing cryopreservation protocols will result in further improvements to the survival and implantation rates.

In conclusion, oocyte cryopreservation's potential has been acknowledged now and numerous worldwide publications validate it. In October 2012, ASRM formally changed its view on oocyte cryopreservation from "research" to a clinically-accepted treatment modality. With time, it is likely that oocyte cryopreservation will be incorporated as an essential element of almost all IVF programs.

KEY ISSUES

- Oocyte cryopreservation represents a promising fertility preservation option.
- Remarkable progress has been made in oocyte cryopreservation.
- Vitrification appears to be an efficient and safe oocyte cryopreservation methodology.
- Though limited, the current data on the safety of oocyte cryopreservation is reassuring.
- Well-designed, randomized controlled trials are necessary in order to compare the effectiveness and long-term safety of slow-freezing and vitrification methodologies for oocyte cryopreservation.

REFERENCES

1. Sherman JK, Lin TP. Survival of unfertilized mouse eggs during freezing and thawing. Proc Soc Exp Biol Med. 1958;98:902-5.
2. Whittingham DG. Fertilization in vitro and development to term of unfertilized mouse oocytes previously stored at --196 degrees C. J Reprod Fertil. 1977;49:89-94.
3. Van Blerkom J. Maturation at high frequency of germinal-vesicle-stage mouse oocytes after cryopreservation: alterations in cytoplasmic, nuclear, nucleolar and chromosomal structure and organization associated with vitrification. Hum Reprod. 1989;4: 883-98.
4. Candy CJ, Wood MJ, Whittingham DG, et al. Cryopreservation of immature mouse oocytes. Hum Reprod. 1994;9:1738-42.
5. Aono N, Abe Y, Hara K, et al. Production of live offspring from mouse germinal vesicle-stage oocytes vitrified by a modified stepwise method, SWEID. Fertil Steril. 2005;84:1078-82.
6. Chen C. Pregnancy after human oocyte cryopreservation. Lancet. 1986;1:884-6.
7. Kuleshova L, Gianaroli L, Magli C, et al. Birth following vitrification of a small number of human oocytes: case report. Hum Reprod. 1999;14:3077-79.
8. Toth TL, Lanzendorf SE, Sandow BA, et al. Cryopreservation of human prophase I oocytes collected from unstimulated follicles. Fertil Steril. 1994;61:1077-82.
9. Toth TL, Baka SG, Veeck LL, et al. Fertilization and in vitro development of cryopreserved human prophase I oocytes. Fertil Steril. 1994;61: 891-4.
10. Tucker MJ, Wright G, Morton PC, Massey JB. Birth after cryopreservation of immature oocytes with subsequent in vitro maturation. Fertil Steril. 1998;70:578-9.
11. Al-Hasani S, Diedrich K, van der Ven H, Krebs D. [Initial results of the cryopreservation of human oocytes]. Geburtshilfe Frauenheilkd. 1986;46:643-4.
12. Al-Hasani S, Diedrich K, van der Ven H, et al. Cryopreservation of human oocytes. Hum Reprod. 1987;2:695-700.
13. van Uem JF, Siebzehnrubl ER, Schuh B, et al. Birth after cryopreservation of unfertilized oocytes. Lancet. 1987;1:752-3.
14. Tucker M, Wright G, Morton P, et al. Preliminary experience with human oocyte cryopreservation using 1,2-propanediol and sucrose. Hum Reprod. 1996;11:1513-15.
15. Porcu E, Fabbri R, Seracchioli R, et al. Birth of a healthy female after intracytoplasmic sperm injection of cryopreserved human oocytes. Fertil Steril. 1997;68:724-6.
16. Polak de Fried E, Notrica J, Rubinstein M, et al. Pregnancy after human donor oocyte cryopreservation and thawing in association with intracytoplasmic sperm injection in a patient with ovarian failure. Fertil Steril. 1998;69:555-7.
17. Porcu E, R F, P C. Cycles of human oocyte cryopreservation and intracytoplasmic sperm injection; results of 112 cycles. Fertil Steril. 1999;72:S2.
18. Wurfel W, Schleyer M, Krusmann G, et al. [Fertilization of cryopreserved and thawed human oocytes (Cryo-Oo) by injection of spermatozoa (ICSI)--medical management of sterility and case report of a twin pregnancy]. Zentralbl Gynakol. 1999;121:444-8.
19. Porcu E, Fabbri R, Seracchioli R. Obstetric, perinatal outcome and follow up of children concieved from cryopreserved oocytes. Fertil Steril. 2000;74:S48.
20. Fabbri R, Porcu E, Marsella T, et al. Human oocyte cryopreservation: new perspectives regarding oocyte survival. Hum Reprod. 2001;16:411-6.
21. Winslow K, D Y, P B. Oocyte cryopreservation; a three year follow up of sixteen births. Fertil Steril. 2001;76:S120.
22. Quintans CJ, Donaldson MJ, Bertolino MV, Pasqualini RS. Birth of two babies using oocytes that were cryopreserved in a choline-based freezing medium. Hum Reprod. 2002;17:3149-52.
23. Borini A, Bonu MA, Coticchio G, et al. Pregnancies and births after oocyte cryopreservation. Fertil Steril. 2004;82:601-5.
24. Bianchi V, Coticchio G, Fava L, et al. Meiotic spindle imaging in human oocytes frozen with a slow freezing procedure involving high sucrose concentration. Hum Reprod. 2005;20:1078-83.

25. Chen SU, Lien YR, Chen HF, et al. Observational clinical follow-up of oocyte cryopreservation using a slow-freezing method with 1,2-propanediol plus sucrose followed by ICSI. Hum Reprod. 2005;20:1975-80.
26. Borini A, Sciajno R, Bianchi V, et al. Clinical outcome of oocyte cryopreservation after slow cooling with a protocol utilizing a high sucrose concentration. Hum Reprod. 2006;21:512-7.
27. Levi Setti PE, Albani E, Novara PV, et al. Cryopreservation of supernumerary oocytes in IVF/ICSI cycles. Hum Reprod. 2006;21:370-5.
28. De Santis L, Cino I, Rabellotti E, et al. Oocyte cryopreservation: clinical outcome of slow-cooling protocols differing in sucrose concentration. Reprod Biomed Online. 2007;14:57-63.
29. Parmegiani L, Cognigni GE, Bernardi S, et al. Freezing within 2 h from oocyte retrieval increases the efficiency of human oocyte cryopreservation when using a slow freezing/rapid thawing protocol with high sucrose concentration. Hum Reprod. 2008;23:1771-77.
30. Katayama KP, Stehlik J, Kuwayama M, et al. High survival rate of vitrified human oocytes results in clinical pregnancy. Fertil Steril. 2003;80:223-4.
31. Liebermann J, Tucker MJ, Sills ES. Cryoloop vitrification in assisted reproduction: analysis of survival rates in >1000 human oocytes after ultra-rapid cooling with polymer augmented cryoprotectants. Clin Exp Obstet Gynecol. 2003;30:125-9.
32. Kuwayama M, Vajta G, Kato O, Leibo SP. Highly efficient vitrification method for cryopreservation of human oocytes. Reprod Biomed Online. 2005;11:300-8.
33. Lucena E, Bernal DP, Lucena C, et al. Successful ongoing pregnancies after vitrification of oocytes. Fertil Steril. 2006;85:108-11.
34. Antinori M, Licata E, Dani G, et al. Cryotop vitrification of human oocytes results in high survival rate and healthy deliveries. Reprod Biomed Online. 2007;14:72-9.
35. Yoon TK, Lee DR, Cha SK, et al. Survival rate of human oocytes and pregnancy outcome after vitrification using slush nitrogen in assisted reproductive technologies. Fertil Steril. 2007;88:952-6.
36. Cobo A, Domingo J, Perez S, et al. Vitrification: an effective new approach to oocyte banking and preserving fertility in cancer patients. Clin Transl Oncol. 2008;10:268-73.
37. Cobo A, Bellver J, Domingo J, et al. New options in assisted reproduction technology: the Cryotop method of oocyte vitrification. Reprod Biomed Online. 2008;17:68-72.
38. Keskintepe L, Agca Y, Sher G, et al. High survival rate of metaphase II human oocytes after first polar body biopsy and vitrification: determining the effect of previtrification conditions. Fertil Steril. 2009; 92(5):1706–15.
39. Sher G, Keskintepe L, Mukaida T, et al. Selective vitrification of euploid oocytes markedly improves survival, fertilization and pregnancy-generating potential. Reprod Biomed Online. 2008;17:524-9.
40. Ghetler Y, Yavin S, Shalgi R, Arav A. The effect of chilling on membrane lipid phase transition in human oocytes and zygotes. Hum Reprod. 2005;20:3385-89.
41. Ford P, Merot J, Jawerbaum A, et al. Water permeability in rat oocytes at different maturity stages: aquaporin-9 expression. J Membr Biol. 2000;176:151-8.
42. Jackowski S, Leibo SP, Maxur P. Glycerol permeabilities of fertilized and unfertilized mouse ova. J Exp Zool. 1980;212:329-41.
43. Sereni E, Bonu M, Borini A. High survival rates after cryopreservation of human prophase oocytes. Fertil Steril. 2000;74(Suppl 1)S161.
44. Senn A, Vozzi C, Chanson A, et al. Prospective randomized study of two cryopreservation policies avoiding embryo selection: the pronucleate stage leads to a higher cumulative delivery rate than the early cleavage stage. Fertil Steril. 2000;74:946-52.
45. Maneiro E, Ron-Corzo A, Julve J, Goyanes VJ. Surface area/volume ratio and growth equation of the human early embryo. Int J Dev Biol. 1991;35:139-43.
46. Fabbri R, Porcu E, Marsella T, et al. Technical aspects of oocyte cryopreservation. Mol Cell Endocrinol. 2000;169:39-42.
47. Dumoulin JC, Bergers-Janssen JM, Pieters MH, et al. The protective effects of polymers in the cryopreservation of human and mouse zonae pellucidae and embryos. Fertil Steril. 1994;62:793-8.
48. Nottola SA, Macchiarelli G, Coticchio G, et al. Ultrastructure of human mature oocytes after slow cooling cryopreservation using different sucrose concentrations. Hum Reprod. 2007;22:1123-33.
49. Nottola SA, Coticchio G, De Santis L, et al. Ultrastructure of human mature oocytes after slow cooling cryopreservation with ethylene glycol. Reprod Biomed Online. 2008;17:368-77.
50. Gook DA, Osborn SM, Johnston WI. Cryopreservation of mouse and human oocytes using 1,2-propanediol and the configuration of the meiotic spindle. Hum Reprod. 1993;8:1101-09.
51. Van Blerkom J, Davis PW. Cytogenetic, cellular, and developmental consequences of cryopreservation of immature and mature mouse and human oocytes. Microsc Res Tech. 1994;27:165-93.
52. Gook DA, Schiewe MC, Osborn SM, et al. Intracytoplasmic sperm injection and embryo development of human oocytes cryopreserved using 1,2-propanediol. Hum Reprod. 1995;10:2637-41.
53. Kazem R, Thompson LA, Srikantharajah A, et al. Cryopreservation of human oocytes and fertilization by two techniques: in-vitro fertilization and intracytoplasmic sperm injection. Hum Reprod. 1995;10:2650-54.
54. Magistrini M, Szollosi D. Effects of cold and of isopropyl-N-phenylcarbamate on the second meiotic spindle of mouse oocytes. Eur J Cell Biol. 1980;22:699-707.
55. McWilliams RB, Gibbons WE, Leibo SP. Osmotic and physiological responses of mouse zygotes and human oocytes to mono- and disaccharides. Hum Reprod. 1995;10:1163-71.
56. Stachecki JJ, Cohen J, Willadsen S. Detrimental effects of sodium during mouse oocyte cryopreservation. Biol Reprod. 1998;59:395-400.
57. Johnson MH, Pickering SJ. The effect of dimethylsulphoxide on the microtubular system of the mouse oocyte. Development 1987;100:313-24.
58. Pickering SJ, Braude PR, Johnson MH. Cryoprotection of human oocytes: inappropriate exposure to DMSO reduces fertilization rates. Hum Reprod. 1991;6:142-3.
59. Pickering SJ, Johnson MH. The influence of cooling on the organization of the meiotic spindle of the mouse oocyte. Hum Reprod. 1987;2:207-16.
60. Pickering SJ, Braude PR, Johnson MH, et al. Transient cooling to room temperature can cause irreversible disruption of the meiotic spindle in the human oocyte. Fertil Steril. 1990;54:102-8.
61. Sathananthan AH, Kirby C, Trounson A, et al. The effects of cooling mouse oocytes. J Assist Reprod Genet. 1992;9:139-48.
62. Boiso I, Marti M, Santalo J, et al. A confocal microscopy analysis of the spindle and chromosome configurations of human oocytes cryopreserved at the germinal vesicle and metaphase II stage. Hum Reprod. 2002;17:1885-91.
63. Rienzi L, Martinez F, Ubaldi F, et al. Polscope analysis of meiotic spindle changes in living metaphase II human oocytes during the freezing and thawing procedures. Hum Reprod. 2004;19:655-9.
64. Coticchio G, De Santis L, Rossi G, et al. Sucrose concentration influences the rate of human oocytes with normal spindle and chromosome configurations after slow-cooling cryopreservation. Hum Reprod. 2006;21:1771-76.

65. Cobo A, Rubio C, Gerli S, et al. Use of fluorescence in situ hybridization to assess the chromosomal status of embryos obtained from cryopreserved oocytes. Fertil Steril. 2001;75:354-60.
66. Ruppert-Lingham CJ, Paynter SJ, Godfrey J, et al. Developmental potential of murine germinal vesicle stage cumulus-oocyte complexes following exposure to dimethylsulphoxide or cryopreservation: loss of membrane integrity of cumulus cells after thawing. Hum Reprod. 2003;18:392-8.
67. Cha KY, Koo JJ, Ko JJ, et al. Pregnancy after in vitro fertilization of human follicular oocytes collected from nonstimulated cycles, their culture in vitro and their transfer in a donor oocyte program. Fertil Steril. 1991;55:109-13.
68. Tucker MJ, Morton PC, Wright G, et al. Clinical application of human egg cryopreservation. Hum Reprod. 1998;13:3156-59.
69. Wu J, Zhang L, Wang X. In vitro maturation, fertilization and embryo development after ultrarapid freezing of immature human oocytes. Reproduction. 2001;121:389-93.
70. Park SE, Son WY, Lee SH, et al. Chromosome and spindle configurations of human oocytes matured in vitro after cryopreservation at the germinal vesicle stage. Fertil Steril. 1997;68:920-6.
71. Fawole AO, Oladapo OT. An evaluation of embryo, zygote and oocyte cryopreservation in assisted reproductive technology. Afr J Med Med Sci. 2007;36:325-34.
72. Minasi MG, Casciani V, Iacobelli M, et al. Evaluation of slush nitrogen vitrification on cumulus enclosed or cumulus free human oocytes. Abstracts of the 24th Annual Meeting of the ESHRE, Barcelona, Spain, 7–9 July, 2008.
73. Imoedemhe DG, Sigue AB. Survival of human oocytes cryopreserved with or without the cumulus in 1,2-propanediol. J Assist Reprod Genet. 1992;9:323-7.
74. Paynter SJ. A rational approach to oocyte cryopreservation. Reprod Biomed Online. 2005;10:578-86.
75. Vajta G, Nagy ZP. Are programmable freezers still needed in the embryo laboratory? Review on vitrification. Reprod Biomed Online. 2006;12:779-6.
76. Ambrosini G, Andrisani A, Porcu E, et al. Oocytes cryopreservation: state of art. Reprod Toxicol. 2006;22:250-62.
77. Porcu E, Bazzocchi A, Notarangelo L, et al. Human oocyte cryopreservation in infertility and oncology. Curr Opin Endocrinol Diabetes Obes. 2008;15:529-35.
78. Coticchio G, Bonu MA, Sciajno R, et al. Truths and myths of oocyte sensitivity to controlled rate freezing. Reprod Biomed Online. 2007;15:24-30.
79. Yoon TK, Kim TJ, Park SE, et al. Live births after vitrification of oocytes in a stimulated in vitro fertilization-embryo transfer program. Fertil Steril. 2003;79:1323-26.
80. Chian RC, Huang JY, Gilbert L, et al. Obstetric outcomes following vitrification of in vitro and in vivo matured oocytes. Fertil Steril. 2009;91(6):2391-8.
81. Bielanski A, Bergeron H, Lau PC, Devenish J. Microbial contamination of embryos and semen during long term banking in liquid nitrogen. Cryobiology. 2003;46:146-52.
82. Bielanski A, Nadin-Davis S, Sapp T, Lutze-Wallace C. Viral contamination of embryos cryopreserved in liquid nitrogen. Cryobiology. 2000;40: 110-16.
83. Kuwayama M, Vajta G, Ieda S, Kato O. Comparison of open and closed methods for vitrification of human embryos and the elimination of potential contamination. Reprod Biomed Online. 2005;11:608-14.
84. Cobo A, Perez S, De los Santos MJ, et al. Effect of different cryopreservation protocols on the metaphase II spindle in human oocytes. Reprod Biomed Online. 2008;17:350-9.
85. Camus A, Clairaz P, Ersham A, et al. The comparison of the process of five different vitrification devices. Gynecol Obstet Fertil. 2006;34: 737-45.
86. Mullen SF, Li M, Li Y, et al. Human oocyte vitrification: the permeability of metaphase II oocytes to water and ethylene glycol and the appliance toward vitrification. Fertil Steril. 2008;89:1812-25.
87. Stachecki JJ, Garrisi J, Sabino S, et al. A new safe, simple and successful vitrification method for bovine and human blastocysts. Reprod Biomed Online. 2008;17:360-7.
88. Ovarian tissue and oocyte cryopreservation. Fertil Steril. 2004;82: 993-8.
89. Kavoussi SK, Fisseha S, Smith YR, et al. Oocyte cryopreservation in a woman with mosaic Turner syndrome: a case report. J Reprod Med. 2008;53:223-6.
90. Yang D, Brown SE, Nguyen K, et al. Live birth after the transfer of human embryos developed from cryopreserved oocytes harvested before cancer treatment. Fertil Steril. 2007;87:1469 e1461-64.
91. Porcu E, Venturoli S, Damiano G, et al. Healthy twins delivered after oocyte cryopreservation and bilateral ovariectomy for ovarian cancer. Reprod Biomed Online. 2008;17:265-7.
92. Meirow D. Fertility preservation in cancer patients using stored ovarian tissue: clinical aspects. Curr Opin Endocrinol Diabetes Obes. 2008;15:536-47.
93. Bedaiwy MA, El-Nashar SA, El Saman AM, et al. Reproductive outcome after transplantation of ovarian tissue: a systematic review. Hum Reprod. 2008;23(12):2709-17.
94. Bedaiwy MA, Jeremias E, Gurunluoglu R, et al. Restoration of ovarian function after autotransplantation of intact frozen-thawed sheep ovaries with microvascular anastomosis. Fertil Steril. 2003;79: 594-602.
95. Huang JY, Buckett WM, Gilbert L, et al. Retrieval of immature oocytes followed by in vitro maturation and vitrification: a case report on a new strategy of fertility preservation in women with borderline ovarian malignancy. Gynecol Oncol. 2007;105:542-4.
96. Demirtas E, Elizur SE, Holzer H, et al. Immature oocyte retrieval in the luteal phase to preserve fertility in cancer patients. Reprod Biomed Online. 2008;17:520-3.
97. Huang JY, Tulandi T, Holzer H, et al. Combining ovarian tissue cryobanking with retrieval of immature oocytes followed by in vitro maturation and vitrification: an additional strategy of fertility preservation. Fertil Steril. 2008;89:567-72.
98. Oktay K, Demirtas E, Son WY, et al. In vitro maturation of germinal vesicle oocytes recovered after premature luteinizing hormone surge: description of a novel approach to fertility preservation. Fertil Steril. 2008;89:228 e219-222.
99. Otte Sv, Thill M, Schöpper B, et al. Fertility preservation in breast cancer: oocyte freezing after IVM & ovarian cortex cryopreservation versus oocyte freezing after modified stimulation. Abstracts of the 24th Annual Meeting of the ESHRE, Barcelona, Spain, 7–9 July, 2008.
100. Chian RC, Gilbert L, Huang JY, et al. Live birth after vitrification of in vitro matured human oocytes. Fertil Steril. 2009;91(2):372–6.
101. Omland AK, Fedorcsak P, Storeng R, et al. Natural cycle IVF in unexplained, endometriosis-associated and tubal factor infertility. Hum Reprod. 2001;16:2587-92.
102. Benagiano G, Gianaroli L. The new Italian IVF legislation. Reprod Biomed Online. 2004;9:117-25.
103. Cil A, Oktem O, Oktay K. A meta-analytic comparison of oocyte vitrification to slow freezing: Time trends and the current state of the technology. Fertil Steril. 2008;90, Suppl (1):S269.
104. Kuwayama M, Leibo SP. Efficiency of the cryotop method to cryopreserve human oocytes: Analysis of in vitro nad in vivo results at eleven IVF clinics. Fertil Steril. 2008;90(1):S281-2.
105. Ovarian tissue and oocyte cryopreservation. Fertil Steril. 2006;86: S142-7.
106. Konc J, Kanyo K, Varga E, et al. Births resulting from oocyte cryopreservation using a slow freezing protocol with propanediol and sucrose. Syst Biol Reprod Med. 2008;54:205-10.

107. Eroglu A, Toner M, Toth TL. Beneficial effect of microinjected trehalose on the cryosurvival of human oocytes. Fertil Steril. 2002;77:152-8.
108. Stachecki JJ, Cohen J, Willadsen SM. Cryopreservation of unfertilized mouse oocytes: the effect of replacing sodium with choline in the freezing medium. Cryobiology. 1998;37:346-54.
109. Boldt J, Tidswell N, Sayers A, et al. Human oocyte cryopreservation: 5-year experience with a sodium-depleted slow freezing method. Reprod Biomed Online. 2006;13:96-100.
110. Petracco A, Azambuja R, Okada L, et al. Comparison of embryo quality between sibling embryos originating from frozen or fresh oocytes. Reprod Biomed Online. 2006;13:497-503.
111. Borini A, Lagalla C, Bonu MA, et al. Cumulative pregnancy rates resulting from the use of fresh and frozen oocytes: 7 years' experience. Reprod Biomed Online. 2006;12:481-6.
112. Bianchi V, Coticchio G, Distratis V, et al. Differential sucrose concentration during dehydration (0.2 mol/l) and rehydration (0.3 mol/l) increases the implantation rate of frozen human oocytes. Reprod Biomed Online. 2007;14:64-71.
113. Borini A, Bianchi V, Bonu MA, et al. Evidence-based clinical outcome of oocyte slow cooling. Reprod Biomed Online. 2007;15:175-81.
114. Antinori M, Licata E, Dani G, et al. Three years of clinical application in human oocytes vitrification: high survival rate and healthy deliveries. Abstracts of the 24th Annual Meeting of the ESHRE, Barcelona, Spain, 7–9 July, 2008.
115. Chang CC, Shapiro DB, Bernal DP, et al. Two successful pregnancies obtained following oocyte vitrification and embryo re-vitrification. Reprod Biomed Online. 2008;16:346-9.
116. Chen GA, Cai XY, Lian Y, et al. Normal birth from cryopreserved embryos after intracytoplasmic sperm injection of frozen semen into vitrified human oocytes. Hum Fertil (Camb). 2008;11:49-51.
117. Cobo A, Kuwayama M, Perez S, et al. Comparison of concomitant outcome achieved with fresh and cryopreserved donor oocytes vitrified by the Cryotop method. Fertil Steril. 2008;89:1657-64.
118. Fioravanti J, Alegretti JR, Hassun PA, et al. Prospective randomized comparison of human oocyte freezing and vitrification: an update. Fertil Steril. 2007;88(Suppl 1):S13.
119. Garcia G, Santos R, Arenas ML, et al. Comparitive study of human oocyte cryopreservation by vitrification or slow freezing. Fertil Steril. 2008;90 (Suppl 1):S291-2.
120. Wang WH, Meng L, Hackett RJ, et al. Limited recovery of meiotic spindles in living human oocytes after cooling-rewarming observed using polarized light microscopy. Hum Reprod. 2001;16:2374-78.
121. Larman MG, Minasi MG, Rienzi L, Gardner DK. Maintenance of the meiotic spindle during vitrification in human and mouse oocytes. Reprod Biomed Online. 2007;15:692-700.
122. Cao YX, Xing Q, Li L, et al. Comparison of survival and embryonic development in human oocytes cryopreserved by slow-freezing and vitrification. Fertil Steril. 2009;92(4):1306-11.
123. Coticchio G, Distratis V, Borini A, et al. Reduced ultrastructural damage in human oocytes cryopreserved after dehydration involving single-step propanediol exposure. Abstracts of the 24th Annual Meeting of the ESHRE, Barcelona, Spain, 7–9 July, 2008.
124. Nottola SA, Coticchio G, Sciajno R, et al. Ultrastructural changes in human metaphase II oocytes cryopreserved by vitrification. Abstracts of the 24th annual meeting of the ESRE, Barcelona, Spain 2008.
125. Borini A, Cattoli M, Mazzone S, et al. Survey of 105 babies born after slow-cooling oocyte cryopreservation. Fertil Steril. 2007;88(Suppl 1):S13.
126. Chavez-Badiola A, Ruvalcaba-Castellon LA, Zheng J, Garcia-Amador MI. Technique safety: Oocyte vitrification. Live Births` , long-term follow-up. Fertil Steril. 2008;90(1):S 205.

10

Embryo Cryopreservation

Bonnie Patel, Candice P Holliday, Mohamed A Bedaiwy

INTRODUCTION

Modern day assisted reproductive technology (ART) has paved a new path for fertility preservation. One of the byproducts of ART is the creation of surplus embryos that can be cryopreserved for later use. Embryo cryopreservation refers to the process of preserving embryos at the embryogenesis stage at sub-zero temperatures for future use.[1] This technology can be used for patients who may wish to preserve future fertility. These patients may suffer from malignancy or other diseases requiring gonadotoxic medical therapy, genetic disorders with predisposition to decreased ovarian reserve, or they simply may want to prolong their reproductive potential for other reasons.[2] Creation and storage of cryopreserved embryos provides assurance of future fertility.

HISTORY

Embryo cryopreservation has been employed since the mid-1980s. The first ever pregnancy derived from a frozen human embryo was reported by Alan Trounson and Linda Mohr in 1983 (although the fetus aborted spontaneously at about 20 weeks of gestation). The first term pregnancy derived from a frozen-thawed embryo was achieved the following year.[3] Since then, an estimated 350,000 to 500,000 births have occurred as a result of embryo cryopreservation. Cryopreserved embryos were used in approximately 17% of all ART cycles performed in 2008 (25,261 cycles).[4] These cycles resulted in 9,164 pregnancies (36%) and 7,123 pregnancies resulted in live births (28%).

INDICATIONS

Fertility preservation for women at risk for premature ovarian failure (POF) has been a concern to gynecologists for over 20 years.[2] POF, defined as ovarian failure before the age of 40, may be attributed to ovarian damage secondary to a myriad of causes. Such damage may be caused by oncologic or autoimmune diseases requiring gonadotoxic chemotherapy, genetic diseases with predisposition to POF, or direct damage by repeat ovarian surgery.

Oncologic Indications

Approximately 60,000 of the cases diagnosed annually in females in the United States occur in women under the age of 40, including over 4,000 cases in pre-pubertal girls and adolescents.[5] Childhood cancers are estimated to occur in 13 of 100,000 children under 15 years of age (Belgian Society of Pediatric Hematology and Oncology, unpublished data), with leukemia and lymphoma being the highest in prevalence (45%). Cancer treatment is the most frequent cause of ovarian damage in girls.[6] Green and colleagues reported that the relative likelihood of female childhood cancer survivors ever conceiving was 0.81 (95% confidence interval 0.73–0.90; $P<0.001$) compared with their female siblings.[6] Toxic effects of chemotherapy and pelvic radiotherapy result in accelerated loss and depletion of gonadal germ cells in these patients. The patient's age, exposure to multiple doses of gonadotoxic therapy and the type of therapy determine the extent of tissue damage.

For radiotherapy, the degree of ovarian impairment depends on the radiation dosage, the radiation field, fractionation schedule and age at the time of treatment.[7] Both external beam radiation (tele-therapy) and intracavitary radiation (brachytherapy) have the potential to damage primordial follicles. In 2005, Wallace and colleagues reported age-related total sterilization dosages.[8] Effective radiotherapy dosages for total sterilization were 20.3 Gy at birth, 18.4 Gy at 10 years of age and 16.5 Gy at 20 years of age. Furthermore, Wallace et al. were able to calculate 95% confidence limits for age at which POF occurs for estimated radiation doses to the ovary, from 1 Gy to the effective sterilization dose and from birth to 50 years of age.

Numerous chemotherapy agents are known to be gonadotoxic, especially alkylating agents such as cyclophosphamide.[9] The extent of tissue damage depends on the age of the patient, the specific type and the dosage of therapy administered. Due to the reduction of the primordial follicle pool with aging, the risk of developing ovarian failure and infertility is higher in older women after a cytotoxic treatment compared with younger women.[10] The type of disease and its associated therapy both determine the risk of diminished ovarian reserve and subfertility in these patients. The risk of POF is about 50% in young women receiving cyclophosphamide at a mean cumulative dose of 9.3 g. Moreover, there is an 11% increase in the risk of POF with each additional 1.4 g/m^2 of cumulative procarbazine.[11,12] Furthermore, it is recommended that women delay child bearing for 6–12 months after cessation of chemotherapy secondary to the higher risk of teratogenesis owing to the DNA toxicity of these agents.[13] Recent data suggest that the risk of teratogenicity in cancer patients undergoing chemotherapy eventually returns to that of the general population.[14] Physicians should make every effort to address the option of fertility preservation with patients with greater than 50% chance of POF.[10] As such, clinical guidelines encouraging fertility preservation amongst reproductive aged women has been published by the American Society of Clinical Oncology.[15]

Non-oncological Indications

Administration of high dose chemotherapy may be necessary in certain benign conditions. Such conditions include myelodysplasia, aplastic anemia, thalassemia, multiple sclerosis, as well as severe rheumatic diseases, such as Wegener's syndrome, polyarthritis and systemic lupus erythematosus.[2]

POF may be related to certain endocrinologic and genetic conditions, such as galactosemia or Turner syndrome. Patients with Turner syndrome (45, X), in particular, have a predisposition to POF. The incidence of Turner syndrome is estimated to be 40 out of 100,000.[16] Only 2–5% of patients with Turner syndrome are able to experience spontaneous menses with the potential to achieve pregnancy without medical intervention.[17] Partial X chromosome deletions and X chromosome mosaicism may account for lesser degrees of ovarian failure.[18] A pre-mutation of the CGG repeats in the Fragile X mental retardation gene (FMR1) accounts for another genetic cause of POF.[19] Expansions of the CGG repeat in *FMR1* over about 200 copies are associated with methylation and subsequent gene inactivation, which causes the Fragile X syndrome. However, the presence of 50–200 unmethylated repeats may predispose a woman to POF.[19] Options to preserve fertility, including embryo cryopreservation, may be offered to these patients.

Repeat ovarian surgery may also predispose a woman to POF. Causes for ovarian surgery include ovarian cysts and mature teratomas, which have a recurrence rate of up to 15%, thus requiring repeat surgery.[2] Physicians should make every attempt to discuss fertility preservation in women with a history of repeat ovarian surgery.

EMBRYO CRYOPRESERVATION

Options for fertility preservation include oocyte cryopreservation, ovarian cortex cryopreservation, ovariopexy and transposition prior to pelvic radiotherapy and embryo cryopreservation. The focus of this chapter will be embryo cryopreservation as other options are discussed elsewhere.

Controlled Ovarian Stimulation

Women desiring fertility preserving measures may opt to undergo controlled ovarian stimulation (COH) with gonadotropins, followed by retrieval and fertilization of oocytes and subsequent cryopreservation of fertilized embryos. Fertilization may be performed with partner or donor sperm, depending on the wishes of the patient. In general, this process may require 2-6 weeks, depending on the phase of the patient's menstrual cycle at the time of initiation of treatment. Oocyte retrieval is undertaken once follicles are deemed "mature," according to their size on transvaginal ultrasonography. The retrieval process is also performed under ultrasound guidance once the patient undergoes sedation or general anesthesia.

The number of oocytes retrieved and their quality are imperative factors predicting the potential efficacy of the embryo preservation procedure. Consequently, patients must be informed of expected ovarian performance after COS. The presence of malignancy may have an adverse effect on oocyte quality and performance.[20] There may be an adverse association of malignancy with an increased metabolic state, increased stress hormones and hypothalamic dysfunction, resulting in infertility.[21, 22] Women with breast and ovarian cancers with *BRCA* mutations may also respond poorly to ovarian stimulation.[23]

Protocols

The ideal COS protocol for fertility preservation is debated. Friedler et al. recently published a meta-analysis detailing the protocols used for controlled ovarian hyperstimulation for the purpose of fertility preservation.[24] The seven studies reviewed included 218 patients who underwent 227 COS cycles before impending chemoradiotherapy for malignancy. Controls included 1253 age-matched patients undergoing 1258 in vitro fertilization/intracytoplasmic sperm injection (IVF/ICSI) cycles for male factor or tubal factor infertility. Most included studies used a gonadotropin releasing hormone (GnRH) antagonist protocol and some studies added an aromatase inhibitor or tamoxifen secondary to concern for elevated estradiol levels in breast cancer patients. Doses of gonadotropin used and peak estradiol levels were lower in the study groups compared to controls, with no differences in the length of stimulation. Significantly fewer mature oocytes were retrieved from study groups as opposed to controls. There were no differences in fertilization rates or cancellations secondary to poor ovarian response. This study led the authors to conclude the presence of local or systemic malignancy may have an adverse effect on ovarian response to COS secondary to poor ovarian reserve and quality. Similarly, the utilization of milder stimulation protocols, as evidenced by lower gonadotropin dosages and peak estradiol levels, may be responsible for comparatively diminished ovarian response. The authors noted that COS protocols per patient were likely used in accordance with the preference of each IVF center. The higher utilization of GnRH antagonist (shortest-term protocol) likely reflects the decreased amount of time available to these patients prior to initiation of chemoradiotherapy. Pregnancy rates are unknown thus far as these studies are relatively recent and most of these patients have not undergone thawing and subsequent transfer of these cryopreserved embryos.

Protocols for Breast Cancer Patients

Breast cancer is the most common cancer in women of reproductive age.[25] Unfortunately, breast cancer in young women exhibits a high ductal infiltrating effect and most of these women are required to undergo highly gonadotoxic chemotherapy for treatment.[26] Endocrine-sensitive tumors are usually treated with adjuvant tamoxifen for at least year years.[27] In women with an estrogen-sensitive tumor, the elevation of circulating estradiol levels during conventional ovulation stimulation with gonadotropins is undesirable and may be potentially harmful. As a result, alternative and potentially safer protocols, including non-stimulated natural cycle IVF and use of SERMs or aromatase inhibitors for ovulation induction alone or in combination with low dose gonadotropins, have been proposed for these patients.[28] Natural cycle IVF usually yields only one oocyte or embryo per cycle and has a high rate of cycle cancellation. This may not be an acceptable option for patients for whom chemotherapy treatment is imminent and thus, may not have a chance for a second cycle of IVF treatment.

Tamoxifen

Tamoxifen is a nonsteroidal triphenylethylene compound and functions as an estrogen agonist antagonist. Tamoxifen has been used in treatment and prevention of estrogen receptor positive breast cancer for nearly three decades and is considered to be a first line drug in hormonal treatment of breast cancer.[29] Similar to clomiphene, tamoxifen may be used during cycles 3–5 to 9 alone or in combination with gonadotropins. Ovarian stimulation using tamoxifen for fertility preservation in cancer patients significantly increases mature oocyte and embryo yield when compared to natural cycle IVF and reduces cycle cancellations.[30] The combination of tamoxifen and gonadotropins for IVF has been shown to further increase the number of oocytes and embryos for cryopreservation.[23] While peak estradiol levels in ovarian stimulation with tamoxifen on day of hCG administration may be significantly higher than in women undergoing natural cycle IVF, the effects of estrogen on breast tissue are mitigated secondary to select blockage at receptor sites.

Aromatase Inhibitors

Aromatase inhibitors have been used in the treatment of breast cancer in postmenopausal women for more than 30 years. Aromatase is a component of the cytochrome P450 complex that catalyzes the conversion of androstenedione and testosterone to estrone and estradiol, respectively. This enzyme is expressed in granulosa cells of the ovary and is stimulated by gonadotropins to convert androgens from thecal cells to estrogens. Aromatase expression also occurs in extragonadal sites such as breast and adipose tissue. Aromatase inhibitors such as letrozole and anastrozole inhibit the enzyme by competitively binding to the active site of the enzyme complex.[31] They may also be used for ovulation induction.[32] Inhibition of the aromatase system increases gonadotropin production by releasing the hypothalamic-pituitary axis from estrogenic negative feedback. Use of aromatase inhibitors yields lower peak estradiol levels compared to natural cycles.[33]

Combined Stimulation Protocols

Combined stimulation protocols with letrozole and gonadotropins are comparable to standard IVF, with the added advantage of less gonadotropin requirements and fewer costs. Combined letrozole and gonadotropin protocols result in significantly lower peak estradiol levels compared to standard IVF.[34] At short-term follow-up, these combined protocols do not show adverse effects on breast cancer recurrence.[35] Although stimulation for IVF may increase the time lapse between surgery and chemotherapy, studies have not found a difference in recurrence and disease free survival rates between patients undergoing combination protocols and controls.[35] Furthermore, delay of chemotherapy initiation by up to 12 weeks after surgery has not been shown to have any adverse effects on recurrence or disease-free survival.[36]

CRYOPRESERVATION

Low temperature banking is now a routine component of ART.[37] Cryopreservation refers to the storage of viable cells at low temperature (normally at –196°C). Cells are prone to damage during the cooling period by three mechanisms: (a) chilling injury that occurs between +15 and –5°C, (b) ice crystal formation between –5 and –80°C, and (c) fracture damage i.e., the mechanical effect of solidified fluid within the cell that occurs between –50 and –150°C.[38] Storage at –196°C is the least harmful aspect of the cryopreservation process. The cell has the potential to experience the same injury during the thawing process. Some strategies to prevent this damage include the avoidance of rapid temperature changes and decreasing the water content of the cells.

Two basic techniques are employed for cooling of embryos: controlled slow freezing and ultra rapid vitrification.[38] Both techniques utilize cryoprotective agents. Cryoprotective agents (CPAs) are used for long-term preservation of fertilized embryos. CPAs like glycerol are small, water-soluble molecules that serve as antifreeze agents by disrupting hydrogen bonds between water.[37] Permeable cryoprotectants prevent ice nucleation inside the cytoplasm of the cells, while extracellular cryoprotectants prevent ice crystal formation from the extracellular medium surrounding the cells. Non-permeable cryoprotectants rely on drawing water from the cytoplasm through osmosis.[38] Unfortunately, permeable cryoprotectants have the potential to damage cells by direct adverse effects and non-permeable cryoprotectants may damage cells via osmotic effects. Cryoprotectant toxicity is proportional to its concentration and the duration of exposure.[39]

Slow freezing involves cooling the cell at strictly controlled slow rates, allowing water to leave the cell after treatment.[37] Low concentrations of cryoprotectants are used in this process. Ultimately, this yields dense cytoplasmic viscosity without ice formation. Programmable freezing machines are used and freezing and thawing may take several hours. The procedure also requires the use of expensive instrumentation.

Conversely, vitrification involves rapid cooling of the cells. Transition from ambient temperature to –196°C occurs in less than a second. The cooling rate is above 15,000–30,000°C/minute.[40] Cells treated with higher doses of cryoprotectants are loaded into a carrier and submerged into liquid nitrogen. Vitrification essentially solidifies the sample into a glass-like state, thus avoiding the formation of both intra- and extracellular ice.[41] While rapid cooling may prevent ice formation and chilling injury, the use of higher doses of cryoprotectants may lead to direct injury. Vitrification is less expensive, as it does not involve expensive instrumentation. Furthermore, this technique is more time-efficient, requiring only several minutes as compared with 1–2 hours with controlled-rate slow freezing.

Kolibianakis and colleagues recently undertook a meta-analysis of randomized trials comparing slow freezing to vitrification.[42] They found that vitrification yielded higher post thaw survival rates for cleavage stage embryos (odds ratio (OR): 6.35, 95% confidence interval (CI): 1.14–35.26) and blastocysts (OR: 4.09, 95% CI: 2.45–6.84). However, overall pregnancy rates did not differ between the two groups (OR: 1.66, 95% CI: 0.98–2.79). Hence, the method of embryo freezing used should depend on the expertise of each ART laboratory.

SUCCESS RATES

Pregnancy rates for non-donor frozen thawed embryos are rapidly improving. According to the Society of Assisted Reproductive Technology, 38.7% of transfers lead to pregnancy in women under 35, yielding a pregnancy rate of 20.4% per transferred embryo.[43] The overall pregnancy rate in all age groups is 27.8% per cycle. These data include all women undergoing frozen thawed embryo transfers, including women undergoing cycles for fertility preservation.

Success rates for embryo yield vary according to the protocol used.[23] In their study of 60 women with breast cancer, Oktay and colleagues reported that women who underwent stimulation with tamoxifen only produced an average of 1.5 mature oocytes and 1.3 embryos during IVF.[23] This was a 2.5 fold increase compared to women who underwent IVF with unstimulated cycles and produced an average of 0.6 embryos per patient. Women taking tamoxifen and FSH produced an average of 5.1 mature oocytes and 3.8 embryos, while women taking letrozole and FSH produced an average of 8.5 mature oocytes and 5.3 embryos.

The researchers also found that breast cancer recurrence rates were similar between the women who underwent IVF and those who did not. After an average of 554 days, the recurrence rate was comparable between patients who underwent IVF (3 of 29 patients) and patients who chose not to undergo the procedure (3 of 31 patients). Unfortunately, the majority of women who have undergone IVF for fertility preservation have not undergone subsequent frozen thawed embryo transfers. Hence, the data with regards to subsequent pregnancy and live birth rates in these women are sparse.

ETHICAL AND LEGAL ISSUES

Prior to undergoing IVF and subsequent embryo cryopreservation, patients should decide upon the fate of the embryos in the event that these embryos are never transferred for any reason, including the failure of the patient to survive treatment. It should be documented whether the remaining partner has rights to future use of these embryos. Alternatively, embryos may be discarded, donated to research, or donated to a third party for reproductive purposes. As expected, these decisions may be difficult considering the life-threatening situation these patients are in and their need to make decisions in an expedient fashion. As such, it is encouraged that these patients be cared for using a multidisciplinary approach, including both psychological and legal counseling.[44]

CONCLUSION

Modern day ART has afforded patients diagnosed with life-threatening illnesses an option of fertility preservation. While numerous methodologies of fertility preservation are available, including oocyte cryopreservation, embryo cryopreservation is a proven and time-tested technique for fertility preservation. The American Society for Reproductive Medicine maintains that embryo cryopreservation is the only firmly established method.[45] Numerous protocols exist to expedite the IVF process, while minimizing the deleterious effects of COS cycles and elevated estradiol levels on the disease process. Success rates are presumably those of frozen thawed cycles. However, long-term studies with regards to pregnancy rates in patients with systemic disease undergoing IVF specifically for fertility preservation remain to be undertaken.

REFERENCES

1. http://en.wikipedia.org/wiki/Embryo_cryopreservation.
2. Jadoul P, Dolmans M, Donnez J. Fertility preservation in girls during childhood: is it feasible, efficient and safe and to whom should it be proposed? Hum Reprod Update. 2010;16(6):617-30.
3. "First Baby Born of Frozen Embryo". The New York Times. April 11, 1984. http://query.nytimes.com/gst/fullpage.html?sec=health&res=9E0DE1DB1738F932A25757C0A962948260.
4. ART data. Retrieved from the World Wide Web. http://www.cdc.gov/art/ART2008/section3.htm#f43.
5. American Cancer Society. Cancer facts and figures-2001. GA: Atlanta; 2001.
6. Green DM, Kawashima T, Stovall M, et al. Fertility of female survivors of childhood cancer: a report from the childhood cancer survivor study. J Clin Oncol. 2009;27:2677-85.
7. Wallace WH, Shalet SM, Hendry JH, et al. Ovarian failure following abdominal irradiation in childhood: the radiosensitivity of the human oocyte. Br J Radiol. 1989;62:995-8.
8. Wallace WH, Thomson AB, Saran F, Kelsey T. Predicting age of ovarian failure after radiation to a field that includes the ovaries. Int J Radiat Oncol Biol Phys. 2005;62(3):738-44.
9. Donnez J, Martinez-Madrid B, Jadoul P, et al. Ovarian tissue cryopreservation and transplantation: a review. Hum Reprod Update. 2006;12:519-35.
10. Wallace WH, Anderson RA, Irvine DS. Fertility preservation for young patients with cancer: who is at risk and what can be offered? Lancet Oncol. 2005;6(4):209-18.
11. De Bruin ML, Huisbrink J, Hauptmann M, et al. Treatment-related risk factors for premature menopause following Hodgkin lymphoma. Blood. 2008;111(1):101-8.
12. Behringer K, Breuer K, Reineke T, et al. Secondary amenorrhea after Hodgkin's lymphoma is influenced by age at treatment, stage of disease, chemotherapy regimen, and the use of oral contraceptives during therapy: a report from the German Hodgkin's Lymphoma Study Group. J Clin Oncol. 2005;23(30):7555-64.
13. Meirow D, et al. Administration of cyclophosphamide at different stages of follicular maturation in mice: effects on reproductive performance and fetal malformations. Hum Reprod (Oxford, England) 2001;16(4):632-7.
14. Langagergaard V, et al. Birth outcome in women with breast cancer. Br J Cancer. 2006;94(1):142-6.
15. Lee SJ, Schover LR, Partridge AH, et al. American Society of Clinical Oncology. American Society of Clinical Oncology recommendations on fertility preservation in cancer patients. J Clin Oncol. 2006;24(18):2917-31.
16. Stochholm K, Juul S, Juel K, et al. Prevalence, incidence, diagnostic delay, and mortality in Turner syndrome. J Clin Endocrinol Metab. 2006;91:3897-902.
17. Saenger P. Turner's Syndrome. N Engl J Med. 1996;335(23):1749-54.
18. Santoro N. Mechanisms of premature ovarian failure. Ann Endocrinol (Paris) 2003;64(2):87-92.
19. Allingham-Hawkins DJ, Babul-Hirji R, Chitayat D, et al. Fragile X premutation is a significant risk factor for premature ovarian failure: the International Collaborative POF in Fragile X study-preliminary data. Am J Med Genet. 1999;83:322-325.
20. Pal L, Leykin L, Schifren JL, et al. Malignancy may adversely influence the quality and behaviour of oocytes. Hum Reprod. 1998;13:1837–40.
21. Agarwal A, Said TM. Implications of systemic malignancies on human fertility. Reprod Biomed Online. 2004;9:673-9.
22. Speroff L, Fritz M. Clinical gynecologic endocrinology and infertility. Philadelphia: Lippincott Williams & Wilkins; 2005.
23. Oktay K, Buyuk E, Libertella N, et al. Fertility preservation in breast cancer patients: a prospective controlled comparison of ovarian stimulation with tamoxifen and letrozole for embryo cryopreservation. J Clin Oncol. 2005;23:4347-53.
24. Friedler S, Koc O, Gidoni Y, et al. Ovarian response to stimulation for fertility preservation in women with malignant disease: a systematic review and meta-analysis. Fertil Steril. 2012;97(1):125-33.
25. Breast cancer statistics. April 2012. www.cdc.gov/cancer/breast/statistics/
26. Rodriguez-Wallberg KA, Oktay K. Options on fertility preservation in female cancer patients. Cancer Treat Rev. 2012;38(5):354-61.
27. Fisher B, Dignam J, Bryant J, Wolmark N. Five versus more than five years of tamoxifen for lymph node-negative breast cancer: updated findings from the National Surgical Adjuvant Breast and Bowel Project B-14 randomized trial. J Natl Cancer Inst. 2001;93(9):684-90.
28. Rodriguez-Wallberg KA, Oktay K. Fertility preservation in women with breast cancer. Clin Obstet Gynecol. 2010; 53(4):753-62.
29. Systemic treatment of early breast cancer by hormonal, cytotoxic, or immune therapy. 133 randomised trials involving 31,000 recurrences and 24,000 deaths among 75,000 women. Early Breast Cancer Trialists' Collaborative Group. Lancet. 1992;339(8785):71-85.
30. Oktay K, Buyuk E, Davis O, et al. Fertility preservation in breast cancer patients: IVF and embryo cryopreservation after ovarian stimulation with tamoxifen. Hum Reprod. 2003;18(1):90-5.
31. Brueggemeier RW, Hackett JC, Diaz-Cruz ES. Aromatase Inhibitors in the Treatment of Breast Cancer. Endocrine Reviews. 2005; 26(3):331-45.
32. Mitwally MF, Casper RF. Use of an aromatase inhibitor for induction of ovulation in patients with an inadequate response to clomiphene citrate. Fertil Steril 2001; 75(2):305-9.
33. Fisher SA, Reid RL, Van Vugt DA, Casper RF. A randomized double-blind comparison of the effects of clomiphene citrate and the aromatase inhibitor letrozole on ovulatory function in normal women. Fertil Steril 2002; 78(2):280-5.
34. Oktay K, Hourvitz A, Sahin G, et al. Letrozole reduces estrogen and gonadotropin exposure in women with breast cancer undergoing ovarian stimulation before chemotherapy. J Clin Endocrinol Metab 2006; 91(10):3885-90.
35. Azim AA, Costantini-Ferrando M, Oktay K. Safety of fertility preservation by ovarian stimulation with letrozole and gonadotropins

in patients with breast cancer: a prospective controlled study. J Clin Oncol. 2008;26(16):2630-5.
36. Cold S, Düring M, Ewertz M, et al. Does timing of adjuvant chemotherapy influence the prognosis after early breast cancer? Results of the Danish Breast Cancer Cooperative Group (DBCG). Br J Cancer. 2005;93(6):627-32.
37. Gosden R. Cryopreservation: a cold look at technology for fertility preservation. Fertil Steril. 2011;96(2):264-8.
38. Ata B, Chian RC, Tan SL. Cryopreservation of oocytes and embryos for fertility preservation for female cancer patients. Best Pract Res Clin Obstet Gynaecol. 2010;24(1):101-12.
39. Vajta G, Kuwayama M, Vanderzwalmen P. Disadvantages and benefits of vitrification. In Tucker MJ & Liebermann J (Eds.). Vitrification in assisted reproduction A user's manual and troubleshooting guide. London: Informa UK, 2007, pp. 33-44.
40. Liebermann J, Nawroth F, Isachenko V, et al. Potential importance of vitrification in reproductive medicine. Biol Reprod. 2002;67:1671-80.
41. Vajta G, Kuwayama M. Improving cryopreservation systems. Theriogenology. 2006;65:236-44.
42. Kolibianakis EM, Venetis CA, Tarlatzis BC. Cryopreservation of human embryos by vitrification or slow freezing: which one is better? Curr Opin Obstet Gynecol. 2009;21(3):270-4.
43. Clinical report summary. Society of Assisted Reproductive Technology. https://www.sartcorsonline.com/rptCSR_PublicMultYear.aspx?ClinicPKID=0
44. Seli E, Agarwal A Fertility Preservation. Emerging Technologies and Clinical applications. New York: Springer; 2012: 424 pages.
45. American Society for Reproductive Medicine. Fertility preservation and reproduction in cancer patients. Fertil Steril. 2005;83(6): 1622-8.

11

The Challenges and Promises of Whole Human Ovary Cryopreservation

Amanda N Kallen, Pasquale Patrizio

CHAPTER OUTLINE

INTRODUCTION

Today, more than ever, young women with childhood cancers are surviving into adulthood. According to the National Cancer Institute's Surveillance, epidemiology and End Results (SEER) Program, the 5-year survival rates for all childhood cancers combined increased from near zero before 1960, to over 80% by 2003. This change can be attributed to improved surgical technique, early diagnosis, chemotherapy and radiotherapy and supportive care.[1] Unfortunately, these therapies are frequently gonadotoxic, leading to premature ovarian failure (POF) and infertility.[2] Some patients will have time to undergo oocyte or embryo preservation prior to beginning cancer treatment; however, others will need to start their treatment immediately.

Options for preservation in patients undergoing immediate gonadotoxic treatments are few. These patients may opt to have ovarian tissue preserved in the form of cortical tissue strips (with the potential for in vitro maturation (IVM) of any oocytes found in the strip prior to freezing) followed by auto-transplantation at a later time, when the cancer is cured. However, despite considerable progress in perfecting the cryopreservation process of cortical strips, in particular with vitrification, the regrafting of ovarian tissue is accompanied by the risk of ischemic damage and thus, short functional lifespan.[2,3] Because these tissues are regrafted without vascular anastomoses, the period between regrafting and establishment of neovascularization (a minimum of 7 days) marks a time of significant ischemic damage and loss of primordial follicles.[4-6] This likely leads to the complete cessation of function seen in these grafts within 2 to 3 years.[7-13] Another option, still unproven in humans, is the in vitro production of follicles from the cultured ovarian cortical strips, either in isolated fragments of cortex or after tridimensional reconstruction in alginate-based artificial follicles.[14,15]

Another option for women requiring immediate intervention to preserve fertility is whole ovary cryopreservation, with an intact pedicle and vascular supply, which provides an alternative form of fertility preservation for patients. This technique can potentially overcome the problem of ischemic damage by providing immediate reperfusion upon regrafting and creation of a vascular anastomosis. The technique is still considered experimental in humans and while the challenges of whole ovary cryopreservation are numerous, the promising results in animal models and the improvement in cryopreservation strategies for whole organs could bode well for its application to human ovaries.

SUCCESSES

Fresh transplantation of the ovary, with intact vasculature, has been performed in rats, rabbits, sheep, dogs and monkeys.[3,16-19] Sheep ovaries in particular, with their high cortical primordial follicle density and dense fibrous stroma, bear strong resemblance to human ovaries, despite being smaller.[20] Studies of whole ovary cyropreservation in sheep is shown in **Table 1**.

Successes in Animals

Animal studies have demonstrated success with whole ovary freezing and re-transplant.[21] Wang et al. (2002) described successful re-transplantation of frozen-thawed rat ovaries, 57% (4 of 7) of which survived for greater than 2 months and were ovulatory. One resulted in a pregnancy.[22] Bedaiwy et al. (2003) successfully transplanted a cryopreserved sheep ovary using the inferior epigastric vessels.[23] Arav et al. (2005) demonstrated progesterone activity in sheep transplanted with frozen/thawed ovaries 36 months after the procedure; ultimately, successful retrieval of oocytes and embryo development occurred.[24] The same group reported successful ovarian re-transplantation with function (as demonstrated by response to exogenous gonadotropins) 6 years post-transplantation in 2 sheep.[20] Lastly, Imhof et al. (2006) followed FSH and progesterone levels after frozen-thawed ovary auto-transplantation in a sheep model, finding that FSH levels reached normal physiologic levels about 6 months after transplantation and delivery of one healthy lamb was reported.[25]

Promising Human Results

Martinez-Madrid and colleagues reported on the viability of frozen/thawed human ovaries and noted promising results. In 3 premenopausal women undergoing oophorectomy, cryopreservation and thawing of the ovary revealed 75.1% live follicles after completion of thawing, as well as live stromal cells and small vessels.[26] Electron microscopy demonstrated well-preserved ultrastructure, healthy-appearing primordial and primary follicles, and normal endothelial cells. In subsequent studies, no primordial or primary follicles were found to be positive for markers of apoptosis.[26] Others have since confirmed these results.[23]

Solving the Problem of Freezing

One challenge in particular that has been successfully addressed lies in the preservation of the ovary itself. A standardized freezing protocol does not yet exist and approaches range from

Table 1 Summary of whole ovary cryopreservation experiments in sheep.

	N=	*Surgical method*	*Freezing method*	*Cryoprotectant*	*Retransplanted?*	*Outcomes measured*	*Endocrine function?*	*pregnancy?*
Bedaiwy et al. 2003	11	Laparoscopy	Slow Cooling	DMSO	Yes	Blood flow, Apoptosis, Follicular viability, Endocrine function, Histology	Yes (3/11)	No
Revel et al. 2004	8	Laparotomy	Slow Cooling	Ethylene Glycol	Yes	Cyclic progesterone	Yes (3/8)	No
Courbiere et al. 2005	15	Laparotomy	Vitrification	DMSO/ acetamide/ propylene glycol or DMSO/ formamide/ propylene glycol	No	Follicle viability, Histological examination of ovary and vessels	N/A	N/A
Imhof et al. 2006	9	Laparotomy	Slow Cooling	DMSO	Yes	Histology, FSH and progesterone	Yes (4/9)	Yes (1/9)
Grazul-Bilska et al. 2008	4	Laparoscopy	Slow Cooling	DMSO	Yes	No. of follicles, No. of fertilized, morphology, vessel viability, cellular proliferation, apoptosis	Yes (2/4)	No
Courbiere et al. 2008	5	Laparotomy	Vitrifi-cation	DMSO/ formamide/ propylene glycol	Yes	Progesterone levels, Histology	1/5	No

slow-freezing with rapid thawing, to vitrification, to ultrarapid-freezing. Slow-freezing is typically done over several hours, using either dimethyl sulphoxide (DMSO) or propanediol (PROH) as a cryoprotectant. However, attempts to cryopreserve large organs, including ovaries, have frequently been unsuccessful due to uneven cooling temperatures. During freezing, latent heat is released causing a rise in the temperature of the organ being frozen with subsequent cycles of formation of ice crystals and recrystallization occurring as the temperature drops. Thus, transient thawing and recrystallization occurs, which can lead to tissue damage.[27-29]

Additionally, as ice crystals form and cooling continues, cells may be exposed to a temperature that is actually lower than intended. As the temperature of the surrounding medium is also lowered, release of accumulated latent heat cannot occur, because the gradient between tissue and medium has also been lowered. As a consequence, the temperature of the material being frozen will drop too rapidly and damaging intracellular crystallization can occur.[30,31]

The technique of vitrification avoids formation of ice crystals, but uses high concentrations of cryoprotectants, which cause ovarian toxicity. Additionally, vitrification requires direct contact with liquid nitrogen, which is a potential source of microbial contamination.[32] Isachenco and colleagues demonstrated better preservation of ovarian tissue, with higher quality follicles preserved, by slow freezing as compared to vitrification.[32,33]

A methodolology called directional multithermal gradient freezing has solved the problem of ice crystal formation. This process, which uses a freezing device that moves the sample through the temperature gradient at a uniform speed, rapidly evacuates latent heat and maintains a uniform cooling rate through the periphery and core of the ovary.[3,24] Bromer and Patrizio (2009) and Johnson and Patrizio (2011) have reported on successful whole human ovary cryopreservation using the directional multi-thermal gradient technique.[3,14] Twelve ovaries from premenopausal women undergoing hysterectomy were successfully cannulated for perfusion of cryoprotectant and cryopreserved for up to 5 days after oophorectomy. The contralateral ovaries were used as fresh controls in all cases, and a blinded pathologist was unable to distinguish between the frozen/thawed ovary and control by histological analysis. Immunohistochemistry and Western Blot assays did show some increase in anti-caspace 3 and p53 phosphoserine expression, suggesting some increased level of apoptosis in the frozen-thawed specimen. In 3 cases, the ipsilateral Fallopian tube was also cryopreserved intact with the associated ovary and pedicle. In these cases, the histological architecture was also preserved, suggesting that cryopreservation of the entire adnexa may be technically feasible.[3,14] A summary of these studies is shown in **Table 2**.

CHALLENGES

While many advances have been made in the area of whole ovary cryopreservation, multiple challenges still exist. Preservation of the whole ovary is dependent on multiple factors, including careful removal of the ovary, degree of tissue survival after freeze and thaw, and recreation of the vascular pedicles with prevention of ischemia and thrombosis.[34] Everything must go perfectly; there is no second chance if the ovary is handled, cryopreserved, or thawed and reimplanted improperly.[14]

Removal of the Ovary

Optimum conditions when planning for ovarian preservation at the time of oophorectomy have been described. When the intent is to preserve the whole ovary, great care must be taken to remove the ovary with a large part (at least 5 cm) of the infundibulopelvic ligament in order to allow for dissection of the ovarian vessels and perfusion with a cryoprotective medium. Laparotomy is the traditional approach, though laparoscopy has been shown to be successful. Robotic surgery may provide additional aid when performing the delicate dissection required to preserve the length of the pedicle. For ovarian freezing, the period of ischemia between ligation of the ovarian pedicle and ovarian cryopreservation must be as short as possible.[35]

To Freeze or not to Freeze?

Two cases of successful fresh ovarian transplantation has been described (the details of which will be reviewed below); however, many patients desiring fertility preservation will require freezing of the ovary until they have completed treatment and are ready for transplantation. Successes of whole ovary cryopreservation in animals have been reviewed, but no successful case of frozen-thawed human ovarian transplantation has been reported. Notably, freezing techniques such as traditional cryopreservation and vitrification are known to cause endothelial cell damage and result in poor follicular survival. Imhof et al. (2006) demonstrated

Table 2 Summary of whole ovary cryopreservation experiments in humans.

	N=	*Surgical method*	*Freezing method*	*Cryoprotectant*	*Outcomes measured*
Martinez-Madrid et al., 2004	3	Laparoscopy	Slow Cooling	DMSO	Follicle, stromal cell, vascular viability, histological morphology
Bedaiwy et al., 2006	2	Laparoscopy	Slow Cooling	DMSO	Follicle viability, apoptosis
Martinez-Madrid et al., 2007	3	Laparoscopy	Slow Cooling	DMSO	Apoptosis, ultrastructural assessment
Bromer and Patrizio, 2009 Johnson and Patrizio, 2011	12	Laparoscopy, laparotomy	Slow Cooling	Ethylene Glycol	Apoptosis, histological morphology

a follicular survival rate of less than 8% within a year and a half after transplantation using traditional freezing techniques.[25] Fortunately, as previously discussed, newer multi-gradient freezing techniques appear to have bypassed this problem.

Reanastomosis and Avoidance of Ischemia and Thrombosis

Avascular ovarian tissue transplantation results in a short graft life due to ischemic injury and subsequent loss of a large proportion of follicles during the period of neovascularization.[36-38] A shorter period of ischemia should lead to improved graft survival, but the exact time required for neovascularization is unclear. For example, animal experiments have demonstrated a neovascularization time of 3 days in mice and up to one week in mice for in vivo for ovarian tissue grafts.[5,39,40] In vitro neovascularlization of human ovarian tissue onto the chorioallantoic membrane of a chick also required 3 days.[41] Thrombosis presents an additional problem. In a series of sheep ovary transplantations, Bedaiwy et al. (2003) reported that 8 of 11 ovaries failed due to thrombosis at the pedicle site.[23] Jeremias et al. (2002) reported that up to 50% of revascularization attempts were compromised in merino sheep due to thrombosis.[42]

Because of the rapid loss of follicles when ischemia occurs, much attention has been focused on whole ovary transplantation with re-creation of the vascular pedicle. Re-creation of the vascular anastomosis is a challenging surgery, requiring meticulous dissection and suturing to ensure the integrity of the vasculature. Sites for revascularization which have been explored include pelvic vessels (the ovarian and iliac vessels), parietal vessels (such as the inferior epigastrics) and estrapelvic vessels such as the carotids.[22,43]

Unfortunately, variation in the ovarian vascular supply can make re-creation of the vascular pedicle impossible for the surgeon attempting whole ovary transplantation. Successful recreation of the ovarian vascular supply requires the presence of a large single draining vein, but in some patients this is not present. Rather, the ovarian vein may be replaced by a meshwork of small venules, making reanastomosis impossible. Indeed, Mhatre et al. (2005) described a case of attempted whole ovarian transplantation, which was converted to avascular ovarian grafting when one such situation was encountered.[44]

With regard to surgical technique, use of fine suture, such as 8-0 or 10-0 prolene, as well as the operating microscope, can aid in success of the procedure.[44] Two authors have described the details of their successful (albeit fresh) ovarian transplantation. Silber et al. (2008) described a case of intact human fresh ovarian auto-transplantation in 38-year-old monozygotic twins discordant for POF.[45] In this case, the donor ovary (from the fertile sister) was removed laparoscopically by dividing the base of the infundibulopelvic ligament in order to maximize length. In a separate publication, Silber explains that, at this point, the specimen is placed in Leibovitz medium at 4°C and the 2 veins and 1 artery are dissected out under the microscope.[46] Returning to the described case, the recipient's ovarian veins, 3.0 mm in diameter, were accessed using mini-laparotomy and anastomosed to the donor's ovarian veins using 9-0 nylon sutures. Similarly, the ovarian arteries, 0.5 mm in diameter, were anastomosed together using 10-0 nylon interrupted sutures. After 100 minutes of ischemia, normal-appearing blood flow was observed through the transplanted vessels. In the following months, the recipient had 11 regular menstrual cycles and 427 days after transplantation she became pregnant. She subsequently delivered a healthy baby girl.[45]

Mhatre and Mhatre (2006) also described a case of orthotopic ovarian transplantation using fresh donor ovaries transplanted into 2 patients with Turner's syndrome. The ovary was removed via a Pfannenstiel incision along with its 6 cm pedicle from the 26-year-old female donor. Upon removal, the ovary was immersed in heparin solution and flushed with 4-degree Ringer's solution to remove donor blood. In the meantime, the 17-year-old sister and intended recipient was administered a bolus of 500 mg of intravenous methylprednisolone and her abdomen opened with a right-sided reversed j-shaped incision parallel to the right inguinal ligament. The ovarian vein was attached in an end-to-side fashion to the external iliac vein with 8-0 continuous prolene, and the ovarian artery was sutured to the inferior epigastric artery using 10-0 prolene interrupted sutures. The ovary was then sutured into a peritoneal window using 3-0 vicryl sutures in the round ligament and peritoneum. For immunosuppression, the patient received a regimen of oral cyclosporine and prednisolone. At 2.5 years post-transplant, the patient reported spontaneous ovulation, menstruation and growth of secondary sexual characteristics.[47] Both of these cases illustrate the need for meticulous surgical technique and planning prior to the procedure; the use of frozen-thawed whole ovaries would present additional challenges with regards to timing.

Tumor Reseeding

Lastly, while it may seem obvious, it is important not to attempt ovarian tissue re-implantation when dealing with tumors that metastasize to the ovary due to the risk of replacing cancer cells.[48] In these situations, the only option is to mature primordial follicles in vitro.[49]

CONCLUSION

While no human studies of whole ovary transplant after cryopreservation have been performed to date, large animal studies have been encouraging. Thus, it is possible that this option for fertility preservation will be a viable treatment option in the future. The surgical techniques described for fresh whole ovary transplantation may be applicable to frozen ovary transplantation as well. Alternatively, some have postulated that due to the excellent results seen with ovarian tissue freezing and grafting, this may be a better tool for fertility preservation. Hopefully, research and continued development in cryoprotectants and surgical techniques will allow for enhancement of vascularization of transplanted tissues to minimize post-transfusion ischemia, which is critical for the viability of ovarian tissue and improved reproductive success in patients who wish to preserve their fertility.

REFERENCES

1. Mariotto AB, Rowland JH, Yabroff KR, et al. Long-term survivors of childhood cancers in the United States. Cancer Epidemiology, Biomarkers & Prevention: A Publication of the American Association for Cancer Research, Cosponsored by the American Society of Preventive Oncology. 2009;18(4),1033-40.
2. Martin J R, Patrizio P. Options for fertility preservation in pediatric populations undergoing cancer chemotherapy. Pediatric Endocrinology Reviews. 2009; 6 Suppl 2:306-14.
3. Bromer JG, Patrizio P. Fertility preservation: The rationale for cryopreservation of the whole ovary. Seminars Reprod Med. 2009; 27(6):465-71.
4. Baird DT, Webb R, Campbell BK, et al. Long-term ovarian function in sheep after ovariectomy and transplantation of autografts stored at -196 °C. Endocrinolog. 1999;140(1):462-71.
5. Israely T, Dafni H, Nevo N, et al. Angiogenesis in ectopic ovarian xenotransplantation: Multiparameter characterization of the neovasculature by dynamic contrast-enhanced MRI. Official J Society Magnetic Resonance Med. 2004; 52(4):741-50.
6. Kim SS. Fertility preservation in female cancer patients: Current developments and future directions. Fertil Steril. 2006; 85(1):1-11.
7. Andersen CY, Rosendahl M, Byskov AG, et al. Two successful pregnancies following autotransplantation of frozen/thawed ovarian tissue. Human Reprod. 2008;23(10):2266-72.
8. Demeestere I, Simon P, Emiliani S, et al. Fertility preservation: Successful transplantation of cryopreserved ovarian tissue in a young patient previously treated for Hodgkin's disease. Oncologist. 2007;12(12): 1437-42.
9. Donnez J, Dolmans MM, Demylle D, et al. Livebirth after orthotopic transplantation of cryopreserved ovarian tissue. Lancet. 2004;364(9443):1405-10.
10. Meirow D, Levron J, Eldar-Geva T, et al. Pregnancy after transplantation of cryopreserved ovarian tissue in a patient with ovarian failure after chemotherapy. New England J Med. 2005;353(3):318-21.
11. Oktay K, Buyuk E. Ovarian transplantation in humans: Indications, techniques and the risk of reseeding cancer. Eur J Obstet Gynecol Reprod Biol. 2004; 113 Suppl 1:S45-7.
12. Oktay K, Buyuk E, Rodriguez-Wallberg KA, Sahin G. In vitro maturation improves oocyte or embryo cryopreservation outcome in breast cancer patients undergoing ovarian stimulation for fertility preservation. Reprod Biomed Online. 2010;20(5):634-8.
13. Radford JA, Lieberman BA, Brison DR, et al. Orthotopic reimplantation of cryopreserved ovarian cortical strips after high-dose chemotherapy for hodgkin's lymphoma. Lancet. 2001;357(9263):1172-5.
14. Johnson J, Patrizio P. Ovarian cryopreservation strategies and the fine control of ovarian follicle development in vitro. Annals New York Academy Sciences. 2011;1221:40-6.
15. Smitz J, Dolmans MM, Donnez J, et al. Current achievements and future research directions in ovarian tissue culture, in vitro follicle development and transplantation: Implications for fertility preservation. Human Reprod Update. 2010;16(4):395-414.
16. Bedaiwy MA, Hussein MR, Biscotti C, Falcone T. Cryopreservation of intact human ovary with its vascular pedicle. Human Reprod 2006; 21(12):3258-69.
17. Israely T, Nevo N, Harmelin A, et al. Reducing ischaemic damage in rodent ovarian xenografts transplanted into granulation tissue. Human Reprod. 2006;21(6):1368-79.
18. Martinez-Madrid B, Dolmans MM, Van Langendonckt A, et al. Freeze-thawing intact human ovary with its vascular pedicle with a passive cooling device. Fertil Steril. 2004;82(5):1390-4.
19. Qi S, Ma A, Xu D. Cryopreservation of vascularized ovary: An evaluation of histology and function in rats. Microsurgery. 2008; 28(5):380-6.
20. Arav A, Gavish Z, Elami A, et al. Ovarian function 6 years after cryopreservation and transplantation of whole sheep ovaries. Reprod Biomed Online. 2010; 20(1):48-52.
21. Silber SJ, Lenahan KM, Levine DJ, et al. Ovarian transplantation between monozygotic twins discordant for premature ovarian failure. New Eng J Med. 2005;353(1):58-63.
22. Wang X, Chen H, Yin H, et al. Fertility after intact ovary transplantation. Nature. 2002;415(6870):385.
23. Bedaiwy MA, Jeremias E, Gurunluoglu R, et al. Restoration of ovarian function after autotransplantation of intact frozen-thawed sheep ovaries with microvascular anastomosis. Fertil Steril. 2003;79(3):594-602.
24. Arav A, Revel A, Nathan Y, et al. Oocyte recovery, embryo development and ovarian function after cryopreservation and transplantation of whole sheep ovary. Human Reprod. 2005;20(12): 3554-59.
25. Imhof M, Bergmeister H, Lipovac M, et al. Orthotopic microvascular reanastomosis of whole cryopreserved ovine ovaries resulting in pregnancy and live birth. Fertil Steril. 2006;85 Suppl 1:1208-15.
26. Martinez-Madrid B, Camboni A, Dolmans MM, et al. Apoptosis and ultrastructural assessment after cryopreservation of whole human ovaries with their vascular pedicle. Fertil Steril. 2007;87(5): 1153-65.
27. Balasubramanian SK, Coger RN. Heat and mass transfer during the cryopreservation of a bioartificial liver device: A computational model. Am Society Artificial Internal Organs. 2005; 51(3):184-93.
28. Fong LP, Hunt CJ, Pegg DE. Cryopreservation of the rabbit cornea: Freezing with dimethyl sulphoxide in air or in medium. Current Eye Res. 1987;6(4):569-77.
29. Koshimoto C, Mazur P. Effects of cooling and warming rate to and from -70 degrees C, and effect of further cooling from -70 to -196°C on the motility of mouse spermatozoa. Biol Reprod. 2002; 66(5): 1477-84.
30. Armitage WJ. Cryopreservation of animal cells. Symposia Society Experimental Bio. 1987;41:379-93.
31. Bischof JC. Quantitative measurement and prediction of biophysical response during freezing in tissues. Ann Review Biomed Engineering. 2000;2: 257-88.
32. Isachenko V, Isachenko E, Weiss JM, et al. Cryobanking of human ovarian tissue for anti-cancer treatment: Comparison of vitrification and conventional freezing. Cryo Letters. 2009;30(6):449-54.
33. Isachenko V, Isachenko E, Reinsberg J, et al. Cryopreservation of human ovarian tissue: Comparison of rapid and conventional freezing. Cryobiol. 2007;55(3):261-8.
34. Yin H, Wang X, Kim SS, et al. Transplantation of intact rat gonads using vascular anastomosis: Effects of cryopreservation, ischaemia and genotype. Human Reprod. 2003;18(6):1165-72.
35. Jadoul P, Donnez J, Dolmans MM, et al. Laparoscopic ovariectomy for whole human ovary cryopreservation: Technical aspects. Fertil Steril. 2007;87(4):971-5.
36. Bedaiwy MA, Falcone T. Whole ovary transplantation. Clin Obstet Gynecol. 2010;53(4):797-803.
37. Donnez J, Martinez-Madrid B, Jadoul P, et al. Ovarian tissue cryopreservation and transplantation: A review. Human Reprod Update. 2006;12(5):519-35.
38. Tao T, Del Valle A. Human oocyte and ovarian tissue cryopreservation and its application. J Assisted Reprod Genetics. 2008;25(7): 287-96.
39. Dissen GA, Lara HE, Fahrenbach WH, et al. Immature rat ovaries become revascularized rapidly after autotransplantation and show a gonadotropin-dependent increase in angiogenic factor gene expression. Endocrinol. 1994;134(3):1146-54.

40. Nugent D, Newton H, Gallivan L, Gosden RG. Protective effect of vitamin E on ischaemia-reperfusion injury in ovarian grafts. J Reprod Fertil. 1998;114(2):341-6.
41. Martinez-Madrid B, Donnez J, Van Eyck AS, et al. Chick embryo chorioallantoic membrane (CAM) model: A useful tool to study short-term transplantation of cryopreserved human ovarian tissue. Fertil Steril. 2009;91(1):285-92.
42. Jeremias E, Bedaiwy MA, Gurunluoglu R, et al. Heterotopic autotransplantation of the ovary with microvascular anastomosis: A novel surgical technique. Fertil Steril. 2002;77(6):1278-82.
43. Goding JR. Ovarian autotransplantation with vascular anastomoses, and its application to the study of reproductive physiology in the ewe. J Physiol. 1966;186(2):86P-87P.
44. Mhatre P, Mhatre J, Magotra R. Ovarian transplant: A new frontier. Transplantation Proceedings. 2005;37(2):1396-8.
45. Silber SJ, Grudzinskas G, Gosden RG. Successful pregnancy after microsurgical transplantation of an intact ovary. New Eng J Med. 2008;359(24):2617-8.
46. Silber SJ. Ovary cryopreservation and transplantation for fertility preservation. Molecular Human Reprod. 2012;18(2):59-7.
47. Mhatre P, Mhatre J. Orthotopic ovarian transplant--review and three surgical techniques. Pediatric Transplantation. 2006;10(7): 782-7.
48. Albani E, Bracone G, Biccari S, et al. Human ovarian tissue cryopreservation as fertility reserve. In: Mohan R (Ed.) Topics in Cancer Survivorship. Rijeka: InTech 2012; Chapter 14.
49. Eppig JJ, O'Brien M, Wigglesworth K. Mammalian oocyte growth and development in vitro. Molecular Reprod Development. 1996;44(2): 260-73.

Ovary Transplantation for Fertility Preservation in Cancer Patients: Fresh and Frozen

12

Sherman J Silber

CHAPTER OUTLINE

Successful fresh human ovary transplantation was first reported between monozygotic (MZ) twins discordant for premature ovarian failure (POF) using a cortical grafting technique.[1,2] We have now reported a total of nine consecutive successful fresh ovary transplants in menopausal women, with resumption of normal hormonal cycling and menstruation in all cases and with 12 pregnancies (and nine healthy babies born) from these nine fresh ovary transplants.[3-5] This experience helped us refine the techniques necessary for successful preservation of fertility for cancer patients using ovarian tissue freezing.

The great majority of women enter menopause in their fifth or sixth decade of life, although ~ 1% undergo menopause prematurely i.e., before 40 years of age.[6-9] POF frequently has a genetic etiology and menopausal age normally is strongly heritable, judging by the greater concordance between MZ than dizygotic (DZ) twins.[10-12] However, another common cause for POF is treatment for cancer in young girls and women of reproductive age.[13-21]

It was remarkable to identify a MZ twin pair in which one sister had undergone menopause for unexplained reasons at age 14, whereas the other, aged 24, was still fertile with three naturally conceived children and normal ovulatory cycles and ovarian reserve.[1,3-5] After the sterile twin received a graft of ovarian tissue from her sibling, she conceived naturally after her first menstrual cycle and delivered a healthy baby at full-term. This case of discordant twins is not unique, however, nine other twin pairs have subsequently consulted our center for ovarian transplantation in preference to conventional oocyte donation. The present chapter provides a clinical evaluation of the 9 cases of fresh ovarian transplantation that have already undergone surgery and its application then to 62 cases of ovarian tissue freezing for cancer and three cases of frozen ovary tissue transplantation.[3,5,13, 20-21] Furthermore, it delineates the expected duration of function of these cortical ovarian grafts, both fresh and frozen.

SUBJECT RECRUITMENT AND CONSENT

Ten MZ twin pairs aged 24–40 years presented with discordant ovarian function, one sibling of each pair having undergone POF. Nine of the 10 twin pairs elected to undergo transplantation of an ovary from the normal twin to the twin with POF. POF was diagnosed after more than four years of amenorrhea, accompanied by elevated serum levels of gonadotropins, over 50 miu/ml. Their sisters, in contrast, still had normal menstrual cyclicity, normal gonadotropin levels and 8 of the 9 donors had successful pregnancy histories. None of the twin pairs was actively recruited. Each pair had enquired about treatment to restore normal reproductive endocrine function with fertility potential after hearing reports of the first successful ovarian transplant in a twin pair in 2005, as well as from researching an earlier testis transplant we had reported for anorchia.[1,22,23]

The patients provided many reasons for preferring transplantation to conventional oocyte donation. Many of them had previous failures with donor oocyte cycles and did not want to go through more cycles. Some had the opportunity to donate an ovary at the same time as having surgery they required for other gynecologic problems (such as fibroids or cysts). All of them found the possibility of natural conception more attractive than in vitro fertilization (IVF) and egg donation. In most cases, the twins lived far apart (even in different countries) and the donors preferred to make a single visit for a one-time donation, with the hope that frozen banked tissue could serve as a backup if the first transplant failed.

CLINICAL PROFILE

These studies were carried out with informed consent under a protocol approved by the Institutional Review Board and the Ethics Committee of St. Luke's Hospital, St. Louis, MO. The donors were informed that they might reach menopause slightly earlier than normal based on theoretical models and experimental studies [24,25] and were aware of the relative risks associated with unilateral oophorectomy.

The reproductive history of each twin pair was reviewed and ovarian function was investigated by standard gynecological procedures. Serum from peripheral blood was prepared for immunoassay of FSH, LH and estradiol (E_2) three days after the start of menses in women who were cycling naturally, but not on any specific day in those with POF. The antral follicle count (AFC) was recorded by transvaginal ultrasound scanning. A tiny piece of spare tissue becoming available during oophorectomy of the donor, as well as resected atrophied ovarian cortex of the recipient, was prepared by fixing it in Bouin's fluid, embedding it in paraffin, sectioning it and staining it with hematoxylin and eosin (**Figures 1A** and **B**). Most of the spare donor tissue was cryopreserved for future use.

GENETIC STUDIES

DNA fingerprinting confirmed the genetic identify of all 10 twin pairs, who were also screened for common genetic causes of POF. Peripheral lymphocytes were prepared as DNA for testing genetic polymorphisms at 15 loci (Paternity Testing Corporation, Columbia, MO) and cultures (and in some cases spare ovarian medullary tissue) were karyotyped by the G-banding technique and fluorescent in-situ hybridization. DNA was also screened for the number of CGG repeats in the *FMR1* gene using Southern blot analysis or the polymerase chain reaction for fragile X syndrome.[1] In addition, genomic DNA and lymphoblastoid cell lines were prepared for future genetic studies of all the twin pairs in the hope of one day identifying the loci responsible for POF.

FRESH CORTICAL OVARIAN TISSUE TRANSPLANTATION

The patients were scheduled for surgery within two weeks of confirming negativity for the HIV type 1 and hepatitis B and

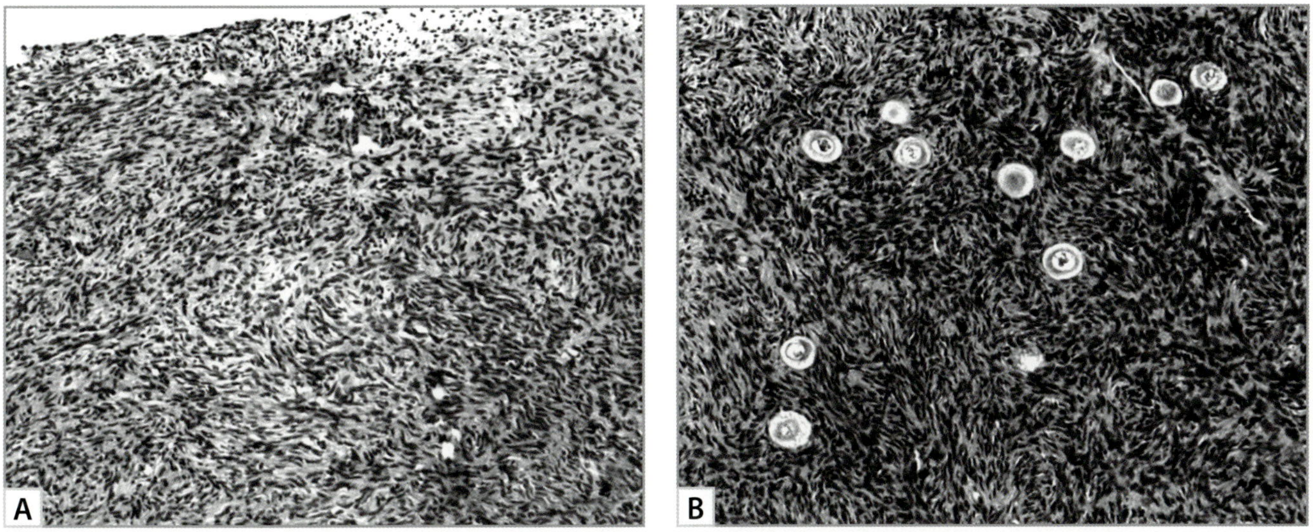

FIGURES 1A AND B Showing the absence of primordial or preantral follicles in ovarian biopsies of this candidate for ovarian transplantation compared with that in her fertile sister.

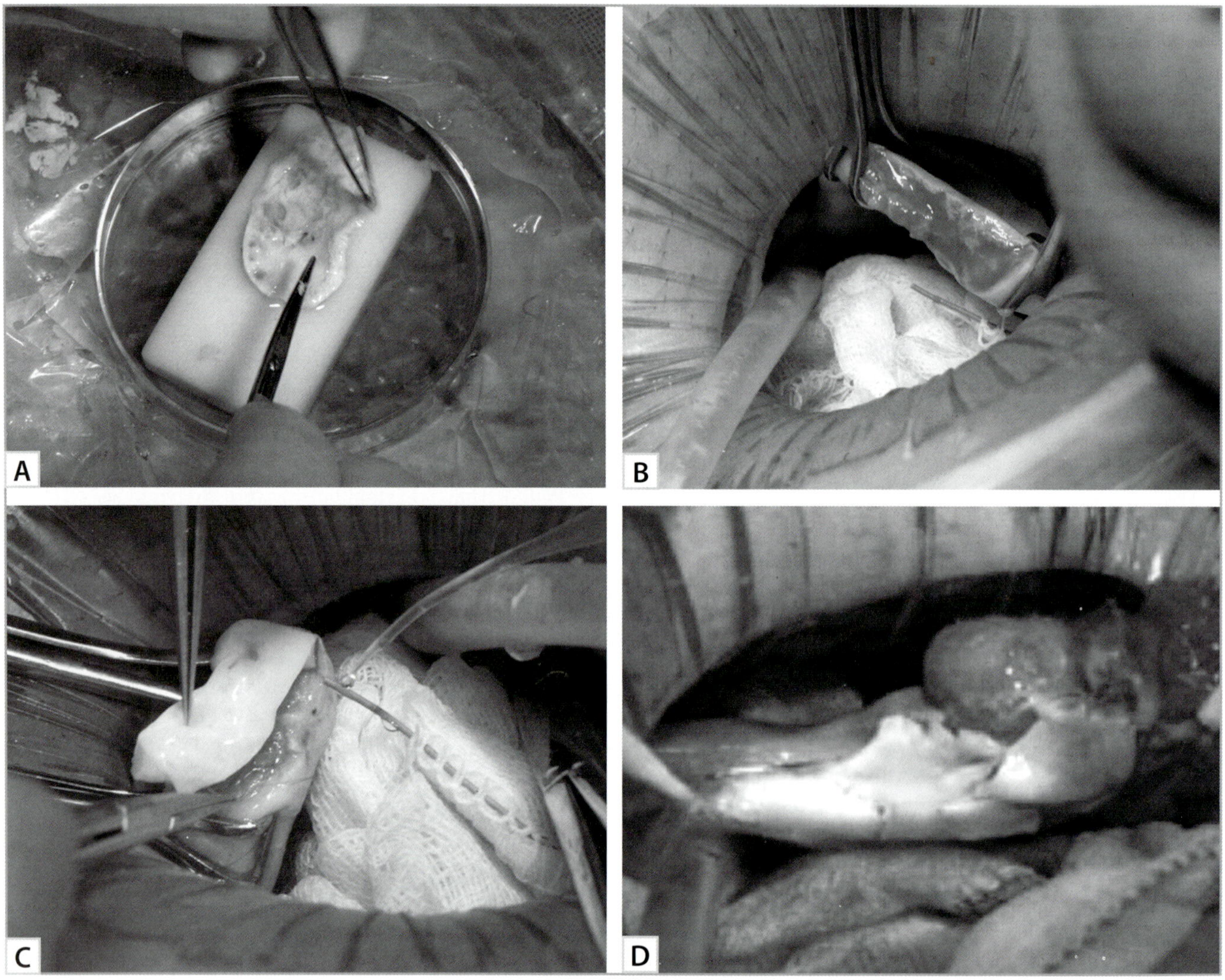

FIGURES 2A TO D Steps in the procedure of ovarian transplantation between MZ twin sisters: (A) Preparation of donor ovarian cortex by dissection in a petri dish on ice; (B) Preparation of recipient ovarian medulla; (C) Attaching donor cortical tissue to recipient ovarian medulla; (D) Attaching thawed donor cortical tissue for retransplant to the recipient.

C viruses. Nine of the presenting identical twin pairs actually underwent the surgery. Under general anesthesia, one ovary was removed from the donor using laparoscopy or mini-laparotomy. For the 8 women undergoing cortical tissue harvesting (excluding the intact whole ovary case), the whole ovary was transferred to a Petri dish for dissection by hand with a scalpel and toothed forceps. It was felt important to prepare a cortical tissue slice no thicker than ~ 1.5 mm to facilitate rapid revascularization while keeping the tissue constantly irrigated with ice-cold Leibovitz L-15 medium (**Figure 2A**). We now recommend a special microtome tissue slicer rather than dissecting by hand, in order to get a thinner slice of only 0.75 mm. But for these initial fresh cases, the hand pared cortex was divided into 3 or 4 pieces of approximately equal size for grafting, one piece to each recipient ovary. The remaining one-half to two-thirds of the cortical tissue was cryopreserved in 1.5 M, 1.2-propanediol and 0.2 M sucrose by slow freezing to liquid nitrogen temperatures.[26,27] Remnants of the trimmed tissue were set aside for histology and genetic studies.

The recipients were prepared by mini-laparotomy via a 3.5 cm incision above the pubis. For cortical tissue transplantation, the recipient ovarian cortex was resected to completely expose medullary tissue (**Figure 2B**); hemostasis was controlled with microbipolar forceps and irrigation with heparinised saline was performed to avoid adhesion formation or a hematoma between donor and recipient tissues. The tissue graft was trimmed to the dimensions of the exposed surface of the recipient organ and attached using 9–0 interrupted sutures under an operating microscope (**Figure 2C**). Very importantly, the medullary bed was also sutured to the under surface of the cortical graft with 9–0 sutures to maintain tight tissue approximation, again to avoid microhematoma formation under the cortical grafts. Irrigation and meticulous pinpoint hemostasis were rigorous to avoid adhesion formation. The same procedure was used for frozen-thawed tissue to replace the first graft that may have ceased to function (**Figure 2D**), and also for the cancer cases. After removing the first graft or the old cortex of the cancer patients to accommodate the new one, all discarded tissue was prepared by histology and found to be completely devoid of follicles. All patients were released from the hospital the same day or the following morning and had a rapid and uneventful recovery. In the one case of bilateral absence of ovary and ampulla, the graft was attached to the Fallopian tube isthmus.

Whole-Ovary Transplantation

To transplant an intact whole ovary, the donor ovary was removed by clamping the infundibular pelvic ligament at its base in order to obtain maximum length. The veins (3–5 mm) were easily identified, but the ovarian artery (0.3 mm) was not grossly visible. The entire specimen was placed in Leibovitz medium at 4°C and 2 veins and 1 artery were dissected and isolated under the operating microscope. Germinal vesicle oocytes were aspirated from antral follicles for in vitro maturation (IVM) and vitrification at the metaphase II stage. Meanwhile, the recipient's infundibular pelvic ligament was clamped at the base and transected close to her nonfunctioning ovary. The donor's ovarian veins were then anastomosed to the recipient's with 9–0 nylon interrupted sutures and the ovarian arteries were anastomosed with 10–0 nylon interrupted sutures (**Figures 3A to D**). When the microvascular clamps were removed, blood flow was observed by fresh bleeding from the surface of the ovary where a cortical slice had been taken for cryopreservation as a backup.

Details on the original chorionicity at birth of these identical twin sisters were available for 6 of the 10 twin pairs consulting our center. Two were monochorionic-diamniotic, 1 was dichorionic-diamniotic and 3 (50%) were monochorionic-monoamniotic, which was a surprisingly high incidence since the incidence of mono/mono is normally only ~ 2% (P<0.0005). It is clear that late splitting, for whatever reason, predisposes otherwise identical twins to discordant germ cell deficiency.

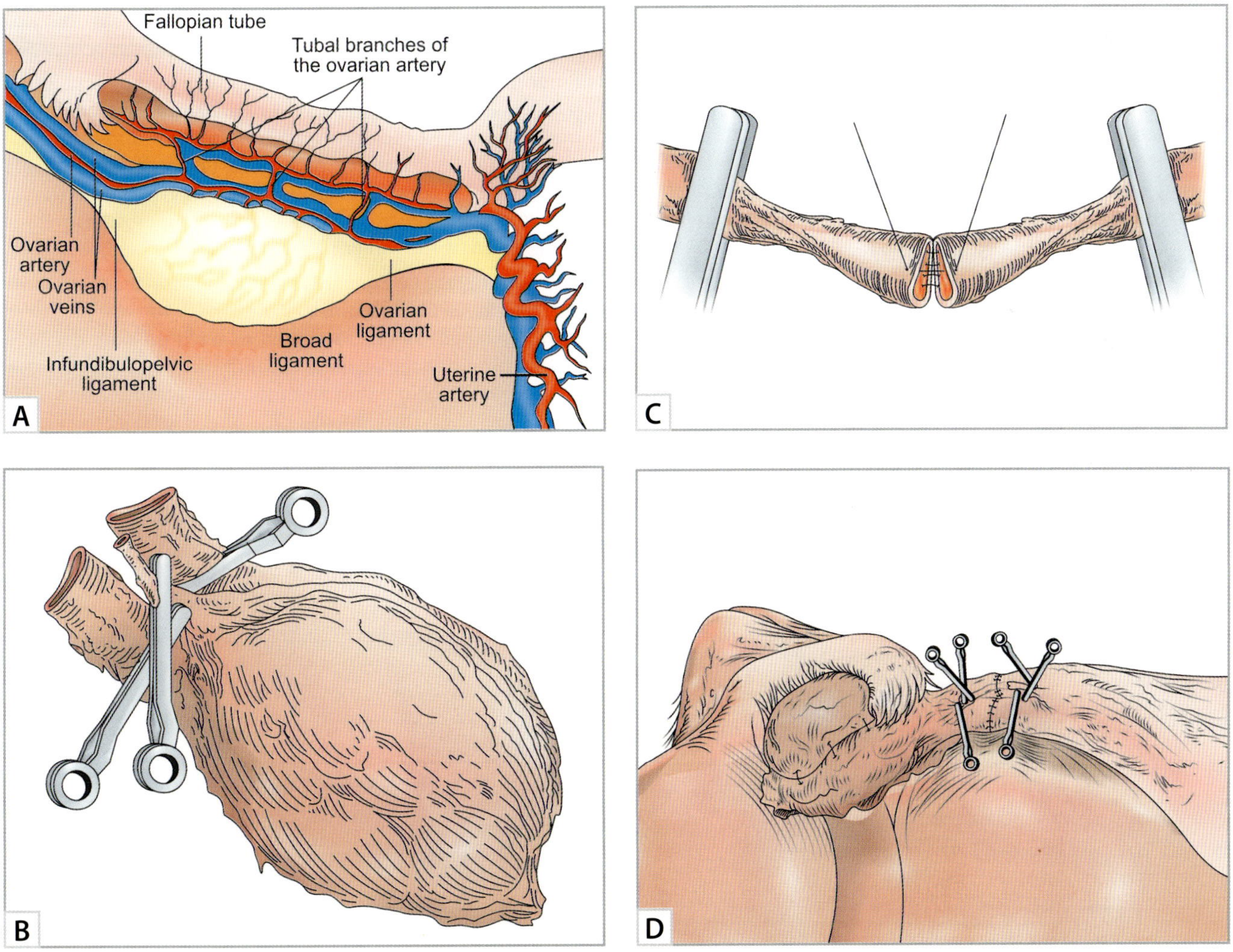

FIGURES 3A TO D Steps in the procedure of intact ovary microvascular transplantation: (A) Depiction of donor oophorectomy; (B) Microsurgical isolation of donor ovary blood supply; (C) End-to-end anastomosis of ovarian blood vessel; (D) Completed anastomosis of ovarian artery and veins.

Postoperative Results

All 9 twin pairs underwent orthotopic ovarian isotransplantation between April 2004 and April 2008. The recipients, for the most part, continued to cycle for over three years to six years or more, although two of them whose donor had low AFC of less than 10, only functioned for two years. However, even these two cases had spare frozen cortical tissue that was available for further transplants. One has not yet done this, but in the other, the frozen transplant was successful and so she also has had more than three years of ovarian function. Day three FSH levels returned to normal by 4.5 months of surgery in all cases (**Figure 4A**), soon after ovulation had recommenced (judging by the results of BBT or home ovulation detection kits monitored by the patients themselves). The refractory period for resuming menses after transplantation was 63-100 days, with the majority of subsequent cycles in the normal range of duration.

The first case, a 25-year old recipient, became pregnant the first time after her second menses without medical assistance and subsequently delivered a healthy baby girl in 2005 following an uneventful pregnancy. After nursing for several months, she resumed menses and during the seventh cycle conceived naturally a second time, but this pregnancy miscarried. Over three years after her transplant, she ceased cycling and hormone levels, which were measured monthly and became post-menopausal again (82mIU/ml FHS, 34mIU/ml LH and 13 pg/ml E_2). After transplanting cryopreserved spare tissue, her hormones again returned to premenopausal levels after four months, a delay identical to her fresh transplant (**Figure 4B**). She conceived again without any intervening menses and without any medical treatment approximately five months after her retransplant and delivered another healthy baby.

The second case became pregnant at 39 years of age without medical assistance after her fifth menses, eight months after transplantation. She too delivered a healthy baby girl at full-term. She then conceived again at age 41 and delivered a healthy baby boy, again at full-term. Her ovary was still functioning after six years.

Only 1 patient failed to conceive, but she had a marginal AFC and was 41-years-old at the time of the transplant. However, the ovary continued to function despite her age for over four years. One case had a microvascular transplant and continued to cycle regularly. Her Day 3 FSH and LH fell to the lowest levels of all the recipients (3.4 and 0.4 mIU/mL, respectively) and her post-operative ultrasound appeared normal. She became pregnant and delivered a healthy baby two years later.

All patients remain pleased with their decision to have undergone transplantation and even the patient requiring IVF preferred this option. Overall, there have been 14 pregnancies and ten healthy live births in this group of nine transplants.

FROZEN CORTICAL OVARIAN TRANSPLANTATION

Since 1996, we have frozen ovary tissue for 62 young women with solid organ cancer, or with great risk for POF, of whom 16 had spare frozen tissue subjected to detailed viability testing before cryopreservation and after thaw. All 62 had histologic review and only one had evidence of ovarian metastasis, a young woman with breast cancer. With the classical slow freeze technique, only 41% of oocytes survived the thaw.[20,21,28,29] However, with vitrification there was no difference between fresh unfrozen controls and frozen tissue.[21] It seemed likely, therefore, that vitrified ovarian tissue would give better results after transplantation than tissue cryopreserved by slow-freeze.

It is naturally to be expected that it could be a decade or more before patients with frozen tissue come back to have it thawed and re-implanted. Firstly, they need to see if they are declared "cured" by their oncologist and secondly, in the modern era, it could be a while before they meet the right partner and decide

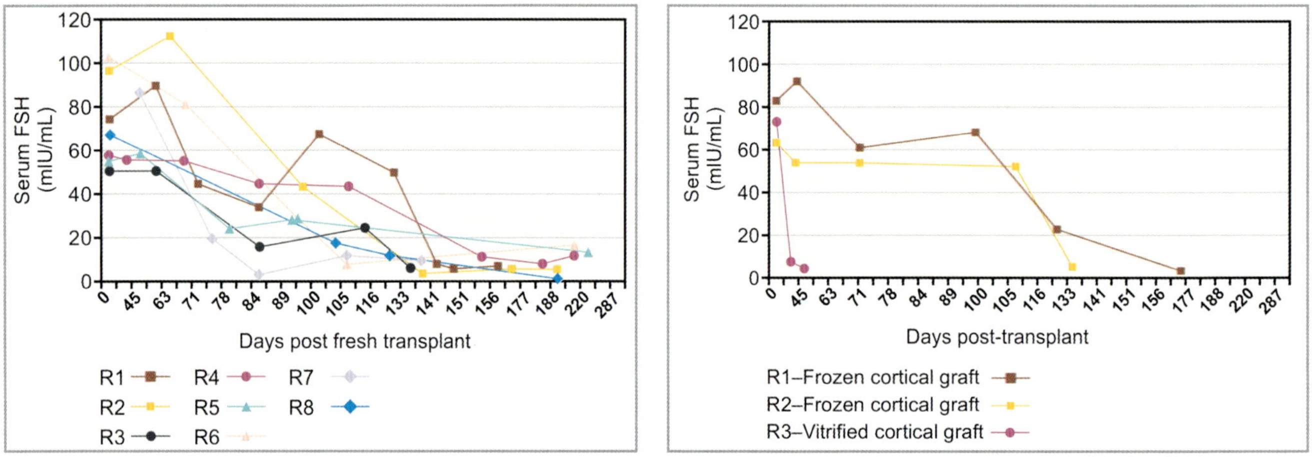

FIGURES 4A AND B (A) The 8 fresh transplant cases showed a dramatic decline in Day 3 serum FSH by 80–140 days postoperatively corresponding approximately to the resumption of menses. The results of the microvascular whole-ovary transplant are not significantly different from cortical grafts; (B) After a frozen cortical retransplant, serum FSH declined again to normal levels, similar to those of fresh transplants.

to have children. Thus, far, only three of our patients have had their frozen tissue transplanted back. In two cases, the tissue was cryopreserved with slow freeze and, in one case, with vitrification.

In addition to these 62 pathologic cases, seven women have had ovarian tissue frozen simply to allow them the possibility of having children at an older age because they had to delay childbearing for strong personal and economic reasons. All of these women are more recent cases and had their ovarian tissue frozen with vitrification.[20, 21]

The method we use for vitrification of ovarian tissue has already been described in detail,[21] but to summarize: Using a "Cryotissue" knife and silicone template, a ¾ mm deep slice is taken off the cortical surface of the ovary, measuring the centimeter wide by two centimeters long. Then, similar cortical slices are removed from the surface of the rest of the ovary and usually 10 to 16 slices can be obtained. The cortical slices are placed in a large test tube containing 7.5% ethylene glycol (EG) and 7.5% dimethyl sulfoxide (DMSO) in hepes buffered media containing 20% synthetic serum substitute for 25 minutes. This is called ES, or equilibrium solution. The thin tissue slices are then transferred to a large test tube containing 20% EG, 20% DMSO, and 0.5M sucrose and kept there until the tissue slices sink to the bottom, which is usually less than 15 minutes. They are then blotted dry and placed on a perforated copper grid (Kitazato, Japan) and plunged directly into liquid nitrogen. A protective cover is then screwed on and the vitrified tissue is transferred to a liquid nitrogen storage tank. The speed of cooling and warming is approximately 20,000°C per minute and successful vitrification is easily observed by the absence of ice crystal formation on the tissue.

For thawing, the copper grid is plunged into a large test tube containing thaw media at 37°C for 5 minutes. Thaw media contains 1.0 M sucrose. The tissue then is transferred to 0.5 M sucrose at room temperature for 5 minutes, following which it is transferred to standard isotonic hepes buffered transfer media. The technique for transplantation of the thawed tissue is no different from that which we described for fresh tissue.

Of the three cases of frozen transplanted tissue thus far, all have had a robust return of ovulatory menstrual cycles with spontaneous pregnancy, but the case with vitrified tissue had the quickest return of function with her first period occurring at just 42 days post-transplant.

DISCUSSION

Including the first MZ twin pair presenting for ovarian transplantation in 2004, there have been eight more comparable cases using fresh ovary so far. There have been three additional frozen cases, for a total of 12 auto- or homo-transplants. The MZ twin cases were characterized by ovarian discordancy, a phenomenon that is not as rare as first assumed.[30] The ovaries with POF were diminutive, fibrous and completely lacking follicles at any stage, while serum gonadotropins were correspondingly elevated and E_2 was low. None of the medical histories provided an explanation for POF with afollicular ovaries in the recipients, except for one who had received chemotherapy. The clinical histories of POF in the other nine MZ cases were idiopathic and consistent with congenital deficiency of germ cells. According to a mathematical model,[25] the follicle reserve at birth must be very small to account for POF as early as adolescence or young adulthood.

With a single exception, the reproductive tracts of the recipients were structurally normal and both ovaries were present, albeit as "streaks" in some cases. In the agonadal case, the ovaries and the tubal ampullae were bilaterally absent, indicating a concurrent Mullerian anomaly.[31]

There may be non-genetic explanations for discordancy in ovarian reserve since MZ twins, like animal clones, are not phenotypically identical and other, non-ovarian discordancies were observed in three twin pairs. One clue to ovarian discordancy might be the monoamniotic, monochorionic twin pregnancies, which were more frequent than expected.[30,32,33] The MZ twin embryos are presumed to arise from late splitting post-implantation, perhaps as late as the primitive streak. If so, late splitting may be a risk factor for decreased ovarian reserve through misallocation of germ cell precursors. Also perhaps, epigenetic factors may affect the ovarian follicle reserve, since we know that there is an excess of imprinting defects in MZ twin pregnancies.[33]

Conventional oocyte donation is the first line of treatment for patients with POF who want to become pregnant. Nevertheless, the robust results obtained in every case of this series of isogenetic twins provide confidence in ovarian transplantation as an alternative strategy for overcoming sterility. Although the surgery might seem more burdensome than oocyte retrieval, it is a straightforward and uneventful outpatient procedure, which has been effective in all nine cases in restoring menstrual cycles and enabling establishment of viable pregnancies.

It has been equally uneventful in the three frozen cases. After ovarian transplantation, the patients were able to attempt natural conception every month without medical assistance. Except the risks of surgery, the procedure avoids the specific risks associated with IVF, notably ovarian hyperstimulation syndrome and multiple pregnancy and moreover, allows spare tissue to be cryopreserved in the event of graft failure. The number of successful retransplants will depend on the age of the patient and the number of follicles surviving, but the results of fresh and frozen cortical tissue from the first few patients suggest that fertility potential may be restored cumulatively for over 15 years by serial transplantation.

Ovarian cortical grafting was chosen for eight of the procedures in preference to vascular anastomosis of the intact ovary because it is less invasive, carries minimal operative risk and reduces recovery time. The peripheral location of primordial follicles is advantageous for rapid revascularization, as well as for successful cryopreservation.[1-4,34-36] The thinner slices used for vitrification may also allow for more rapid revascularization than the thicker slices used in earlier efforts. Heterotopic sites have produced no successful pregnancies to date and our patients preferred the chance of natural conception.[26,27,37,38] The whole-ovary microvascular approach was adopted at one patient's request in the hope of maximizing the functional longevity of her transplant. We suspect follicle ischemia was minimal, as predicted from transplants of intact rat ovaries using vascular anastomosis.[6] However, the long duration of function of our ovarian cortical grafts suggests that ischemia may not be problematic, if very thin cortical slices are used.

There was remarkable consistency between subjects in the return of menses after ovarian transplantation. The refractory period of about three months was similar to auto-transplants in the sheep model[2] and consistent with estimates of the time taken for small follicles to grow to ovulatory size in humans.[39] There was one exception of an extraordinarily rapid return of function in the one patient who had vitrified tissue transplanted and this could very well be due to the exceptional thinness of the slice (0.75mm) and the fact that vitrification in itself causes no tissue or cellular damage. In some case reports of transplantation in cancer patients, a longer refractory period of up to nine months has been reported,[35,36,39] but it is not clear whether the difference is due to technical aspects of surgery, the type of cryopreservation, or patient selection, any of which could influence the speed of recovery and duration of graft function. While this evidence suggests that follicle dynamics are relatively normal once the transplant is fully active, the follicle reserve might be compromised by ischemia. Graft longevity might be affected by graft ischemia time or by cryopreservation damage. This is now the subject of intense study.[20, 21]

This is the most extensive clinical series of orthotopic ovarian transplantation of which we are aware. Twins are unlikely to be the main candidates for this procedure in the future and the major application is likely to be for fertility preservation in cancer patients and possibly other women who need to delay childbearing. While neither ovarian autografts nor isografts should present any problem of histocompatability, allografts are potentially at risk. However, allografts might occasionally be considered if ovarian tissue is available from a young woman who previously donated bone marrow to the same patient, or if mild immunosuppression proves adequate to prevent rejection, which we are currently studying. Reassuringly, well-matched (HLA) kidney transplant recipients on immunosuppression have favorable obstetric outcomes.[40]

At the time of this writing, we are only aware of a small number of other births or ongoing pregnancies after re-implanting frozen ovarian tissue and these were all for cancer patients.[35,36,41-44] This is not surprising for a new procedure involving patients who must delay transplantation until they are assured of long-term remission or await confirmation that their frozen tissue is free of malignant cells. We had no such concern in our series, which offers a better chance to rapidly evaluate this technique in both fresh and frozen grafts from the same individual. No such concerns applied to the healthy twins and the evidence from this series of the effectiveness of both fresh and frozen transplants gives hope that cryopreserved ovarian tissue for cancer patients should no longer be considered experimental.

REFERENCES

1. Silber SJ, Lenahan KM, Levine DJ, et al. Ovarian transplantation between monozygotic twins discordant for premature ovarian failure. New Eng J Med. 2005;353:58-63.
2. Gosden RG, Baird DT, Wade JC, Webb R. Restoration of fertility to oophorectomized sheep by ovarian autografts stored at -196 degrees C. Human Reprod. 1994;9:597-603.
3. Silber SJ, Gosden RG. Ovarian transplantation in a series of monozygotic twins discordant for ovarian failure. New Eng J Med. 2007;356:1382-4.
4. Silber SJ, DeRosa M, Pineda J, et al. A series of monozygotic twins discordant for ovarian failure: ovary transplantation (cortical versus microvascular) and cryopreservation. Human Reproduction. 2008;23:1531-7.
5. Silber SJ, Grudzinskas G, Gosden RG. Successful pregnancy after microsurgical transplantation of an intact ovary. New Eng J Med. 2008;359:2617-8.
6. Coulam CB, Adamson SC, Annegers JF. Incidence of premature ovarian failure. Obstet Gynecol. 1986;67:604-6.
7. Riboli E, Hunt KJ, Slimani N, et al. European Prospective Investigation into Cancer and Nutrition (EPIC): study populations and data collection. Public Health Nutrition. 2002;5:1113-24.
8. Luborsky JL, Meyer P, Sowers MF, et al. Premature menopause in a multi-ethnic population study of the menopause transition. Human Reprod. 2003;18:199-206.
9. Goswami D, Conway GS. Premature ovarian failure. Human Reproduction Update. 2005;11:391-410.
10. Snieder H, MacGregor AJ, Spector TD. Genes control the cessation of a woman's reproductive life: a twin study of hysterectomy and age at menopause. J Clin Endocrinol Metab. 1998;83:1875-80.
11. de Bruin JP, Bovenhuis H, van Noord PA, et al. The role of genetic factors in age at natural menopause. Human Reprod. 2001;16:2014-8.
12. van Asselt KM, Kok HS, Pearson PL, et al. Heritability of menopausal age in mothers and daughters. Fertil Steril. 2004;82:1348-51.
13. Bleyer WA. The impact of childhood cancer on the United States and the world. CA Cancer. 1990;40:355-67.
14. Ries LAG. Cancer incidence and survival among children and adolescents: United States SEER program. 1976-1995. 1999.
15. Jeruss JS, Woodruff TK. Preservation of fertility in patients with cancer. N Engl J Med. 2009;360:902-11.
16. Anderson RA, Themmen AP, Al-Qahtani A, et al. The effects of chemotherapy and long-term gonadotropin suppression on the ovarian reserve in premenopausal women with breast cancer. Hum Reprod. 2006;21:2583-92.
17. Anderson RA, Cameron DA. Assessment of the effect of chemotherapy on ovarian function in women with breast cancer. J Clin Oncol. 2007;25:1630-1. author reply 1632.
18. Larsen EC, Muller J, Schmiegelow K, et al. Reduced ovarian function in long-term survivors of radiation and chemotherapy-treated childhood cancer. J Clin Endocrinol Metab. 2003;88:5307-14.
19. Lee SJ, Schover LR, Partridge AH, et al. American Society of Clinical Oncology. American Society of Clinical Oncology recommendations on fertility preservation in cancer patients. J Clin Oncol. 2006;24:2917-31.
20. Silber S, Kagawa N, Kuwayama M, Gosden R. Duration of fertility after fresh and frozen ovary transplantation. Fertil Steril. 2010;94(6): 2191-6.
21. Kagawa N, Silber S, Kuwayama M. Successful vitrification of bovine and human ovarian tissue. Reprod Biomed Online. 209;18:568-77.

22. Bedaiwy MA, Falcone T. Harvesting and autotransplantation of vascularized ovarian grafts: approaches and techniques. Reprod Biomed Online. 2007;14:360-71.
23. Silber SJ. Transplantation of a human testis for anorchia. Fertil Steril. 1978;30:181-7.
24. Gosden RG, Telfer E, Faddy MJ, Brook DJ. Ovarian cyclicity and follicular recruitment in unilaterally ovariectomized mice. J Reprod Fertil. 1989;87:257-64.
25. Faddy MJ, Gosden RG, Gougeon A, et al. Accelerated disappearance of ovarian follicles in mid-life: implications for forecasting menopause. Human Reprod. 1992;7:1342-6.
26. Oktay K, Buyuk E, Veeck L, et al. Embryo development after heterotopic transplantation of cryopreserved ovarian tissue. Lancet. 2004;363:837-40.
27. Rosendahl M, Loft A, Byskov AG, et al. Biochemical pregnancy after fertilization of an oocyte aspirated from a heterotopic autotransplant of cryopreserved ovarian tissue: case report. Human Reprod. 2006;21:2006-9.
28. Newton H, Aubard Y, Rutherford A, et al. Low temperature storage and grafting of human ovarian tissue. Human Reprod. 96;11:1487-91.
29. Gook DA, Edgar DH, Stern C. Effect of cooling rate and dehydration regimen on the histological appearance of human ovarian cortex following cryopreservation in 1, 2-propanediol. Human Reprod. 1999;14:2061-8.
30. Gosden RG, Treloar SA, Martin NG, et al. Prevalence of premature ovarian failure in monozygotic and dizygotic twins. Human Reprod. 2007;22:610-5.
31 Dueck A, Poenaru D, Jamieson MA, Kamal IK. Unilateral ovarian agenesis and fallopian tube maldescent. Ped Surg Intl 2001;17:228-9.
32. Su LL. Monoamniotic twins: diagnosis and management. Acta Obstet Gynecol Scandinavica. 2002;81:995-1000.
33. Weksberg R, Shuman C, Caluseriu O, et al. Discordant KCNQ1OT1 imprinting in sets of monozygotic twins discordant for Beckwith-Wiedemann syndrome. Human Molecular Genetics. 2002;11:1317-25.
34. Salle B, Demirci B, Franck M, et al. Normal pregnancies and live births after autograft of frozen-thawed hemi-ovaries into ewes. Fertil Steril. 2002;77:403-8.
35. Donnez J, Dolmans MM, Demylle D, et al. Livebirth after orthotopic transplantation of cryopreserved ovarian tissue. Lancet. 2004;364: 1405-10.
36. Meirow D, Levron J, Eldar-Geva T, et al. Pregnancy after transplantation of cryopreserved ovarian tissue in a patient with ovarian failure after chemotherapy. New Eng J Med. 2005;353:318-21.
37. Hilders CG, Baranski AG, Peters L, et al. Successful human ovarian autotransplantation to the upper arm. Cancer. 2004;101:2771-8.
38. Kim SS, Hwang IT, Lee HC. Heterotopic autotransplantation of cryobanked human ovarian tissue as a strategy to restore ovarian function. Fertil Steril. 2004;82:930-2.
39. Donnez J, Martinez-Madrid B, Jadoul P, et al. Ovarian tissue cryopreservation and transplantation: a review. Human Reprod Update. 2006;12:519-35.
40. Armenti VT, Radomski JS, Moritz MJ, et al. Report from the National Transplantation Pregnancy Registry (NTPR): outcomes of pregnancy after transplantation. Clin Transplants. 2000:123-34.
41. Andersen CY, Rosendahl M, Byskov AG, et al. Two successful pregnancies following autotransplantation of frozen/thawed ovarian tissue. Human Reprod. 2008;23:2266-72.
42. Demeestere I, Simon P, Emiliani S, et al. Fertility preservation: successful transplantation of cryopreserved ovarian tissue in a young patient previously treated for Hodgkin's disease. Oncologist. 2007;12:1437-42.
43. Sanchez-Serrano M, Crespo J, Mirabet V, et al. Twins born after transplantation of ovarian cortical tissue and oocyte vitrification. Fertil Steril. 2010;93:268.e11-3.
44. Piver P, Aniot C, Agnani G, et al. Two pregnancies obtained after a new technique of autotransplantation of cryopreserved ovarian tissue. Hum Reprod. 2009;24:10-35.

13

In Vitro Maturation of Oocytes as a Fertility Preservation Strategy

Baris ATA, Hai Ying Chen, Ayse Seyhan,
Alper Mumcu, Seang Lin Tan

CHAPTER OUTLINE

- In Vitro Maturation of Human Oocytes
  - Overview of an IVM cycle for Fertility Preservation
- Embryology Laboratory Procedures
- IVM Treatment Outcome
  - Chromosomal Constitution of IVM Embryos
  - Pregnancy Rates
  - Pregnancy Loss
  - Obstetric Outcome
  - Congenital Abnormalities, Physical and Neuromotor Development
- IVM for Fertility Preservation for Women with Medical Conditions
- IVM for Social Fertility Preservation

INTRODUCTION

Female reproductive potential usually does not last much beyond the end of the fourth decade of life. This has implications for many modern women who postpone child bearing until their late thirties or early forties. Over the last thirty years in industrialized societies, there has been a significant delay in starting a family.[1] Extended life expectancy together with increasing involvement of women in the workforce are the most likely reasons of this delay. Advanced female age not only impacts fecundity, but also decreases the chances of achieving a pregnancy following assisted reproductive technology (ART) if the need arises. In the year 2008, decreased ovarian reserve was the sole indication for 14% of all reported ART cycles in the United States. The female partner was older than 35 years of age in over half of all ART cycles performed in the same year.[2] Moreover, the risk of pregnancy loss increases with female age, further decreasing the chance of giving birth to an infant.

The natural decline in fertility is significantly accelerated following gonadotoxic therapy for cancer and other non-oncologic conditions. Cancer is a major health problem and in the United States, the estimated number of women who would be diagnosed with cancer in 2009 was approximately 739,940.[3] Improved treatment methods have resulted in a steady increase in the survival rates over the last few decades.[3] The number of cancer survivors is on the rise and resultantly, an increasing number of women face the risk of infertility following gonadotoxic treatment. Treatment of childhood cancers has improved similarly and it is estimated that 1 in every 250 adults will be a childhood cancer survivor.[4] Moreover, patients who are exposed to gonadotoxic agents for the treatment of non-oncologic diseases such as systemic lupus erythematosus, those who are undergoing major surgery for severe/extensive endometriosis or excision of large endometriomas, as well as women with genetic disorders such as Turner syndrome and fragile-X premutation are faced with similar risks, further increasing the number of women who need fertility preservation procedures.[5-8]

Today, it is possible to preserve the reproductive potential of these women. Advances in reproductive medicine, particularly in cryopreservation methods, have rendered fertility preservation a realistic option. Increased awareness of the options available for fertility preservation among medical professionals and the society at large has led to a greater number of women demanding, being offered and utilizing these technologies.[9] Currently available options for preservation of female fertility are cryopreservation of oocytes or embryos following in vitro fertilization (IVF) or in vitro maturation (IVM), or cryopreservation of ovarian tissue. Although successful transplantation of a fresh whole ovary has been reported in a pair of monozygotic twins, discordant for ovarian failure and encouraging results have been achieved with frozen ovaries in animal models, cryopreservation of the entire ovary has not been successfully performed in humans.[10-11] Administration of gonadotropin releasing hormone analogs or inhibitors of apoptosis have been proposed as alternative strategies for patients undergoing chemotherapy, however, effectiveness of these techniques remains to be proven.[12] The fertility preservation method of choice for any woman is determined by several factors, including the indication for fertility preservation, availability of a male partner, time available and patient preference.

In this chapter, we will review the role of IVM as a strategy for fertility preservation. An overview of IVM will be followed by the role of IVM in fertility preservation for patients with medical conditions and for social fertility preservation.

IN VITRO MATURATION OF HUMAN OOCYTES

Classical IVF involves collection and in vitro fertilization of in vivo matured oocytes at the metaphase II (MII) stage. In IVM cycles, however, immature oocytes present in the small antral follicles are collected. Immature oocytes are arrested at the prophase stage of meiotic division and are not amenable to fertilization by sperm before they complete maturation and reach the MII stage. The immature oocytes have the potential to resume meiosis upon removal from the meiotic inhibiting environment of the follicle and can be fertilized in vitro. More than 80% of oocytes were reported to resume meiosis independent of the menstrual cycle day and gonadotropin support in IVM medium.[13] Collection and IVM of these immature oocytes provides multiple MII oocytes that can be fertilized in vitro. Although the term "IVM" refers to the maturation of oocytes collected at the germinal vesicle (GV) stage, in the clinical context "IVM" means performing oocyte collection while the leading follicle is still ≤14 mm. Therefore, some in vivo matured oocytes can also be harvested in some IVM cycles. In theory, an ideal IVM program would provide the high pregnancy rates of conventional stimulated IVF without the risks and costs associated with controlled ovarian hyperstimulation (COH).

Although research on immature oocytes dates as far back as the 1930s, the first pregnancy and live birth from in vitro matured oocytes in humans was only reported in 1983.[14-15] Veeck et al. reported 2 pregnancies resulting from IVM of immature oocytes collected alongside mature oocytes in gonadotropin stimulated IVF cycles.[15] However, IVF with COS had already become the norm and IVM did not attract attention until 1991 when Cha and colleagues first reported intentional collection of immature oocytes from women undergoing gynecological surgery.[16] The immature oocytes donated by these women were matured in vitro and the resulting embryos were transferred to a recipient with premature ovarian failure.[16] The recipient delivered healthy triplet girls.

Three years later, Trounson et al. reported the collection of immature oocytes from women with polycystic ovarian syndrome (PCOS) for their own use. The immature oocytes collected were matured in vitro with gonadotropin-enriched medium, then fertilized and a healthy live birth following transfer of resultant embryos was reported.[17] Unfortunately, the initial pregnancy rates were low and it took another 5 years for success rates to exceed 35% per cycle in selected patients.[18-19]

Currently, IVM is not only a recognized treatment alternative for couples who need ART, but also is considered as an innovative fertility preservation method that extends the options for patients with various diseases that preclude treatment with conventional methods. However, compared to widespread application of IVF, IVM is still practiced by relatively few clinics worldwide.

Overview of an IVM cycle for fertility preservation

Monitoring starts with a baseline scan performed in the early follicular phase of the menstrual cycle, preferably between days 2 to 5 of a natural menstrual cycle or a withdrawal bleed, induced with progesterone administration in amenorrheic women. The number and size of the antral follicles are recorded. The uterus and ovaries are examined for any abnormalities. A second scan is performed about a week later when it is anticipated that the largest follicle has reached 10–12 mm. The presence of a dominant follicle does not require cancellation of the treatment cycle because smaller follicles are found to contain viable oocytes, even in the presence of a dominant follicle.[20-21] Based on our own experience and a favorable trend observed in trials of HCG priming, the current routine IVM protocol at the authors' institution involves HCG administration 10,000 IU IM 38 hours before oocyte collection.[22] Although, the decision regarding timing of the HCG injection and therefore oocyte retrieval requires that both the follicle size and endometrial thickness be taken into consideration in a regular IVM cycle, endometrial thickness is ignored in fertility preservation cycles as there will not be an embryo transfer in the same cycle.

The immature oocyte collection procedure is easily tolerated by most patients under conscious sedation with intravenous midazolam and fentanyl. The vagina is cleaned with sterile saline and paracervical block is achieved with 1% bupivacain injection. As the follicles are smaller than mature follicles aspirated in IVF cycles, a smaller-gauge needle (19–20 G) with a shorter bevel is used. The aspiration pressure is set at 75–80 mmHg, approximately half the conventional IVF aspiration pressure, in order to minimize the risk of oocyte denudation during aspiration. Multiple ovarian punctures are usually required to collect the follicles, which are often widespread throughout the ovarian stroma. Moreover, the fine-bore needle may be occasionally blocked with bloodstained aspirate and ovarian stroma. The needle lumen is flushed with heparinized saline between punctures. Patients with difficult-to-reach ovaries or poor pain control may do better under short general anesthesia with propofol.

EMBRYOLOGY LABORATORY PROCEDURES

Identification of small immature oocytes surrounded by fewer granulosa cells is more difficult compared to mature oocytes collected in an IVF cycle and they can be overlooked. The follicular aspirate is first examined under a stereomicroscope to identify cumulus-oocyte complexes (COC). Following the removal of initially identified COCs, the follicular aspirate is filtered through a nylon mesh strainer with 70 micrometer pores. The filtered aspirate is re-examined after washing with HEPES buffered human serum albumin containing medium. The maturation status of the oocytes is assessed immediately after collection. Oocytes reaching the MII stage on the day of collection are denuded and cryopreserved/fertilized together with any in-vivo matured oocytes, while immature oocytes are cultured in IVM medium and periodically assessed for maturation status. They are denuded and cryopreserved/fertilized upon completion of nuclear maturation.

Although similar implantation and pregnancy rates have been reported following fertilization of in vitro matured oocytes with intracytoplasmic sperm injection (ICSI) or IVF, ICSI has been commonly practiced in IVM cycles due to a theoretical risk of zonal hardening during the in vitro culture period.[23-24] In fact, fertilization rates with ICSI were shown to be higher than with IVF in the same study (84.1% versus 56.3%).[24] Another reason for preferring ICSI over IVF in IVM cycles is that some immature oocytes were denuded for assessment of polar-body extrusion. Oocytes devoid of cumulus cells may have decreased chemotactic potential for sperm in the medium.[25] We routinely perform ICSI at 2-4 hours after polar-body extrusion. Culture conditions for fertilized oocytes and cleavage-stage embryos derived from in vitro matured oocytes are similar as those in IVF cycles.

IVM TREATMENT OUTCOME

Chromosomal Constitution of IVM Embryos

We recently compared the incidence of chromosomal abnormality (CA) in embryos from IVM and IVF cycles.[26] The copy numbers of chromosomes 13, 15, 16, 18, 21, 22, X and Y were assessed with fluorescence in-situ hybridization (FISH) in single blastomeres biopsied from cleavage stage embryos. IVM and IVF groups comprised 6 and 30 couples, with mean (standard deviation—SD) embryos with FISH result of 8.0 (4.4) and 11.7(3.8), respectively. All women in the IVM group had either polycystic ovaries (PCO) or PCOS and the vast majority of women in both groups had a history of either recurrent miscarriage or recurrent implantation failure. The incidence of CA per FISH result was similar in IVM and IVF embryos (58.7% versus 57.4%, respectively). When embryos were categorized based on maturation time of oocytes in IVM cycles, embryos derived from oocytes that matured 48 hours after collection had a higher CA rate compared with embryos derived from in-vivo matured oocytes and to embryos derived from oocytes that matured in the first 24 hours after collection.

Requena et al. reported a similar 60% aneuploidy rate following FISH analysis of the same set of 8 chromosomes in 20 cleavage stage IVM embryos from 11 oocyte donors with a mean age of 22.1 years.[27] Compared with 33% chromosome abnormality rate in IVF embryos from women under risk of sex chromosome linked diseases, but without fertility problems (mean age 33 years), the difference was not statistically significant.

While women in our cohort were comprised of comparatively older (mean age 33 years) women with fertility problems such as PCOS, recurrent miscarriage or IVF failure, women in the other study were young healthy oocyte donors (women with PCOS were excluded) with mean age of 22 years. Importantly, while all women in our cohort had a HCG injection 36–38 hours before immature oocyte collection, an HCG injection was not given to donors in the other study. Intuitively, the incidence of CA in embryos from healthy oocyte donors could be expected to be lower than that in embryos from older infertile patients who were on average ten years older. While, in theory, differences between IVM protocols such as HCG injection preceding immature oocyte collection can affect aneuploidy rates, it is not clearly supported with data yet.

Pregnancy Rates

Female age and the number of oocytes collected are the two most important determinants of pregnancy following an IVM cycle. Young women with PCO are the best candidates for IVM treatment. In 2009, we achieved an embryo implantation rate of 19.5% and a clinical pregnancy rate per embryo transfer (CPR) of 55.2% in women with PCO or PCOS with an average age of 32.6 ± 3.6 years. Successful results have been reported by other centers around the world.[28] Pregnancy rates seem to be significantly higher when an in vivo matured oocyte has been collected as well.

Pregnancy Loss

In a retrospective analysis of 1,581 women who had a positive pregnancy test following ART with IVM, IVF or ICSI in our unit during a 5-year period, we found biochemical pregnancy loss rates to be similar among these patients (17.5% for IVM pregnancies, 17% for IVF and 18% for ICSI pregnancies, $p = 0.08$).[29] However, the clinical miscarriage rate was significantly higher in IVM pregnancies (25.3%) than in IVF (15.7%) and ICSI (12.6%) pregnancies ($p < 0.01$). It is known that women with PCOS have higher miscarriage rates, regardless of the method of conception. Miscarriage rates reaching 25% after ovulation induction and ranging from 25 to 37% following IVF, have been reported in such women.[30-32] Therefore, the higher miscarriage rate observed in the IVM group can be explained by the higher incidence of PCOS in these patients. Indeed, while only 8%

and <1% of women in the IVF and ICSI groups had PCOS, respectively, the incidence of PCOS in the IVM group was 80%. Importantly, miscarriage rates were not different between IVM and IVF pregnancies among women with PCOS, 24.5% versus 22.8%, respectively.[29]

Obstetric Outcome

We further analyzed obstetric outcomes of pregnancies following ART and compared them with those of spontaneous conceptions.[33] The study population consisted of all pregnancies delivered at the McGill University Health Centre after ART (IVM, IVF or ICSI) with a birth weight of at least 500 g at the time of confinement, from January 1, 1998, to December 31, 2003. IVM pregnancies comprised 15.9% of 344 ART pregnancies during the study period. The reason for the relatively low number of ART deliveries is that many women who conceived with ART at the McGill Reproductive Center delivered at other hospitals in Québec or outside the province. Therefore, inclusion of these externally delivered cases and reporting all conceptions was impossible. However, this has enabled all assessment of obstetrical and neonatal outcome to be done by the same group of physicians and prevented varying interpretations of congenital abnormalities.

The incidence of twin and high-order multiple pregnancies were not different among IVM (21% and 5%), IVF (20% and 3%) and ICSI (17% and 3%) pregnancies. The incidence of Cesarean delivery was similar among singleton pregnancies conceived with different treatments (IVM 39%, IVF 36% and ICSI 36%). Likewise, the mean birth weights of all infants conceived with ART were similar among all ART groups. The proportion of low birth weight and very low birth weight infants was similar across ART children. Apgar scores at 1 and 5 minutes, the proportion of infants with an Apgar score ≤ 6 at 1 and 5 minutes and the incidence of acidosis were all similar among IVM, IVF, ICSI and spontaneous-conception deliveries. Our figures compare favorably with results reported by other IVM programs, supporting our conclusions.[34-36]

Congenital Abnormalities, Physical and Neuromotor Development

In our series of 55 IVM newborns, there were only 2 major congenital abnormalities; one case of ventriculoseptal defect and one of omphalocele.[33] There were 9 major congenital abnormalities (2 hydronephroses, 1 Fallot's tetralogy, 1 single ventricle, 2 atrio-septal defects, 1 hydrocephaly and intraventricular hemorrhage and 2 trisomies) and 14 minor abnormalities among 350 infants born to the 344 age- and parity-matched spontaneously-conceived controls. Compared with spontaneous conceptions, the observed odds ratios (ORs) for any congenital abnormality were 1.42 (95% confidence interval [CI] 0.52–3.91) for IVM, 1.21 (95% CI 0.63–2.32) for IVF and 1.69 (95% CI 0.88–3.26) for ICSI, respectively. None of these were statistically significant.[33] Interestingly, the OR was lower for IVM than for ICSI, even though ICSI was used for all IVM cases. This can be regarded as indirect evidence of the reported high congenital abnormality rate with ICSI being due to poor sperm per se, because ICSI with normal sperm did not increase the odds of congenital abnormality.

The chromosomal constitution and mental development of 21 children conceived through IVM were compared with those of spontaneously conceived children.[37] All of the IVM children were found to have normal karyotype and mean developmental index score, similar to controls. Another study of 46 IVM babies reported similar findings.[35] In the latter study, the neuropsychological development of children was assessed until 24 months and was found to be within population standards. The physical growth of IVM children also appears to be similar to that of spontaneously conceived children.[35, 37] Currently available data seem reassuring and do not suggest an increased risk of congenital malformations, physical, or neurological developmental delay in IVM children.

IVM FOR FERTILITY PRESERVATION FOR WOMEN WITH MEDICAL CONDITIONS

When the threat to gonads is limited to direct radiotherapy, surgically positioning the ovaries out of the irradiation field is an effective method and can be combined with other methods if deemed necessary.[38] However, in the case of systemic administration of gonadotoxic agents, the gametes at risk should be removed from the body and preserved in some form until they can be re-implanted or used for reproduction upon completion of treatment for the underlying disease. Besides gonadotoxicity, advancing age during treatment is another concern. In some cases, treatment of the underlying disease may require several years, meaning that the natural decline in fertility may become an issue even in the absence of direct gonadotoxicity.[39-40] At present, embryo cryopreservation following IVF is the only method endorsed by the American Society of Clinical Oncology (ASCO) and the American Society of Reproductive Medicine (ASRM), while the other methods are still considered experimental.

The successful cryopreservation of surplus embryos after IVF and resultant pregnancy following frozen-thawed embryo transfer (FET) was first reported in 1983 and the first child after embryo freezing was born in 1984.[41-42] It is estimated that almost one quarter of the children born after ART are born following cryopreservation of mostly cleavage-stage embryos and, less commonly, blastocysts and oocytes.[43] However, several points raise concern about IVF–embryo freezing in cancer patients. These are: (1) a possible delay of 2 to 5 weeks in treatment of the primary disease due to ovarian stimulation, depending on the timing of the first consultation with the reproductive endocrinologist in relation to onset of the next menstrual cycle; (2) exposure to supraphysiologic estrogen levels induced by ovarian stimulation; (3) the requirement for a male partner or willingness to use donor sperm for embryo production; and (4) legal ethical, and religious issues related to cryopreservation of embryos in general. These issues and alternatives provided with IVM are discussed below.

Problems with Ovarian Stimulation in Cancer Patients

Two major concerns about ovarian stimulation in cancer patients are (a) a possible delay in commencing anticancer therapy while waiting for completion of ovarian stimulation and (b) effect of elevated estrogen levels during stimulation on the prognosis of the underlying malignancy.

The time required for completion of the fertility preservation procedure, which starts with the initial reproductive medicine consultation and technically ends with oocyte collection, depends on the conditions of any particular clinic. Ovarian stimulation takes between 2 and 5 weeks, depending on the stimulation protocol employed and the timing of the following menstrual cycle of the patient. This is a matter of concern for both the patients and treating physicians. The effect of such a delay in treatment obviously depends on the underlying disease and must be evaluated on a case-by-case basis together with the treating oncology team.

Serum estradiol (E2) levels are increased during ovarian stimulation for IVF and can reach levels twenty times higher than those of a natural cycle.[44] Breast cancer remains the most common cancer in females, representing 27% of all female cancers. Between 2002 and 2006, 12.4% of all breast cancer cases were diagnosed in women younger than 45 years, who are in their reproductive period.[45] The risk of breast cancer is consistently found to be associated with persistently elevated blood estrogen levels.[46] Although the effect of a temporary increase in serum E2 levels on the risk of recurrence of breast cancer is controversial, this remains another factor causing concern among both physicians and patients. Such concerns are not limited to women with estrogen receptor positive breast cancer, because recent findings also suggest the presence of an indirect mitogenic effect of estrogen on hormone receptor negative breast cancer.[47] Increased E2 levels can be relevant for patients undergoing fertility preservation treatment due to other oncologic or non-oncologic diseases considered to be estrogen sensitive, such as desmoid tumors, systemic lupus erythematosus or severe endometriosis. Special stimulation protocols involving aromatase inhibitors in order to limit the rise in estradiol levels have been developed for such patients.[48] Despite encouraging results with regard to disease free survival and recurrence rates reported by the authors, it is interesting to note that 63.3% of breast cancer patients referred for reproductive endocrinology and infertility consultation at the same center declined ovarian stimulation and IVF due to concerns about delay of chemotherapy, effect of ovarian stimulation on cancer, or costs associated with treatment.[48]

While most fertility preservation procedures for breast cancer patients used to be performed in the 2–4 week interval between surgery and initiation of adjuvant chemotherapy, neoadjuvant chemotherapy is increasingly being given to women who are likely to have micrometastases.[49] Such practice narrows the window for fertility preservation to the period between diagnosis and initiation of neoadjuvant therapy and requires COS be done while the tumor is in place, a fact which is disconcerting for both the oncologists and the patients.[49]

Recently, Sonmezer et al. described a random start COS protocol utilizing letrozole together with gonadotropins to prevent both the delay and the rise in estrogen levels associated with conventional COS.[50] The authors reported 3 women diagnosed with breast cancer, who were referred on menstrual cycle days 11, 14 and 17 and did not have time to wait until the onset of the next menstrual period before chemotherapy. Letrozole and recombinant FSH were started immediately on the day of referral with the aim of promoting the growth of another follicular recruitment wave in the same menstrual cycle. GnRH antagonists were used to prevent a premature LH surge. COH lasted between 9 and 11 days, peak estradiol levels were between 478–988 pg/ml and 7 to 11 MII oocytes were collected. Two to 7 immature oocytes at metaphase I and GV stages were also collected. The women had 7 to 9 embryos frozen. IVM of immature oocytes contributed 1 or 2 additional embryos per woman. This new approach certainly deserves further investigation with regard to acceptability by patients and treating oncologists, effect on prognosis of underlying disease and implantation potential of the embryos obtained from these oocytes. Occurrence of a clinical pregnancy from embryos obtained from stimulation of a second follicular wave during ovarian stimulation has been recently reported.[51]

Advantages of IVM

IVM avoids these two important concerns, which prevent a substantial amount of patients at risk of infertility from using ART.

Immature oocyte retrieval in an unstimulated menstrual cycle or from ovarian tissue biopsies followed by IVM and oocyte or embryo cryopreservation provides a novel fertility preservation strategy.[52-53] Avoiding ovarian stimulation provides several important advantages for cancer patients. Compared to 2–5 weeks required for a stimulated IVF cycle, immature oocyte retrieval can be done within 2–10 days, depending on the patient's menstrual status.[53] Immature oocytes can be collected even in the luteal phase. We reported 3 women without male partners seeking fertility preservation prior to chemotherapy, who presented for the first time in the luteal phase of their menstrual cycle and were to undergo gonadotoxic treatment immediately. Five to 7 immature oocytes were recovered by luteal-phase oocyte retrieval from these women. Three to 5 metaphase II (MII) oocytes were vitrified following IVM. Two of the 3 women later underwent 1 and 2 more collections, respectively, in the follicular phase of the next cycle(s) and additional immature oocytes were vitrified following IVM.[54]

Recently, Maman et al. reported luteal phase oocyte collection in 5 women seeking emergency fertility preservation and compared the number of cryopreserved oocytes/embryos with 13 women who underwent IVM oocyte collection in the follicular phase.[55] Women who presented in the luteal phase were given 10,000 IU HCG and oocyte collection was performed 34–36 hours later. Women who underwent regular IVM cycle for fertility preservation were given HCG when the leading follicle size reached 12–14 mm. All women were chemotherapy naive and under 35-years-old. Mean age was comparable between the groups (23.4 vs. 24.1 years). It should be noted that mean

(SD) Anti-Müllerian hormone (AMH) level was lower, albeit not significantly, in women who underwent luteal collection, than women who underwent follicular phase collection (3.7 (2.2) vs. 6.4 (6.9) ng/ml). The mean number (SD) of oocytes collected (12.8 (8.4) vs. 17.3 (13.5)), the mean number of MII oocytes in the first 24 hours after collection (4.0 (5.7) vs. 4.5 (3.8)), the mean total number of MII oocytes (7 (7.6) vs. 9.5 (7.7)), the oocyte maturation rate (48.6% vs. 57.8%), the fertilization rates (69.2% vs. 63.2%) and the mean total number of oocytes and embryos available (6.4 (6.6) vs. 7.8 (7.5)) were comparable between the luteal collection and follicular collection groups.[55]

Moreover, immature oocyte collection in the luteal phase provides a rescue option for a patient who experiences a premature LH surge during ovarian stimulation.[56] Although cancelling the treatment cycle can be an option for the regular patient, cancer patients undergoing fertility preserving treatment usually do not have time for a new treatment cycle and require immediate solutions. We were able to collect 4 immature oocytes in a breast cancer patient who had a premature LH surge during an ovarian stimulation cycle started for fertility preservation. She had experienced an abrupt increase in serum LH level on the 7th day of stimulation. Progesterone level reached 8.38 ng/ml on the 10th day of stimulation. On the same day, leading follicle size was 20 mm and there was no sonographic finding suggesting ovulation. Ten thousand IU HCG was administered and collection was scheduled 35 hours later. At the time of collection, there were approximately 10 follicles sized ≥ 10 mm, and 4 of them had the appearance of corpus lutei accompanied by free fluid around the ovaries. Nevertheless, all follicles were aspirated resulting in collection of 4 immature oocytes at the GV stage from follicles smaller than 10 mm in average diameter. Two GV oocytes were matured in vitro and fertilized successfully, resulting in vitrification of 2 embryos .

In addition to avoiding potential delay in treatment and rise in estradiol levels, IVM eliminates the risk of ovarian hyperstimulation syndrome (OHSS). OHSS is a major complication of COS, characterized with increased vascular permeability.[57] Clinically, it manifests as ascites, pleural effusion, hypovolemia, hemoconcentration and hypercoagulability. Severe cases could be complicated by thromboembolism and even death. When superimposed on cancer, OHSS can have serious consequences on the health of these patients and can cause further delay in pending oncologic treatment.

Collection of Immature Oocytes from Ovarian Tissue Specimens for Cryopreservation

Immature oocytes can also be harvested from ovarian biopsy specimens and fertilized or vitrified following IVM.[52] This combination of ovarian-tissue cryobanking and IVM represents a new strategy for fertility preservation. We retrieved 11 immature oocytes from a wedge resection specimen in a 16-year-old patient with mosaic Turner syndrome. Eight of these oocytes were vitrified following IVM.[7] In 4 women with cancer (2 Hodgkin's lymphoma, 1 breast cancer and 1 rectal cancer), we harvested 11 immature oocytes from wedge biopsy specimens collected for ovarian tissue cryopreservation. The patients' ages ranged between 18 and 38 years. In 2 patients, surgery was performed in early follicular phase whereas 2 women underwent surgery in the luteal phase of the menstrual cycle. Median number of immature oocytes collected was 3. Eight of the 11 immature oocytes reached MII stage following IVM and were vitrified.[52]

IVM – Oocyte Vitrification

Requirement for a male partner and ethical/legal/religious issues associated with embryo cryopreservation are other aspects that require attention when IVF-embryo cryopreservation is considered as a fertility preservation measure. Although infertility affects a couple in general, cancer affects the individual. Fertility preservation should aim to preserve not only the individual's germ line, but also her autonomy for her own reproductive potential. For single women, generating then freezing embryos conceived with donor sperm is obviously not the same as cryopreserving unfertilized oocytes for possible use with a future partner. On the other hand, while donor sperm is not required for women who have a partner, freezing embryos means sharing the control over embryos with him. Unfortunately, some couples split up in the face of cancer. In case of separation, the former male partner also has rights over the embryos, with all possible legal and ethical implications. The ex-male partner may disagree to the use of the embryos to conceive a child.[58-59] If there is any doubt, it seems better to freeze oocytes since oocytes belong to the woman, while embryos belong to the couple. We believe that in contrast to embryo cryopreservation, oocyte cryopreservation provides the most effective means of ensuring the reproductive autonomy of the patient. Another advantage of oocyte cryopreservation is that it avoids the ethical and religious quandaries associated with the storage and disposal of embryos.

Oocyte cryopreservation is considered an investigational procedure in the ASCO and ASRM reports as well as in a working-party report of the royal colleges of physicians, radiologists and obstetricians and gynecologists on the management of cancer patients undergoing gonadotoxic treatment.[60-63] The major motivation behind this opinion is that a relatively better clinical outcome is being reported with embryo cryopreservation than with oocyte cryopreservation.

However, these opinions by ASRM, ASCO and the royal colleges are based on data published prior to 2005, 2006 and 2007, respectively. A meta-analysis of the efficiency of oocyte cryopreservation published in 2006 reported live-birth rates of 1.9% and 2% per oocyte thawed after slow freezing and vitrification, respectively.[64] The vast majority of data on oocyte cryopreservation were from experience with slow freezing at that time and a substantial amount of relevant data favoring vitrification has subsequently been published.[65-70] In a clinical trial at the McGill Reproductive Center involving 38 infertile women who underwent oocyte collection in a gonadotropin stimulated cycle, oocyte vitrification (OV) using the McGill Cryoleaf resulted in a mean survival rate of 81% post-thawing, a 76% fertilization rate, a CPR per cycle of 45%, a live birth rate of 40% and 22 healthy babies.[71] In a review of 165 pregnancies and 200 infants conceived following oocyte vitrification, the birth weight and the incidence of congenital anomalies (2.5%) were comparable to those following spontaneous conception or IVF treatment.[71] A more recent review corroborates our observations.[72]

Similar to in vivo matured oocytes, in vitro matured oocytes can be successfully cryopreserved with vitrification, further expanding the choices for women who wish to preserve their fertility potential. Although smaller sized immature oocytes without the meiotic spindle can be anticipated to better survive cryopreservation, laboratory and clinical outcomes of cryopreservation of oocytes at the GV stage by slow-freezing or vitrification have not been as good as those achieved with mature oocytes.[65] Despite similar survival rates for GV and MII oocytes after vitrification (85.4% versus 86.1% respectively), the maturation rate of vitrified warmed GV oocytes is significantly lower than that of fresh GV oocytes (50.8% versus 70.4% respectively).[65] However, fertilization rate and embryo development are similar for vitrified or fresh GV oocytes once they reach MII stage.

Given these facts, it seems cryopreservation of immature oocytes after they have matured to MII stage appears to be a better strategy. In a pilot study at the McGill Reproductive Center on IVM- oocyte vitrification, a live birth rate of 20 % per cycle was achieved, including the world's first 4 live births from vitrified IVM oocytes.[71] Compared to in vivo matured oocytes collected following ovarian stimulation, IVM oocytes had significantly lower survival (81.4% vs. 67.5%) and fertilization (75.6% vs. 64.2%) rates following vitrification-warming. Despite a trend towards lower implantation (19.1% vs. 9.6%), CPR (44.7% vs. 20.0%) and live birth rates (39.5% vs. 20%) with IVM-oocyte vitrification, none of the differences were statistically significant.[71] The clinical outcome of IVM- oocyte vitrification is regarded as satisfactory for patients whose conditions preclude ovarian stimulation for any reason.

A suggested algorithm for cancer patients is presented in **Figure 1**.

IVM FOR SOCIAL FERTILITY PRESERVATION

Both the ASRM and European Society of Human Reproduction and Embryology recommendations are against ovarian tissue cryopreservation in healthy women who are not faced with an "immediate threat to fertility".[60, 73] Similar to ovarian tissue freezing, oocyte cryopreservation is also regarded as an experimental procedure and both societies find it too early to "recommend" or "encourage" oocyte freezing without a medical indication.[60, 73] Risk-to-benefit ratio of the procedure is one of the major concerns. IVM provides the unique opportunity of oocyte freezing without ovarian stimulation for women who wish to delay child bearing for social reasons. IVM-oocyte vitrification avoids the risk of OHSS and inconvenience of daily gonadotropin injections for these healthy women. The direct and indirect costs of treatment i.e., cost of gonadotropins, loss of working days for monitoring scans, etc. are less with IVM. Based on these benefits, IVM can be considered a simpler and safer procedure and regarded as more acceptable.

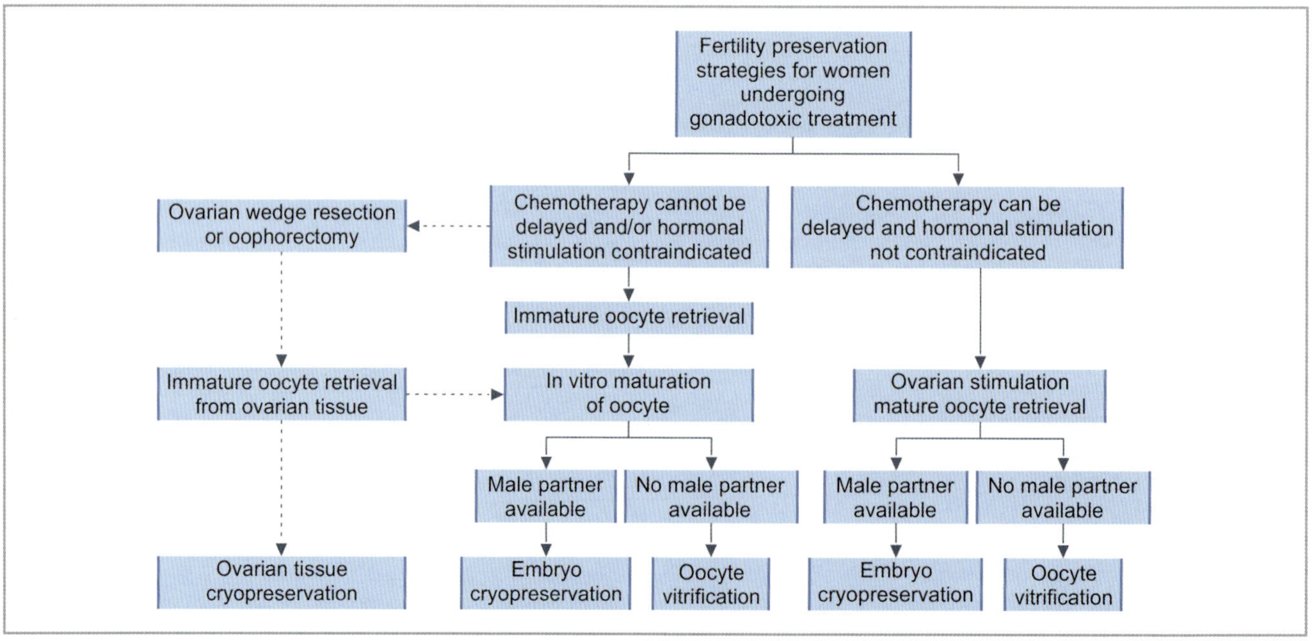

FIGURE 1 Suggested algorithm for fertility preservation
Reprinted with permission from Chian et al. Fertility Sterility 2009; 91(6):2391–8.

CONCLUSION

In conclusion, IVM combined with embryo or oocyte vitrification provides previously unavailable options for some patients and improves the services provided by a fertility preservation program. Primary-care physicians and oncologists need to be made aware of the available fertility preservation options in order to allow early discussion with their patients followed by referral, if desired, to an ART center that offers the full range of fertility preservation options. This is contingent on the long term achievement of comparable pregnancy rates with IVM-oocyte vitrification and IVF-oocyte vitrification.

REFERENCES

1. Martin J, Hamilton B, Sutton P, et al. National vital statistics reports. National Vital Statistics Reports. 2009;57.
2. Society of Assisted Reproductive Technology. https://www.sartcorsonline.com/rptCSR_PublicMultYear.aspx?ClinicPKID=0.
3. The American Cancer Society. Cancer Facts and Figures 2009. http://www.cancerorg/docroot/STT/STT_0asp.
4. Bleyer WA. The impact of childhood cancer on the United States and the world. CA Cancer J Clin. 1990;40:355-67.
5. Elizur S, Chian R, Pineau C, et al. Fertility preservation treatment for young women with autoimmune diseases facing treatment with gonadotoxic agents. Rheumatology. 2008;47:1506-9.
6. Elizur SE, Chian RC, Holzer HE, et al. Cryopreservation of oocytes in a young woman with severe and symptomatic endometriosis: a new indication for fertility preservation. Fertil Steril. 2009;91:293e1-3.
7. Huang J, Tulandi T, Holzer H, et al. Cryopreservation of ovarian tissue and in vitro matured oocytes in a female with mosaic Turner syndrome: Case Report. Human Reprod. 2008;23:336.
8. Lau N, Huang J, MacDonald S, et al. Feasibility of fertility preservation in young females with Turner syndrome. Reprod BioMedicine Online. 2009;18:290-5.
9. Stoop D, Nekkebroeck J, Devroey P. A survey on the intentions and attitudes towards oocyte cryopreservation for non-medical reasons among women of reproductive age. Hum Reprod. 2011;26:655-61.
10. Silber SJ, Grudzinskas G, Gosden RG. Successful Pregnancy after Microsurgical Transplantation of an Intact Ovary. N Engl J Med. 2008;359:2617-8.
11. Wang X, Chen H, Yin H, et al. Fertility after intact ovary transplantation. Nature. 2002;415:385.
12. Georgescu ES, Goldberg JM, du Plessis SS, Agarwal A. Present and future fertility preservation strategies for female cancer patients. Obstet Gynecol Surv. 2008;63:725-32.
13. Edwards RG. Maturation in vitro of human ovarian oocytes. Lancet. 1965;2:926-9.
14. Pincus G, Enzmann E. The comparative behaviour of mammalian eggs in vivo and in vitro: I. The activation of ovarian eggs. J Exp Med. 1935;62:665-75.
15. Veeck LL, Wortham Jr JW, Witmyer J, et al. Maturation and fertilization of morphologically immature human oocytes in a program of in vitro fertilization. Fertil Steril. 1983;39:594.
16. Cha KY, Koo JJ, Ko JJ, et al. Pregnancy after in vitro fertilization of human follicular oocytes collected from nonstimulated cycles, their culture in vitro and their transfer in a donor oocyte program. Fertil Steril. 1991;55:109-13.
17. Trounson A, Wood C, Kausche A. In vitro maturation and the fertilization and developmental competence of oocytes recovered from untreated polycystic ovarian patients. Fertil Steril. 1994;62:353-62.
18. Chian RC, Gulekli B, Buckett WM, Tan SL. Priming with human chorionic gonadotropin before retrieval of immature oocytes in women with infertility due to the polycystic ovary syndrome. N Engl J Med. 1999;341:1624-6.
19. Chian RC, Buckett WM, Tulandi T, Tan SL. Prospective randomized study of human chorionic gonadotrophin priming before immature oocyte retrieval from unstimulated women with polycystic ovarian syndrome. Human Reprod. 2000;15:165-70.
20. Chian RC, Buckett WM, Abdul Jalil AK, et al. Natural-cycle in vitro fertilization combined with in vitro maturation of immature oocytes is a potential approach in infertility treatment. Fertil Steril. 2004;82:1675-8.
21. Elizur SE, Chian RC, Pineau CA, et al. Fertility preservation treatment for young women with autoimmune diseases facing treatment with gonadotoxic agents. Rheumatology (Oxford). 2008;47:1506-9.
22. Son WY, Chung JT, Chian RC, et al. A 38 h interval between hCG priming and oocyte retrieval increases in vivo and in vitro oocyte maturation rate in programmed IVM cycles. Hum Reprod. 2008;23:2010-6.
23. Nagy ZP, Cecile J, Liu J, et al. Pregnancy and birth after intracytoplasmic sperm injection of in vitro matured germinal-vesicle stage oocytes: case report. Fertil Steril. 1996;65:1047-50.
24. Soderstrom-Anttila V, Makinen S, Tuuri T, Suikkari AM. Favourable pregnancy results with insemination of in vitro matured oocytes from unstimulated patients. Hum Reprod. 2005;20:1534-40.
25. Oren-Benaroya R, Orvieto R, Gakamsky A, et al. The sperm chemoattractant secreted from human cumulus cells is progesterone. Hum Reprod. 2008;23:2339-45.
26. Zhang XY, Ata B, Son WY, et al. Chromosome abnormality rates in human embryos obtained from in-vitro maturation and IVF treatment cycles. Reprod Biomed Online. 2010;21:552-9.
27. Requena A, Bronet F, Guillen A, et al. The impact of in-vitro maturation of oocytes on aneuploidy rate. Reprod Biomed Online. 2009;18:777-83.
28. Chian RC, Buckett WM, Tan SL. In-vitro maturation of human oocytes. Reprod Biomed Online. 2004;8:148-66.
29. Buckett WM, Chian RC, Dean NL, et al. Pregnancy loss in pregnancies conceived after in vitro oocyte maturation, conventional in vitro fertilization, and intracytoplasmic sperm injection. Fertil Steril. 2008;90:546-50.
30. Homburg R. Pregnancy complications in PCOS. Best Pract Res Clin Endocrinol Metab. 2006;20:281-92.
31. Balen AH, Tan SL, MacDougall J, Jacobs HS. Miscarriage rates following in-vitro fertilization are increased in women with polycystic ovaries and reduced by pituitary desensitization with buserelin. Hum Reprod. 1993;8:959-64.
32. Kousta E, White DM, Franks S. Modern use of clomiphene citrate in induction of ovulation. Hum Reprod Update. 1997;3:359-65.
33. Buckett WM, Chian RC, Holzer H, et al. Obstetric outcomes and congenital abnormalities after in vitro maturation, in vitro fertilization, and intracytoplasmic sperm injection. Obstet Gynecol. 2007;110:885-91.
34. Cha KY, Chung HM, Lee DR, et al. Obstetric outcome of patients with polycystic ovary syndrome treated by in vitro maturation and in vitro fertilization-embryo transfer. Fertil Steril. 2005;83:1461-5.

35. Soderstrom-Anttila V, Salokorpi T, Pihlaja M, et al. Obstetric and perinatal outcome and preliminary results of development of children born after in vitro maturation of oocytes. Hum Reprod. 2006;21:1508-13.
36. Mikkelsen AL. Strategies in human in-vitro maturation and their clinical outcome. Reprod Biomed Online. 2005;10:593-9.
37. Shu-Chi M, Jiann-Loung H, Yu-Hung L, et al. Growth and development of children conceived by in-vitro maturation of human oocytes. Early Hum Dev. 2006;82:677-82.
38. Tulandi T, Huang J, Tan S. Preservation of Female Fertility: An Essential Progress. Obstet Gynecol. 2008; 112: 1160-72.
39. Heffner LJ. Advanced maternal age--how old is too old? N Engl J Med. 2004;351:1927-9.
40. Tan SL, Royston P, Campbell S, et al. Cumulative conception and livebirth rates after in-vitro fertilisation. Lancet. 1992;339:1390-4.
41. Trounson A, Mohr L. Human pregnancy following cryopreservation, thawing and transfer of an eight-cell embryo. Nature. 1983;305:707-9.
42. Zeilmaker GH, Alberda AT, van Gent I, et al. Two pregnancies following transfer of intact frozen-thawed embryos. Fertil Steril. 1984;42:293-6.
43. ICMART. Presentation of preliminary data for 2004. Human Reprod 2008;Supplement.
44. Cahill DJ, Wardle PG, Harlow CR, et al. Expected contribution to serum oestradiol from individual ovarian follicles in unstimulated cycles. Hum Reprod. 2000;15:1909-12.
45. National Cancer Institute. SEER Cancer Statistics Review. 1975-2006.
46. Yager JD, Davidson NE. Estrogen carcinogenesis in breast cancer. N Engl J Med. 2006;354:270-82.
47. Gupta PB, Kuperwasser C. Contributions of estrogen to ER-negative breast tumor growth. J Steroid Biochem Mol Biol. 2006;102:71-8.
48. Azim AA, Costantini-Ferrando M, Oktay K. Safety of fertility preservation by ovarian stimulation with letrozole and gonadotropins in patients with breast cancer: a prospective controlled study. J Clin Oncol. 2008;26:2630-5.
49. Kim SS, Klemp J, Fabian C. Breast cancer and fertility preservation. Fertil Steril. 2011;95(5):1535-43.
50. Sonmezer M, Turkcuoglu I, Coskun U, Oktay K. Random-start controlled ovarian hyperstimulation for emergency fertility preservation in letrozole cycles. Fertil Steril. 2011;95(6):2125.e9-11.
51. Bentov Y, Esfandiari N, Gokturk A, et al. An ongoing pregnancy from two waves of follicles developing during a long follicular phase of the same cycle. Fertil Steril. 2010;94:350 e8-11.
52. Huang J, Tulandi T, Holzer H, et al. Combining ovarian tissue cryobanking with retrieval of immature oocytes followed by in vitro maturation and vitrification: an additional strategy of fertility preservation. Fertil Steril. 2008;89:567-72.
53. Rao G, Chian R, Son W, et al. Fertility preservation in women undergoing cancer treatment. Lancet. 2004;363:1829-30.
54. Demirtas E, Elizur SE, Holzer H, et al. Immature oocyte retrieval in the luteal phase to preserve fertility in cancer patients. Reprod Biomed Online. 2008;17:520-3.
55. Maman E, Meirow D, Brengauz M, et al. Luteal phase oocyte retrieval and in vitro maturation is an optional procedure for urgent fertility preservation. Fertil Steril. 2011;95:64-7.
56. Oktay K, Demirtas E, Son WY, et al. In vitro maturation of germinal vesicle oocytes recovered after premature luteinizing hormone surge: description of a novel approach to fertility preservation. Fertil Steril. 2008;89:228 e19-22.
57. Ata B, Tulandi T. Pathophysiology of ovarian hyperstimulation syndrome and strategies for its prevention and treatment. Expert Review Obstet Gynecol. 2009;4:299-311.
58. Caroline M. Evans v. United Kingdom: Paradigms Of Parenting. Modern Law Review. 2007;70:992-1002.
59. Demeestere I, Simon P, Emiliani S, et al. Fertility preservation: successful transplantation of cryopreserved ovarian tissue in a young patient previously treated for Hodgkin's disease. Oncologist. 2007;12:1437-42.
60. The Practice Committee of the American Society for Reproductive Medicine, Practice Committee of the Society for Assisted Reproductive Technology. Ovarian tissue and oocyte cryopreservation Fertil Steril. 2008;90:S241-6.
61. Royal College of Physicians, Royal College of Radiologists, Royal College of Obstetricians and Gynaecologists. The effects of cancer treatment on reproductive functions. Guidance on management. Report of a working party. Available at http://wwwrcogorguk/womens-health/clinical-guidance/effects-cancer-treatment-reproductive-function-guidance-management 2007.
62. Lee SJ, Schover LR, Partridge AH, et al. American Society of Clinical Oncology recommendations on fertility preservation in cancer patients. J Clin Oncol. 2006;24:2917-31.
63. American Society of Reproductive Medicine. Fertility preservation and reproduction in cancer patients. Fertil Steril. 2005;83:1622-8.
64. Oktay K, Cil AP, Bang H. Efficiency of oocyte cryopreservation: a meta-analysis. Fertil Steril. 2006;86:70-80.
65. Cao Y, Xing Q, Zhang ZG, et al. Cryopreservation of immature and in-vitro matured human oocytes by vitrification. Reprod Biomed Online. 2009;19:369-73.
66. Huang J, Chen H, Park J, et al. Comparison of spindle and chromosome configuration in in vitro-and in vivo-matured mouse oocytes after vitrification. Fertil Steril. 2008;90:1424-32.
67. Kuwayama M. Highly efficient vitrification for cryopreservation of human oocytes and embryos: the Cryotop method. Theriogenology. 2007;67:73-80.
68. Fadini R, Brambillasca F, Renzini M, et al. Human oocyte cryopreservation: comparison between slow and ultrarapid methods. Reprod BioMedicine Online. 2009;19:171-80.
69. Rienzi L, Romano S, Albricci L, et al. Embryo development of fresh 'versus' vitrified metaphase II oocytes after ICSI: a prospective randomized sibling-oocyte study. Hum Reprod. 2010;25(1):66–73.
70. Cobo A, Kuwayama M, Perez S, et al. Comparison of concomitant outcome achieved with fresh and cryopreserved donor oocytes vitrified by the Cryotop method. Fertil Steril. 2008;89:1657-64.
71. Chian RC, Huang JY, Gilbert L, et al. Obstetric outcomes following vitrification of in vitro and in vivo matured oocytes. Fertil Steril. 2009;91:2391-8.
72. Noyes N, Porcu E, Borini A. Over 900 oocyte cryopreservation babies born with no apparent increase in congenital anomalies. Reprod Biomed Online. 2009;18:769-76.
73. Shenfield F, Pennings G, Cohen J, Devroey P, Sureau C, Tarlatzis B. Taskforce 7: Ethical considerations for the cryopreservation of gametes and reproductive tissues for self use. Hum Reprod. 2004;19:460-2.

Fertility Preservation in Women with Breast Cancer

14

Wayne Lin, Elizabeth Ginsburg

CHAPTER OUTLINE

THE EPIDEMIOLOGY OF BREAST CANCER

There are more than 2.6 million breast cancer survivors in the United States. About 1 in 8 women in the United States will develop invasive breast cancer over the course of her lifetime. Based on that estimate, in 2012, 226,870 new cases of invasive breast cancer will be diagnosed, 63,300 new cases of carcinoma in situ will be diagnosed and 39,510 women will die from breast cancer. Breast cancer is the second leading cause of cancer death in women, next to lung cancer.[1,2] The death rate from breast cancer has been declining since 1990, with large decrease in women younger than 50-years-old, which is attributed to early detection, increased awareness and advances in treatments. Therefore, the proportion of young breast cancer survivors in the population has significantly increased.

Although breast cancer risk increases with age, approximately 35% of breast cancers occur during the reproductive and perimenopausal years:1.9% below age 35, 10.2% between the ages of 35 and 44 and 22.6% between the ages of 45 and 54.[2] At earlier ages of diagnosis, women who have not completed childbearing are potentially affected and fertility becomes an important concern.

Fifty-seven percent of women who had a diagnosis of breast cancer before age 40, recalled concerns about fertility. Of those women, 29% reported that fertility concerns actually influenced their treatment decisions.[3] In a survey in 2005, only 68% of women who had a diagnosis of breast cancer before age 50 recalled discussion of early menopause with their physician, and only 34% recalled discussion of infertility risk.[4]

Fortunately, with rising awareness, in 2006 the American Society of Clinical Oncology published recommendations on fertility preservation in people treated for cancer.[5] These recommendations have become the standard of care in providing early fertility counseling for premenopausal breast cancer patients, including infertility risk and possible interventions to preserve fertility prior to the treatments.

BREAST CANCER TREATMENT

Treatment modality depends on stage, tumor type and response to therapy. It can be divided into major categories of surgery, radiation, chemotherapy, hormone therapy and targeted therapy. It is important to be familiar with potential treatment regimens in order to individualize counseling regarding the likelihood of infertility and the potential fertility preservation approach.[6] The choices of adjuvant therapy are listed in **Table 1**.

Surgery

Surgery to remove the primary cancer lesions from the breast is usually the first step in treatment. Based on the staging, surgery may range from breast-conserving surgery (lumpectomy or partial mastectomy) to total mastectomy (with or without lymph node dissection) or modified radical mastectomy (often with simultaneous or interval breast reconstruction). However, in some circumstances neoadjuvant chemotherapy prior to surgery is performed.

Radiation

Radiation of breast cancer does not affect the pelvic organs directly. However, later complications from radiation may include radiation pneumonitis and the risk of second malignancies, such as thyroid cancer.

Chemotherapy

The stage and molecular features of breast cancers determine the need for chemotherapy, the agents used and the choice of modalities used. Chemotherapy generally includes cyclophosphamide and may involve doxorubicin, paclitaxel, fluorouracil, or methotrexate. There are single agent regimens and multiple combination regimens in use, including AC (doxorubicin and cyclophosphamide), AC-T (doxorubicin, cyclophosphamide, and paclitaxel) and CAF (cyclophosphamide, doxorubicin and fluorouracil). Older regimens such as CMF (cyclophosphamide, methotrexate and fluorouracil) and FEC (fluorouracil, epirubicin, and cyclophosphamide) cause high rates of ovarian failure and are not used as front-line treatment at this time.

Adjuvant trastuzumab is indicated in Her2 overexpression patients. Monoclonal antibodies, trastuzumab (Herceptin), block the effects of Her2, a growth factor protein related to breast cancer. One-fourth of breast cancers are related to Her2. Tyrosine kinase inhibitors, lapatinib, also block the effects of the Her2 protein and may be used in Her2-positive patients who have progressed after treatment with trastuzumab.

TABLE 1 National Cancer Institute (NCI) Breast cancer adjuvant systemic therapy treatment strategy

A: Risk categories for women with node—negative breast cancer

	Low risk (has all listed factors)	***Intermediate risk (Risk classified between the other two categories)***	***High risk (Has at least one listed factor)***
Tumor size	≤ 1cm	1–2 cm	>2 cm
ER or PR status	positive	positive	negative
Tumor grade	grade 1	grade 1–2	grade 2–3

ER = estrogen receptor; PR = progesterone receptor

B: Adjuvant systemic treatment options for premenopausal women with axillary node—negative breast cancer

Patient group	***Low risk***	***Intermediate risk***	***High risk***
ER (+) or PR (+)	None or tamoxifen	1. Tamoxifen + chemotherapy, or 2. Tamoxifen alone, or 3. Ovarian ablation, or 4. GnRH[a]	1. Chemotherapy + tamoxifen, or 2. Chemotherapy + ablation or GnRH analog[a], or 3. Chemotherapy + tamoxifen + ovarian ablation or GnRH[a], or 4. Ovarian ablation alone or with tamoxifen or GnRH alone or with tamoxifen
ER (-) or PR (-)	—	—	Chemotherapy

AI = aromatase inhibitor; ER = estrogen receptor; GnRH = gonadotropin-releasing hormone; PR = progesterone receptor,
[a]Note: This treatment option is under clinical evaluation.

C: Treatment options for premenopausal women with axillary node—Positive Breast Cancer

Patient group	***Treatments***
ER (+) or PR (+)	1. Chemotherapy + tamoxifen, or 2. Chemotherapy + ovarian ablation/GnRH analog, or 3. Chemotherapy + tamoxifen + ovarian ablation/ GnRH analog,[a] or 4. Ovarian ablation alone or with tamoxifen or GnRH alone or with tamoxifen
ER (-) or PR (-)	Chemotherapy

AI= aromatase inhibitors; ER = estrogen receptor; GnRH = gonadotropin-releasing hormone; PR = progesterone receptor;
[a]Note: This treatment option is under clinical evaluation.

Hormonal Treatment

Hormonal therapy is recommended for estrogen receptor and/or progesterone receptor positive patients. The selective estrogen receptor modulator Tamoxifen (20 mg/d for 5 years) is often used in early stages of breast cancer, metastatic breast cancer, for chemoprevention in *BRCA* carriers and particularly estrogen receptor positive (ER+) invasive tumors. Raloxifene (60mg/d for 5 years), on the other hand, is considered for reduction in risk of invasive breast cancer in postmenopausal women with osteoporosis. However, in triple negative breast cancer patients, adjuvant therapy relies on chemotherapeutic regimens in combination with experimental targeted therapy.

In summary, most patients will proceed to surgical intervention to different extents based on the staging, with or without chemotherapy and then to chemoprevention. Traditionally, complete cancer treatment and delay in attempting conception is recommended after the diagnosis of breast cancer. Some patients might opt to conceive prior to completing five years of tamoxifen treatment. This choice in turn creates a dilemma between the incomplete cancer treatment and diminished ovarian reserve, which in turn may reduce the likelihood of pregnancy as the woman ages.

CHEMOTHERAPY AND OVARIAN RESERVE

There is a fixed pool of primordial follicles, which is maximal at 6–7 million at five months of gestational age. Thereafter, the size of the follicular pool decreases with age in a bi-exponential fashion through the mechanism of apoptosis to 300,000 at menarche and eventually burnout of the pool at menopause (**Figure 1**). When the ovaries are exposed to different chemotherapy agents, there are differential impacts observed on primordial, dormant and growing follicles. Through accelerated follicular apoptosis and cortical fibrosis, the primordial follicle pool diminishes, leading to ovarian atrophy and disrupted ovarian blood vasculature.[7,8] Female fertility can be compromised through loss of ovarian function, decrease in primordial follicle number and affected hormonal balance after chemotherapy or radiation therapy.[9]

Amenorrhea in premenopausal breast cancer patients is defined as the absence of menses for more than three cycles or six months. Menopause is defined as the absence of menstrual cycles with menopausal levels of FSH and estradiol one year after the end of chemotherapy. The amenorrhea may be temporary or permanent. In some cases, fertility and menstrual cycles might return after months to years of completion of the therapy.[10,11] Therefore, it is important to clarify the etiology of amenorrhea. The key factors involved are chemotherapy agent, drug regimen and patient age.

Age and Amenorrhea

Age at diagnosis and the type of breast cancer treatment play a crucial role in the risk of ovarian failure (**Figure 2**). Older patients and those patients with lower ovarian reserve are at much higher risk of permanent amenorrhea/premature ovarian failure due to chemotherapy.[12] Patients who maintained ovarian function post-treatment were much younger(27.4 +/–8.3 years) than those who lost ovarian function (34.7 +/–8 years) in one study.[13]

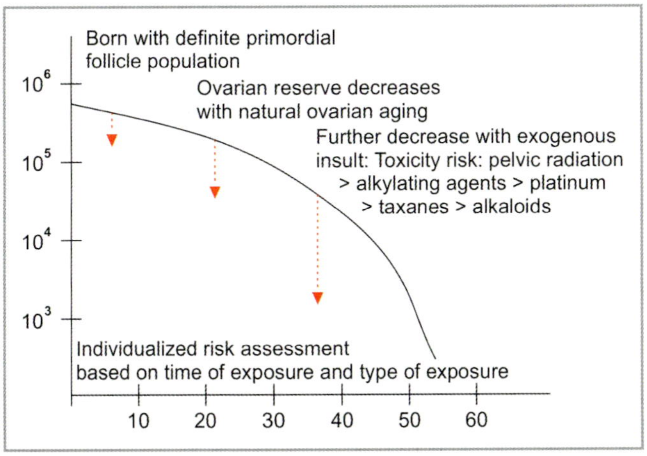

FIGURE 1 Women are born with a definite pool of primordial follicles which decrease with natural ovarian aging. However, with exposure to chemotherapy or pelvic radiation, the toxicity may deplete the ovarian reserve and decrease the primordial follicle numbers. The toxicity risk of pelvic radiation and alkylating agents are the highest [Adapted from Clin Obstet Gynecol. 2010 Dec;53(4):727-39].

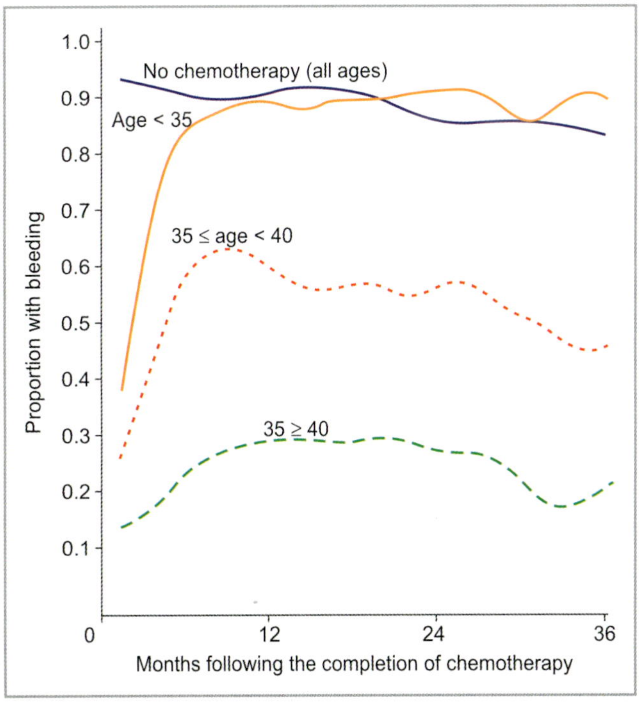

FIGURE 2 Patient age was significantly related to the proportion of recovery of menstrual bleeding after chemotherapy. 85% recovery was observed in patients younger than 35-years-old, 45–61% recovery in 35–40 years-old, and low in those older than 40-years-old [Adapted from Journal of Clinical Oncology. American Society of Clinical Oncology 2006;24:1045-51].

For breast cancer patients younger than 35 years old, 85% recovered their periods, while only 45-61% of those aged 35-40 years recovered their periods.[13] For women, who were 40 years or older, only less than 30% recovered their periods.[14] In other words, younger patients were less affected. The doses of cyclophosphamide that caused all women to have amenorrhea were 5.2 grams in women 40 years or older, but 9.5 grams in younger women.[15-17]

Effect of Chemotherapy and Tamoxifen on Amenorrhea

Chemotherapy agents and tamoxifen may both lead to amenorrhea. The effect from tamoxifen may be temporary through its reversible effect on estrogen receptors. It does not appear to cause permanent effect or infertility. However, the length of tamoxifen treatment itself may compromise fertility through the ageing process, as women are typically five years older at the end of treatment. Chemotherapy may lead to temporary amenorrhea from destruction of maturing follicles and/or permanent amenorrhea by depletion of primordial follicles.[18]

In breast cancer treatment, different treatment regimens pose significant differences in risk of amenorrhea and may be stratified to different ovarian failure risk profiles.[19] Among the major categories of chemotherapy agents (alkylating agents, platinum derivatives, antibiotics, antimetabolites, plant alkaloids and taxanes), a wide variance in the extent of ovarian damage is observed (**Figure 3**). Alkylating agents (for example, cyclophosphamide) are one of the primary agents used in combination therapy for breast cancer. Alkylating agents lead to DNA cross links and introduce single strand DNA breaks. Cyclophosphamide is associated with particularly high levels of premature ovarian failure with an odds ratio (OR) of 3.98.[13]

Some studies have demonstrated that the risk of ovarian failure was greater with the use of CMF than with AC.[20] Petrek et al. prospectively observed the menstrual pattern after completion of chemotherapy in 500 breast cancer patients.[14] When comparing AC alone, AC combined with taxol (ACT), or CMF, it was noted that 16% of those receiving the AC regimen soon recovered monthly menstruation, compared to 48% in the CMF group. In the AC group, a slow recovery phase followed by a plateau at 50% was noted, while there was no recovery phase and a continual decline to approximately 18% in the CMF group in the end of study (**Figure 4**). Tamoxifen use increased the risk of amenorrhea between months 12 and 24 after chemotherapy by 15%.[14]

Abusief et al. showed that there is no significant effect of amenorrhea from paclitaxel use, dose density, and/or trastuzumab on treatment-related amenorrhea in premenopausal women with breast cancer.[21] But again, amenorrhea was associated significantly with tamoxifen use and with age at diagnosis.

FERTILITY AFTER CHEMOTHERAPY

Resumption of menstrual cycles in breast cancer patients implies the recovery of ovarian function. However, in combination with FSH and estradiol levels, it does not necessarily imply fertility potential, as most infertile women still have menstrual periods. Amenorrhea is therefore not a good indicator for menopause or fertility.

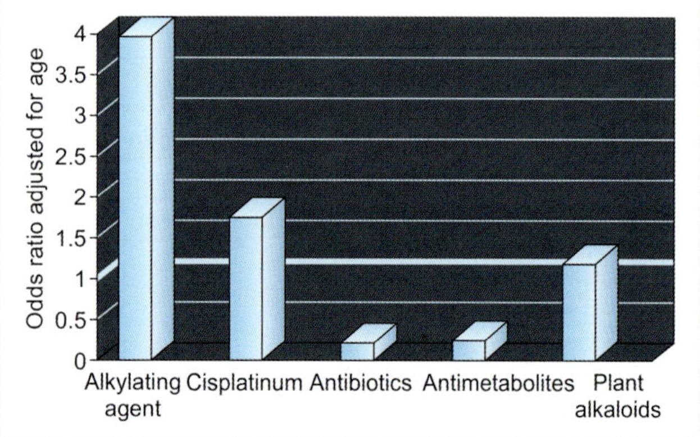

FIGURE 3 Age adjusted odds ratio of ovarian failure after exposure to different chemotherapy agents with the highest odds ratio of 3.98 in alkylating agents and 1.77 in platinum derivatives. There was no significant impact of ovarian failure observed in antibiotics or antimetabolites (Adapted from Mol Cell Endocrinol. Elsevier. 2000;169:123-31).

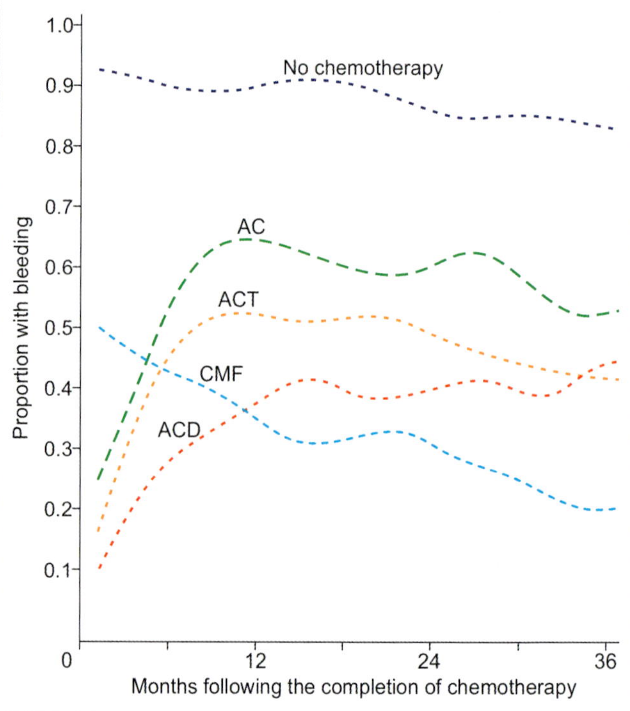

FIGURE 4 Type of combination of chemotherapy agents was significantly related to the proportion of recovery of menstrual bleeding after chemotherapy. (AC, doxorubicin and cyclophosphamide; ACT, doxorubicin, cyclophosphamide, paclitaxel; CMF, cyclophosphamide, methotrexate, fluorouracil; ACD, doxorubicin, cyclophosphamide, docetaxel.) (Adepted from Journal of Clinical Oncology. American Society of Clinical Oncology. 2006; 24:1045-1051).

Anti-Müllerian hormone (AMH) and primordial follicle counts can be helpful in evaluating the risk of undergoing amenorrhea.[22] In a study of ovarian tissue cryopreservation for fertility preservation, lower primordial follicle counts in chemotherapy patients compared to the control group who had not received chemotherapy (5.4+/-1.3 versus 9.6+/-2.2) and lower counts in the alkylating agent groups than in the non-alkylating agent groups (2.9+/-1 versus 7.9+/-1.6) were seen.[23] Another study, comparing 20 breast cancer survivors and 20 control women demonstrated that antral follicle count (AFC) and AMH levels were highly correlated (r = 0.72) and were better indicators of ovarian reserve than FSH and inhibin B.[24] Interestingly, it also showed that survivors on tamoxifen had lower AFC, AMH and inhibin B and higher estradiol levels than non-tamoxifen-treated survivors. AMH, which is not cycle-day dependent, is indeed a better predictor of ovarian reserve and more accurately differentiates normal from abnormal ovarian reserve after chemotherapy than do FSH and estradiol levels. However, more prospective studies are needed to determine the predictive value of these tests for pregnancy after chemotherapy.

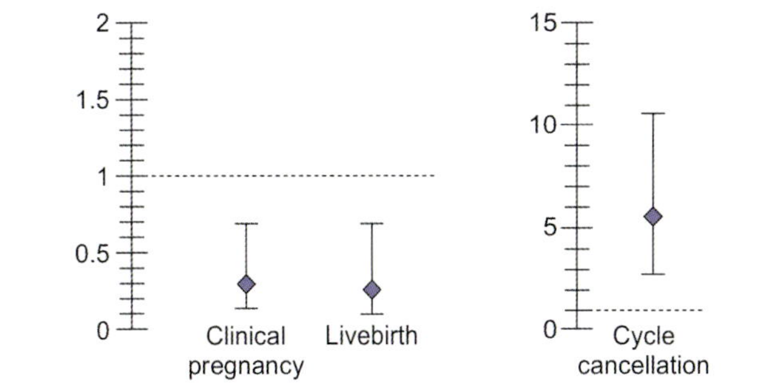

	Clinical pregnancy	Livebirth	Cycle cancellation
◆ Odds ratio	0.30	0.27	5.60
—95% confidence interval	(0.13-0.68)	(0.10-0.69)	(2.94-10.66)

FIGURE 5 The odds ratio of both clinical pregnancy and livebirth were both significantly lower and odds ratio of cycle cancellation is significantly higher in cancer survivors compared to all other who received IVF/ICSI treatment (Adapted from Barton, Fertil Steril. 2012; 97(2):381-6).

Pregnancy after Chemotherapy

Overall, the fertility potential among female cancer survivors is compromised after chemotherapy. But subsequent pregnancy after early stage breast cancer does not adversely affect the prognosis.[25] Patients are generally advised to wait at least two years to be free of disease before attempting to conceive after chemotherapy. The first two years after diagnosis are when recurrence rates are the highest. In addition, this delay allows the developing follicles with theoretical DNA damage from chemotherapy to be cleared from the ovary and new follicles to be recruited from surviving primordial follicles.[26]

A recent mice study raised concern that some anticancer drugs might result in transgeneration algenomic instability manifesting in their offspring in mice model.[27] However, there had been several large scale studies looking into pregnancy outcomes in childhood cancer survivors who were able to conceive and who received chemotherapy and/or radiation therapy. There were no significant differences in pregnancy outcomes, including stillbirth, miscarriages, abortions, live birth, and birth weight.[28-30]

Fertility Outcome with IVF/ICSI after Chemotherapy

In a recent retrospective study comparing cancer survivors receiving in vitro fertilization and intracytoplasmic sperm injection (IVF/ICSI), to other IVF/ICSI patients, the cancer survivors: (1) had fewer oocytes retrieved and embryos available for transfer; (2) were more likely to have a cancelled cycle (OR 5.60, 95%CI 2.94–10.66); and (3) had lower pregnancy (OR 0.30, 95%CI 0.13–0.68, and live birth rates (OR. 0.27, 95%CI 0.10–0.69) (**Figure 5**).[31]

Various studies have shown pregnancy rates ranging from 5% to 57% in breast cancer survivors, with varying ages and treatment modalities.[32,33] In young women with malignancy prior to chemotherapy, ovarian reserve, response to gonadotropins, oocytes retrieved and oocyte maturity remain unaltered by the neoplastic process.[34-36]

Safety of Fertility Treatment

While the estrogen levels may increase up to 10 fold in some ovarian stimulation protocols, there is a theoretical concern of tumor growth in estrogen and/or progesterone receptor positive breast cancers. There are no large, randomized clinical trials evaluating the major intervention methods or long-term follow-up of outcomes of fertility treatment on cancer survivors. A small study of 79 patients who underwent ovarian stimulation for cryopreservation of oocytes or embryos prior to adjuvant chemotherapy compared to 136 patients who did not undergo fertility treatments or ovarian stimulation showed that the breast cancer patients who underwent ovarian stimulation with letrozole and gonadotropins did not appear to have an increase of mortality or cancer recurrence.[37]

Timing of Fertility Preservation

Between the completion of breast cancer surgery and the initiation of chemotherapy, there is usually a 4 to 6 week interval. It is important to initiate fertility counseling early and to make use of the interval before chemotherapy initiation, which is adequate for at least 1 cycle of ovarian stimulation.[38,39] Timing of ovarian stimulation is, however, difficult and sometimes not possible in patients with chemotherapy planned prior to surgery. In these cases, short stimulations with retrieval of immature oocytes, or ovarian tissue freezing, may be considered.

FERTILITY PRESERVATION OPTIONS

Current fertility preservation treatment is built on the assisted reproduction technology framework with IVF/ICSI and embryo or oocyte cryopreservation, through the ovarian stimulation with letrozole/FSH protocol. The preferred timing is the 4 to 6 week window between the initial surgical intervention and chemotherapy. For those who need to start chemotherapy imminently, in vitro maturation (IVM) and random start cycle can be considered. Based on the individual situation and the timing of breast cancer treatment, different options could be considered before chemotherapy, including embryo cryopreservation, oocyte cryopreservation and ovarian tissue banking. During the chemotherapy, methods of ovarian suppression and protection are being investigated, but no consistent result has been established yet.

Ovarian Stimulation Regimens—Letrozole/FSH Protocol

Ovarian stimulation with aromatase inhibitors and gonadotropins are the current preferred regimen. In the letrozole/FSH protocol, letrozole is initiated on the second day of the menstrual cycle and gonadotropins are started two days later. When Estradiol levesl reach above 250 pg/mL or the lead follicle size reaches 14mm, a gonadotropin-releasing hormone (GnRH) antagonist is administered to prevent premature ovulation prior to retrieval. Human chorionic gonadotropin (hCG) is administered to induce ovulation when the leading follicle reaches 19 to 20 mm in diameter. Letrozole treatment is restarted after oocyte retrieval until the estradiol levels are lower than 50 pg/mL (**Figure 6**).[37]

The Letrozole-FSH protocol yields peak estradiol levels close to the levels in natural cycles,[40] which is lower than the level in anastrozole cycles.[41] The letrozole/low dose FSH protocol results in higher embryo yield (5.3 +/–0.8) when compared to tamoxifen/low-dose FSH (3.8 +/–0.8) or to tamoxifen alone(1.3 +/–0.2), and also the lowest peak estradiol levels.[42] The risk of ovarian hyperstimulation syndrome is also significantly decreased.[43]

The safety of the letrozole-FSH protocol was studied in a small study of 79 breast cancer patients receiving stimulation for the purpose of oocyte retrieval, embryo cryopreservation, or oocyte cryopreservation. Although the duration between surgery and chemotherapy in the letrozole-FSH group was longer than that of the control group without fertility treatment (45 versus 34 days), there was no difference in cancer recurrence or survival (hazard ratio 0.56, 95% CI 0.17–1.9).[37]

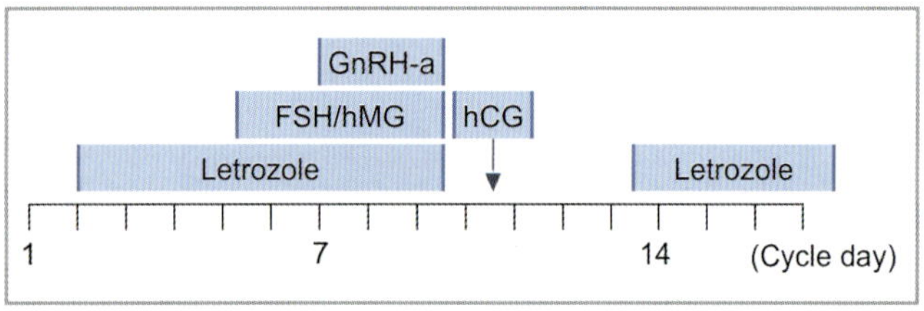

FIGURE 6 Letrozole/FSH protocol—Letrozole is initiated on day 2. Gonadotropins are started 2 days later. GnRH antagonist (GnRH-a) is started when estradiol>250 pg/mL or lead follicle size >14 mm. hCG was used in the triggering. Letrozole is restarted after oocyte retrieval until estradiol <50 pg/mL. [Adapted from J Clin Oncol. 2008;26(16): 2630-5].

In Vitro Maturation

For patients who cannot wait until the second day of the next menstrual period to start stimulation, alternative starting points are possible. Germinal vesicle stage (GV) oocyte retrieval during the luteal phase and IVM followed by IVF and cryopreservation of the embryo has been reported.[44] In standard IVF cycles, 12–20% of oocytes retrieved are immature and discarded. The proportion may be even higher due to the harvesting of smaller follicles and the use of letrozole.

In the IVM technique, cumulus is removed after retrieval, and the immature oocytes at GV stage and metaphase I stage are identified. They are placed in IVM medium for 24–48 hours. The medium was supplemented with 75 IU FSH and 75 IU LH[44] or 75 IU/mL FSH, 10 ng/mL epidermal growth factor, 0.5 mg/L insulin, transferrin and selenium. ICSI was performed on all oocytes matured in vitro and embryos were frozen at the pronuclear stage.

In one study, among 32 breast cancer patients, 464 oocytes were retrieved, of which 274 were mature. The overall fertilization rate after IVM was statistically significantly higher than the fertilization of already mature oocytes at retrieval (86% versus 73%, respectively, $P < 0.05$). The total number of oocytes and embryos frozen before IVM was 207 (45% of all oocytes retrieved). This number increased to 320 (69% of all oocytes retrieved) following IVM ($P < 0.0001$).[45]

Research on the extraction of immature oocytes from ovarian tissue, followed by IVM before freezing or after thawing is ongoing. One advantage of ovarian tissue harvesting is that it can be performed laparoscopically immediately and it avoids exposing estrogen sensitive tumors to the higher estrogen levels associated with ovarian stimulation.[46–48] It is thought that immature oocytes may resist cryoinjury better than mature oocytes, as there is no metaphase spindle involved. The implantation rate per embryo transferred may still be lower than with conventional IVF. Further investigation of the IVM technique is needed and there have been no deliveries from immature oocytes extracted from ovarian tissue.[49–51]

Random Start Cycle

Recently, there were also case reports of emergency fertility preservation with a random start ovarian hyperstimulation approach, which can be randomly started at any time point without compromising fertility rates. This approach was established based on the thought that multiple major follicle recruitment waves occur during a normal menstrual cycle. With the start of controlled ovarian hyperstimulation (COH) in 3 patients on cycle day 11, 14 and 17, when a letrozole/FSH protocol with GnRH antagonist was administered. After a total duration of 9–12 days of COH, hCG was used to trigger the ovulation. Nine to 17 oocytes were harvested, resulting in 7–10 embryos frozen, with the mean maturity and fertilization rates of 58.8% to 77.7% and 69.2% to 87.5%, respectively.[52] Further investigation is needed, however.

Embryo Cryopreservation

Cryopreservation of embryos is preferable to oocyte cryopreservation when possible, because all IVF programs are capable of embryo cryopreservation, thaw, and transfer, whereas the experience with oocyte cryopreservation, thaw fertilization and transfer is limited. The current live birth rate per transfer in frozen-thawed embryos from non-donor oocytes is 38.7% (SART 2010). The overall live birth rate from frozen-thawed embryos approaches the fecundity rate in natural conception.

Oocyte Cryopreservation

Oocyte cryopreservation is the option for the situations when embryo cryopreservation is not feasible—for example, single women who are uninterested in utilizing donor sperm. ASRM has made recommendations on the informed consent guidelines prior to elective oocyte cryopreservation in general circumstances.[53] On October 22, 2012, ASRM formally lifted the experimental label of mature oocyte cryopreservation technique, published new guidelines and offered this option to all eligible patients.[54]

The first live birth from a cryopreserved oocyte was reported in 1986. In a study in 2009, 936 healthy babies have been reported and verified.[55] There was no difference in the rate of congenital anomalies. Cryopreservation of oocytes has been technically much more challenging, as oocytes are more sensitive than embryos due to potential cryoinjury on the spindles, cytoskeleton, cortical granules and zona pellucida. Past studies showed approximately 70% of the cryopreserved oocytes survived the freeze-thaw process and the implantation rates of embryos generated from thawed oocytes are lower than those from fresh cycles.[56,57] Most recently, the survival rate has been reported to be upto 92%, with a pregnancy rate of 57% in some centers.[58]

As for the freezing technique, vitrification yields more favorable outcomes than slow-freezing protocols. The ongoing pregnancy, top-quality embryo, embryo cleavage, and fertilization rate of vitrification approach is similar to fresh oocyte cycles.[59,60] A systematic review and meta-analysis showed that vitrification yields better oocyte survival rate (OR 2.46, 95% CI 1.82–2.32), higher fertilization rate (22.4% vs. 8.0%, OR 3.32, 95% CI 1.37–8.02), and higher day 3 embryo cleavage rate (53.0% vs. 33.3%, OR 2.25, 95% CI 1.32–2.85) compared to slow-freezing.[59]

A recent prospective blind, randomize-controlled study compared the outcome from 295 fresh donor oocytes and 289 vitrified frozen donor oocytes. The fertilization rate (74.2% vs. 73.3%), implantation rate (39.9% vs. 40.9%), clinical pregnancy per cycle (50.2% vs. 49.8%), ongoing pregnancy rate/cycle (44.4% vs. 43.3%) and twin pregnancy rate (32.4% vs. 37.5%) were all similar[61] randomized, controlled, clinical trial (Electronic. (Of note, the donors were 26-years-old on average, while the recipients were 41-years-old.)

A recent study showed that AMH is the most reliable serum marker to predict the outcome of an embryo/oocyte cryopreservation cycle, together with the biophysical marker of AFC. Low response rate is highly likely when AMH level is $\leq$ 1.2 ng/mL.[62]

Ovarian Tissue Transplantation or Preservation

Ovarian tissue may be cryopreserved, with heterotopic (in a different location of the body) re-implantation, orthotopic (in the area that the tissue was removed from) re-implantation, or even with trans-pedicle and vascular supply, which remains investigational. As compared to immature or mature oocyte preservation, ovarian tissue transplantation cyclic hormonal secretion generally resumes after 60 to 244 days.[63–65] Orthotopic transplantation appears to be more successful than heterotopic transplantation. There have been multiple reports of live birth from transplantation of thawed ovarian tissues or orthotopic implantation. None were from breast cancer patients. No live birth from heterotopic transplantation has been reported as of yet.

It is important to identify the appropriate candidates for ovarian tissue cryopreservation, and to ensure that they have sporadic breast cancer and are not *BRCA1* or *BRCA2* (*BRCA1/2*) carriers, as *BRCA1/2* carriers are at increased risk for ovarian cancer (please refer to the special consideration section at the end of chapter).

OVARIAN SUPPRESSION DURING CHEMOTHERAPY

Some believe that chemotherapy toxicity on ovarian tissues may be reduced by suppression of pituitary-ovarian stimulation with GnRH agonists GnRH agonists initiated before chemotherapy and continued until completion of the chemotherapy.

It is thought that the cytotoxicity of the chemotherapy may lead to decreased estradiol, which in turn increases FSH, follicular recruitment and oocytes exposed to chemotoxicity. Through cessation of hypothalamic GnRH secretion, resulting absent FSH and LH and stimulation to the ovaries, GnRH agonists may cause amenorrhea and hypoestrogenism. This may achieve the effect of ovarian protection. However, this protection may occur with side effects such as hot flashes, night sweats, sleep disruption and with longer term use, vaginal dryness. Regardless, the current evidence of its ovarian protection has been inconsistent.

A randomized trial with 60 patients younger than 46 years old with hormone sensitive breast cancer were allocated to AC-based neoadjuvant chemotherapy with or without goserelin.[66] The goserelin was administered at least two weeks before initiation of chemotherapy, and continued at 3.6 mg subcutaneously every 4 weeks until the end of the last cycle. Six months after the end of chemotherapy, no significance was observed in rate (70% versus 56.7%, p=0.284) and time of resumption of menstruation (6.8 versus 6.1 months, p=0.304).

Another randomized, controlled trial with 281 breast cancer patients tested the intervention of triptorelin administered intramuscularly at a dose of 3.75 mg at least one week before chemotherapy initiation and then every four weeks during chemotherapy.[67] It was shown that the rate of early menopause significantly decreased in the chemotherapy with triptorelin group than the chemotherapy alone group (8.9% versus 25.9%, p<0.001). It suggested that triptorelin-induced temporary ovarian suppression during chemotherapy in premenopause patients with early breast cancer may decrease the rate of primary ovarian insufficiency. However, the pregnancy number remains small and the effect on fertility remains uncertain.

A meta-analysis of six randomized trials showed that GnRH agonist use during chemotherapy, when compared to those without GnRH agonist use, indeed increased the likelihood of preserved ovarian function.[68] It increased the incidence of spontaneous menstruation and spontaneous ovulation, but not spontaneous pregnancy (**Table 2**).

ALTERNATIVES—DONOR EGG, GESTATIONAL CARRIER, AND ADOPTION

If fertility preservation methods above are infeasible or unsuccessful, alternative fertility options including donor egg, gestational carrier, and adoption can be considered. Fresh or frozen donor eggs can be obtained from egg banks or from known or anonymous donor through controlled ovarian hyperstimulaion. After fertilization with IVF/ICSI, the embryos can be either cryopreserved for long-term banking or transferred in the future.

While chemotherapy does not affect the uterine function, the patient can carry the pregnancy herself after disease-free

TABLE 2 Meta-analysis on the possible effect of GnRH antagonist on ovarian protection during chemotherapy. [Adapted from Fertil Steril, 2011; 95(3):906-14]

A: Rate of not having premature ovarian failure

	GnRH		*Control*			*Odds ratio*
Study or subgroup	***Events***	***Total***	***Events***	***Total***	***Weight***	***M-H, Random, 95% CI***
Badaway 2008	35	40	13	40	18.9%	14.54 (4.62, 45.78)
Gilani 2007	15	15	10	15	8.8%	16.24 (0.81, 325.88)
Guiseppe 2007	14	14	8	15	8.8%	25.59 (1.29, 506.45)
Sverrisdottir 2009	8	29	2	28	15.6%	4.95 (0.95, 25.86)
Sverrisdottir 2009	2	37	3	29	14.3%	0.50 (0.08, 3.18)
Waxman 1987	4	8	6	10	14.2%	0.67 (0.10, 4.35)
Zoro 2009	21	30	17	30	19.5%	1.78 (0.62, 5.17)
Total (95% CI)		**173**		**167**	**100.0%**	**3.46 (1.13, 10.57)**
Total events	99		59			

Heterogeneity: $Tau^2 = 1.38$; $Chi^2 = 17.68$, df = 6; $I^2 = 66\%$

Test for overall effect: Z = 2.17

Odds ratio M-H, Random, 95%CI

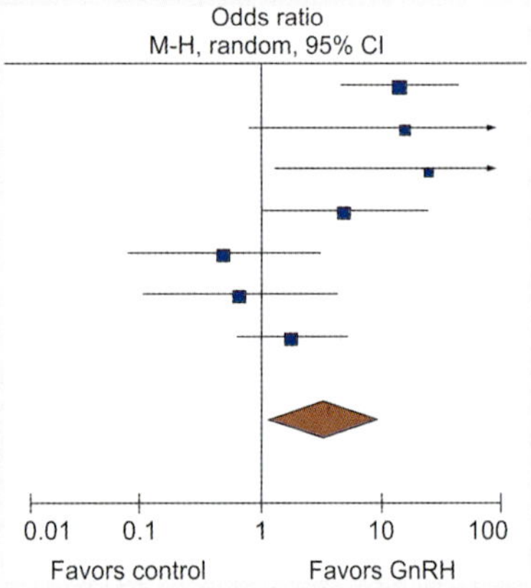

B: Incidence of spontaneous ovulation

	GnRH-a		*Control*			*Odds ratio*
Study or subgroup	***Events***	***Total***	***Events***	***Total***	***Weight***	***M-H, Random, 95% CI***
Badaway 2008	27	40	10	40	87.8%	6.23 (2.35, 16.51)
Waxman 1987	2	8	1	10	12.2%	3.00 (0.22, 40.93)
Total (95% CI)		**48**		**50**	**100.0%**	**5.70 (2.29, 14.20)**
Total events	29		11			

Heterogeneity: $Tau^2 = 0.00$; $Chi^2 = 0.26$, df = 1; $I^2 = 0\%$

Test for overall effect: Z = 3.73

Odds ratio M-H, Random, 95%CI

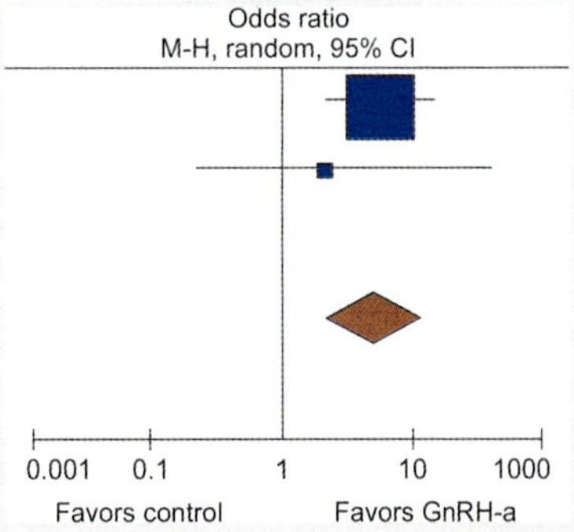

C: Incidence of spontaneous pregnancy

	GnRH-a		***Control***			***Odds ratio***	***Odds ratio***
Study or subgroup	***Events***	***Total***	***Events***	***Total***	***Weight***	***M-H, Random, 95% CI***	***M-H, Random, 95%CI***
Guiseppe 2007	0	14	2	15	32.2%	0.19 (0.01, 4.24)	
Waxman 1987	2	8	1	10	12.2%	0.37 (0/01, 10.43)	
ZORO 2009	1	30	1	30	39.5%	1.00 (0.06, 16.76)	
Total (95% CI)		**52**		**55**	**100.0%**	**0.44 (0.07, 2.59)**	
Total events	1		4				
Heterogeneity: $Tau^2 = 0.00$; $Chi^2 = 0.63$, df = 2; $I^2 = 0\%$							
Test for overall effect: Z = 0.91							

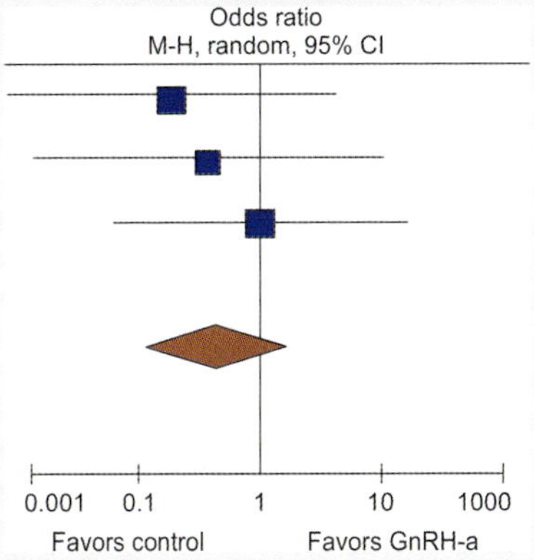

and/or tamoxifen course for at least two years as previously discussed. Medical clearance and maternal-fetal-medicine consultation is required. However, if the patient does not wish to wait or if the general wellness does not allow, a gestational carrier should be considered.

SPECIAL CONSIDERATIONS

Hereditary Breast and Ovarian Cancer Syndromes

The *BRCA1/2* genes operate as tumor suppressor genes and are essential for double-stranded DNA break repair. Although, the prevalence is only 1–2% in the general population and only 5–10% of breast cancers are linked to the *BRCA1/2* gene, the *BRCA* mutation leads to a significantly elevated lifetime risk of 56 to 84% of breast cancer and elevated life-time risks for ovarian cancer (36 to 63% for *BRCA1* and 10 to 27% for *BRCA2*). Effective management options include prophylactic mastectomy, risk reducing salpingo-oophorectomy, chemoprevention with tamoxifen and oral contraception pills, routine surveillance for ovarian cancer with CA-125, pelvic exam and transvaginal ultrasound every 6 months and routine surveillance for breast cancer with mammography, and breast MRI annually.[69]

Among those methods, oral contraceptive pills decrease the risk for ovarian cancer by 60%. Tamoxifen decreases contralateral breast cancer by 75% in affected *BRCA* carriers, and by 62% in unaffected carriers. Prophylactic mastectomy reduces greater than 90% of breast cancer risk. Risk reducing salpingo-oophorectomy has been shown to have a protective effect in reducing the risk of ovarian cancer by 96% and breast cancer by 60%.[70] It may be part of the treatment plan in patients with a breast cancer diagnosis, or in healthy *BRCA* carriers. As there is no consensus for the best timing for this procedure in healthy carriers, generally salpingo-oophorectomy is recommended after completion childbearing.

In healthy carriers, cryopreservation of oocytes and/or embryos may be performed based on the patient's choice. However, they are not appropriate candidates for cryopreservation of ovarian tissue as there is a risk of occult ovarian cancer or a potential risk of developing ovarian cancer.

A recent study by Lin et al. shows that *BRCA1/2* carriers are at significant risk of earlier natural menopause by 3–4 years and those who are current heavy cigarette smokers may undergo even earlier menopause.[71] Moreover, Oktay et al. observed that *BRCA1* carriers diagnosed with breast cancer, when compared to non-carriers, are poorer responders to ovarian stimulation with letrozole/FSH protocol before chemotherapy for breast cancer (3% versus 33%) and yield fewer eggs (7 versus 12).[72] These findings imply occult ovarian insufficiency in *BRCA1/2* carriers. Further studies are undergoing to clarify the association of *BRCA1/2* mutation and diminished ovarian reserve and to investigate the underlying mechanism.

Clinically, although there is no evidence showing differences in natural fertility or miscarriage rates in *BRCA1/2* carriers,[73,74] the findings of occult primary ovarian insufficiency, including poor ovarian stimulation response and early menopause carry important implications. Because the relationship between the ending of natural fertility and age at natural menopause is thought to be approximately 10 years,[75] it is important to provide adequate counseling for *BRCA* carriers and advise early planning of childbearing.

SUMMARY

In summary, the National Comprehensive Cancer Network (NCCN) Guideline[76] recommends that:

- All premenopausal patients should be informed about the potential impact of chemotherapy on fertility and asked about their desire for potential future pregnancies. Patients who may desire future pregnancies should be referred to fertility specialists before chemotherapy.

- Although amenorrhea frequently occurs during or after chemotherapy, it appears that the majority of women younger than 35-years-old resume menses within two years of finishing adjuvant chemotherapy. (Most recover within one year.)
- Menses and fertility are not necessarily linked. Absence of regular menses, particularly if the patient is taking tamoxifen, does not necessarily imply lack of fertility. Conversely, the presence of menses does not guarantee fertility. There is limited data regarding fertility after chemotherapy.
- Patients should not become pregnant during treatment with radiation therapy, chemotherapy, or endocrine therapy.
- Although the data is limited, hormone-based birth control is discouraged, regardless of the hormone receptor status of the patient's breast cancer.
- No therapy has been proven to preserve fertility in patients receiving chemotherapy.
- Breast feeding following breast conserving cancer treatment is not contraindicated. However, the quantity and quality of breast milk produced by the breast conserved may not be sufficient or may be lacking some of the nutrients needed. Breast feeding during active treatment with chemotherapy and endocrine therapy is not recommended.

REFERENCES

1. Society AC. Breast Cancer Facts & Figures 2011-2012. 2012.
2. Institute NC. Surveillance Epidemiology and End Results (SEER) Stat Fact Sheets: Breast Cancer. 2012.
3. Partridge AH, et al. Web-based survey of fertility issues in young women with breast cancer. J Clin Oncol. 2004; 22(20): 4174-83.
4. Duffy CM, Allen SM, Clark MA. Discussions regarding reproductive health for young women with breast cancer undergoing chemotherapy. J Clin Oncol. 2005; 23(4): 766-73.
5. Lee SJ, et al. American Society of Clinical Oncology recommendations on fertility preservation in cancer patients. J Clin Oncol. 2006; 24(18): 2917-31.
6. Lee S, et al. Value of early referral to fertility preservation in young women with breast cancer. J Clin Oncol. 2010; 28(31):4683-6.
7. Meirow D. Reproduction post-chemotherapy in young cancer patients. Mol Cell Endocrinol. 2000;169(1-2):123-31.
8. Meirow D, et al. Toxicity of chemotherapy and radiation on female reproduction. Clin Obstet Gynecol. 2010;53(4):727-39.
9. Schilsky RL, et al. Gonadal dysfunction in patients receiving chemotherapy for cancer. Ann Intern Med. 1980;93(1):109-14.
10. Hershlag A, Schuster MW. Return of fertility after autologous stem cell transplantation. Fertil Steril. 2002;77(2):419-21.
11. Bakri YN, Pederson P, Nassar M. Normal pregnancy after curative multiagent chemotherapy for choriocarcinoma with brain metastases. Acta Obstet Gynecol Scand. 1991;70(7-8):611-3.
12. Walshe JM, Denduluri N, Swain SM. Amenorrhea in premenopausal women after adjuvant chemotherapy for breast cancer. J Clin Oncol. 2006;24(36):5769-79.
13. Meirow D, Nugent D. The effects of radiotherapy and chemotherapy on female reproduction. Hum Reprod Update. 2001;7(6):535-43.
14. Petrek JA, et al. Incidence, time course, and determinants of menstrual bleeding after breast cancer treatment: a prospective study. J Clin Oncol. 2006;24(7):1045-51.
15. Epstein RJ. Drug-induced DNA damage and tumor chemosensitivity. J Clin Oncol. 1990;8(12):2062-84.
16. Koyama H, et al. Cyclophosphamide-induced ovarian failure and its therapeutic significance in patients with breast cancer. Cancer. 1977; 39(4):1403-9.
17. Warne GL, et al. Cyclophosphamide-induced ovarian failure. N Engl J Med. 1973; 289(22):1159-62.
18. Falcone T, et al. Ovarian function preservation in the cancer patient. Fertil Steril. 2004; 81(2):243-57.
19. Sonmezer M, Oktay K. Fertility preservation in female patients. Hum Reprod Update. 2004;10(3):251-66.
20. Bines J, Oleske DM, Cobleigh MA. Ovarian function in premenopausal women treated with adjuvant chemotherapy for breast cancer. J Clin Oncol. 1996;14(5):1718-29.
21. Abusief ME, et al. The effects of paclitaxel, dose density, and trastuzumab on treatment-related amenorrhea in premenopausal women with breast cancer. Cancer. 2010;116(4):791-8.
22. Anderson RA, Cameron DA. Pretreatment serum anti-mullerian hormone predicts long-term ovarian function and bone mass after chemotherapy for early breast cancer. J Clin Endocrinol Metab. 2011;96(5):1336-43.
23. Oktem O,Oktay K. Quantitative assessment of the impact of chemotherapy on ovarian follicle reserve and stromal function. Cancer. 2007;110(10):2222-9.
24. Partridge AH, et al. Ovarian reserve in women who remain premenopausal after chemotherapy for early stage breast cancer. Fertil Steril. 2010;94(2):638-44.
25. Gelber S, et al. Effect of pregnancy on overall survival after the diagnosis of early-stage breast cancer. J Clin Oncol. 2001;19(6): 1671-5.
26. Lawrenz B, et al. Pregnancy after breast cancer: case report and review of the literature. Arch Gynecol Obstet. 2011;283(4):837-43.
27. Glen CD, Dubrova YE. Exposure to anticancer drugs can result in transgenerational genomic instability in mice. Proc Natl Acad Sci. USA. 2012;109(8):2984-8.
28. Green DM, et al. Pregnancy outcome of female survivors of childhood cancer: a report from the Childhood Cancer Survivor Study. Am J Obstet Gynecol. 2002;187(4):1070-80.
29. Chiarelli AM, Marrett LD, Darlington GA. Pregnancy outcomes in females after treatment for childhood cancer. Epidemiology. 2000; 11(2):161-6.
30. Reulen RC, et al. Pregnancy outcomes among adult survivors of childhood cancer in the British Childhood Cancer Survivor Study. Cancer Epidemiol Biomarkers Prev. 2009; 18(8): 2239-47.
31. Barton SE, et al. Female cancer survivors are low responders and have reduced success compared with other patients undergoing assisted reproductive technologies. Fertil Steril. 2012;97(2):381-6.
32. Partridge AH, et al. Fertility and menopausal outcomes in young breast cancer survivors. Clin Breast Cancer. 2008; 8(1):65-9.
33. Ives A, et al. Pregnancy after breast cancer: population based study. BMJ. 2007;334(7586):194.
34. Das M, et al. Ovarian reserve, response to gonadotropins, and oocyte maturity in women with malignancy. Fertil Steril. 2011;96(1):122-5.
35. Knopman JM, et al. Women with cancer undergoing ART for fertility preservation: a cohort study of their response to exogenous gonadotropins. Fertil Steril. 2009; 91(4 Suppl):1476-8.
36. Quintero RB, et al. Ovarian stimulation for fertility preservation in patients with cancer. Fertil Steril. 2010;93(3):865-8.
37. Azim AA, Costantini-Ferrando M, Oktay K. Safety of fertility preservation by ovarian stimulation with letrozole and gonadotropins

in patients with breast cancer: a prospective controlled study. J Clin Oncol. 2008;26(16):2630-5.
38. Ginsburg ES, Yanushpolsky EH, Jackson KV. In vitro fertilization for cancer patients and survivors. Fertil Steril. 2001;75(4):705-10.
39. Dolmans MM, et al. Efficacy of in vitro fertilization after chemotherapy. Fertil Steril. 2005;83(4):897-901.
40. Oktay K. Further evidence on the safety and success of ovarian stimulation with letrozole and tamoxifen in breast cancer patients undergoing in vitro fertilization to cryopreserve their embryos for fertility preservation. J Clin Oncol. 2005;23(16):3858-9.
41. Azim AA, et al. Relative potencies of anastrozole and letrozole to suppress estradiol in breast cancer patients undergoing ovarian stimulation before in vitro fertilization. J Clin Endocrinol Metab. 2007; 2(6):2197-200.
42. Oktay K, et al. Fertility preservation in breast cancer patients: a prospective controlled comparison of ovarian stimulation with tamoxifen and letrozole for embryo cryopreservation. J Clin Oncol. 2005;23(19):4347-53.
43. Oktay K, Turkcuoglu I, Rodriguez-Wallberg KA. GnRH agonist trigger for women with breast cancer undergoing fertility preservation by aromatase inhibitor/FSH stimulation. Reprod Biomed Online. 2010;20(6):783-8.
44. Maman E, et al. Luteal phase oocyte retrieval and in vitro maturation is an optional procedure for urgent fertility preservation. Fertil Steril. 2011;95(1):64-7.
45. Oktay K, et al. In vitro maturation improves oocyte or embryo cryopreservation outcome in breast cancer patients undergoing ovarian stimulation for fertility preservation. Reprod Biomed Online. 2010;20(5):634-8.
46. Huang JY, et al. Combining ovarian tissue cryobanking with retrieval of immature oocytes followed by in vitro maturation and vitrification: an additional strategy of fertility preservation. Fertil Steril. 2008;89(3): 567-72.
47. Telfer EE, McLaughlin M. In vitro development of ovarian follicles. Semin Reprod Med. 2011;29(1):15-23.
48. Jurema MW, Nogueira D. In vitro maturation of human oocytes for assisted reproduction. Fertil Steril. 2006;86(5):1277-91.
49. Smitz JE, Thompson JG, Gilchrist RB. The promise of in vitro maturation in assisted reproduction and fertility preservation. Semin Reprod Med. 2011;29(1):24-37.
50. Chian RC, et al. Obstetric outcomes following vitrification of in vitro and in vivo matured oocytes. Fertil Steril. 2009;91(6):2391-8.
51. Chian RC, et al. Live birth after vitrification of in vitro matured human oocytes. Fertil Steril. 2009;91(2):372-6.
52. Sonmezer M, et al. Random-start controlled ovarian hyperstimulation for emergency fertility preservation in letrozole cycles. Fertil Steril. 2011;95(6):2125 e9-11.
53. Essential elements of informed consent for elective oocyte cryopreservation: a Practice Committee opinion. Fertil Steril. 2007; 88(6):1495-6.
54. Mature oocyte cryopreservation: a guideline. Fertil Steril 2013;99(1): 37-43.
55. Noyes N, Porcu E, Borini A. Over 900 oocyte cryopreservation babies born with no apparent increase in congenital anomalies. Reprod Biomed Online. 2009;18(6):769-76.
56. Ambrosini G, et al. Oocytes cryopreservation: state of art. Reprod Toxicol. 2006; 22(2): 250-62.
57. Jain JK, Paulson RJ. Oocyte cryopreservation. Fertil Steril. 2006;86 (4 Suppl): 1037-46.
58. Grifo JA,Noyes N. Delivery rate using cryopreserved oocytes is comparable to conventional in vitro fertilization using fresh oocytes: potential fertility preservation for female cancer patients. Fertil Steril. 2010;93(2): 391-6.
59. Cobo A, Diaz C. Clinical application of oocyte vitrification: a systematic review and meta-analysis of randomized controlled trials. Fertil Steril. 2011;96(2): 277-85.
60. Oktay K, Cil AP, Bang H. Efficiency of oocyte cryopreservation: a meta-analysis. Fertil Steril. 2006; 86(1):70-80.
61. Cobo A, et al. Use of cryo-banked oocytes in an ovum donation programme: a prospective, randomized, controlled, clinical trial. Hum Reprod. 2010; 25(9): 2239-46.
62. Lee S, et al. Anti-Mullerian hormone and antral follicle count as predictors for embryo/oocyte cryopreservation cycle outcomes in breast cancer patients stimulated with letrozole and follicle stimulating hormone. J Assist Reprod Genet. 2011;28(7):651-6.
63. Bedaiwy MA, et al. Reproductive outcome after transplantation of ovarian tissue: a systematic review. Hum Reprod. 2008;23(12): 2709-17.
64. Bedaiwy MA, Shahin AY, Falcone T. Reproductive organ transplantation: advances and controversies. Fertil Steril. 2008; 90(6): 2031-55.
65. Kim SS, et al. Long-term ovarian function and fertility after heterotopic autotransplantation of cryobanked human ovarian tissue: 8-year experience in cancer patients. Fertil Steril. 2009;91(6): 2349-54.
66. Gerber B, et al. Effect of luteinizing hormone-releasing hormone agonist on ovarian function after modern adjuvant breast cancer chemotherapy: the GBG 37 ZORO study. J Clin Oncol. 2011; 29(17): 2334-41.
67. Del Mastro L, et al. Effect of the gonadotropin-releasing hormone analogue triptorelin on the occurrence of chemotherapy-induced early menopause in premenopausal women with breast cancer: a randomized trial. JAMA 2011;306(3): 269-76.
68. Bedaiwy MA, et al. Gonadotropin-releasing hormone analog cotreatment for preservation of ovarian function during gonadotoxic chemotherapy: a systematic review and meta-analysis. Fertil Steril. 2011;95(3):906-14 e1-4.
69. Robson M, Offit K. Clinical practice. Management of an inherited predisposition to breast cancer. N Engl J Med. 2007;357(2):154-62.
70. Heemskerk-Gerritsen BA, Kriege M, Seynaeve C. Association of risk-reducing surgery with cancer risks and mortality in BRCA mutation carriers. JAMA 2010; 304(24): 2695; author reply 2695-6.
71. Lin WT, et al. Comparison of age at natural menopause in BRCA1/2 mutation carriers with a non-clinic-based sample of women in northern California. Cancer. 2013 May 1;119(9):1652-972.
72. Oktay K, et al. Association of BRCA1 mutations with occult primary ovarian insufficiency: a possible explanation for the link between infertility and breast/ovarian cancer risks. J Clin Oncol. 2010;28(2): 240-4.
73. Pal T, et al. Fertility in women with BRCA mutations: a case-control study. Fertil Steril. 2010;93(6):1805-8.
74. Moslehi R, et al. Impact of BRCA mutations on female fertility and offspring sex ratio. Am J Hum Biol. 2010;22(2):201-5.
75. Evers JL. Female subfertility. Lancet. 2002; 360(9327):151-9.
76. National Comprehensive Cancer Network (NCCN) Guideline 2013.

Section 2

Fertility Preservation Strategies in the Male

15

Pathology Affecting Male Fertility

Edmund Y Ko, Edmund S Sabanegh Jr

CHAPTER OUTLINE

INTRODUCTION

Male factor is found to be responsible in up to 50% of couples presenting for infertility evaluation.[1] The American Urological Association and the American Society for Reproductive Medicine have produced guidelines outlining the optimal evaluation and management of the infertile male.[2]

A thorough male evaluation is performed to identify: (a) potentially reversible conditions, (b) irreversible conditions that are best managed with assisted reproductive techniques (ART) using the male's sperm, (c) irreversible conditions that are not treatable with ART, (d) potentially life/health-threatening conditions that may be the cause of infertility and require intervention and (e) genetic abnormalities that have implications for the health of the male and his offspring if ART are utilized.[2]

The goals of this chapter are to briefly review the evaluation of the male and to discuss the variety of presenting pathology (**Table 1**) that can cause infertility as well as its management.

EVALUATION

History

A history and physical should be performed for every male presenting for infertility evaluation. A detailed discussion should include a thorough reproductive, sexual, infectious disease, childhood and development, medical, surgical, medication, social, gonadotoxin exposure and family history. The purpose of a detailed history is to elucidate any risk factors and to capture any problems that may play a role and be potentially treatable. A detailed history plays an important role because male factor infertility is oftentimes attributable to multifactorial causes.

The reproductive history includes the duration of infertility, any prior pregnancies with the current or previous partners and prior fertility treatments. This history also includes a brief review of the female partner and her prior pregnancy history, contraception use, prior gynecological evaluation, as well as any fertility therapies that she has been or is currently on. The

TABLE 1 Pathology affecting male fertility

• **GU anomalies** – Undescended testis – Varicoceles – Ductal obstruction (EDO, CBAVD) – Ejaculatory disorders (Premature, retrograde, delayed/absent)	• **Genetic anomalies** – Kallmann syndrome – Klinefelter Syndrome – Other (Y-linked microdeletion; 47,XYY; XX male syndrome; mixed gonadal dysgenesis; translocations)
• **Endocrinopathies** – Hyperprolactinemia – Diabetes mellitus – Thyroid abnormalities	• **Malignancies** – Testicular cancer – Other (lymphoma, leukemia, etc.)

sexual history assesses frequency and timing of intercourse, methods used for timing ovulation and use of any lubricants that can be detrimental to sperm function. Libido, erectile and ejaculatory quality should also be noted. Anejaculation, premature ejaculation and decreased ejaculatory volume should prompt additional history taking and investigation. Any previous infections with and treatments of, sexually transmitted diseases, including chlamydia and gonorrhea, can also result in male infertility.

Childhood and developmental histories are both very important in the evaluation of the infertile male. A history of undescended testicles or post-pubertal mumps orchitis can affect future spermatogenesis. Testicular trauma or torsion can result in atrophy of the testes. Timing of puberty should also be noted. Any significant deviation from normal developmental milestones may suggest an underlying endocrine disorder.

Many medical conditions can affect male fertility, including diabetes mellitus, multiple sclerosis, myotonic dystrophy, cirrhosis, recent febrile illnesses, chronic or recurrent upper respiratory infections, cystic fibrosis, hypothyroidism, cancer with prior chemoradiation therapy, chronic prostatitis or epididymitis, urinary tract infections and varicocele. These medical conditions may be indirectly linked to infertility and may only be a single syndrome in a constellation of symptoms.

Medications used to treat underlying chronic medical conditions may have side effects resulting in sexual or testicular dysfunction (**Table 2**). Over-the-counter vitamins and supplements should also be included in the medication list, as some supplements can have detrimental effects on spermatogenesis. It is important to involve the patient's primary physician or specialist overseeing his medical care in order to see if any of these medications can be safely stopped or changed to other acceptable alternatives, which may have less impact on his fertility.

Surgical procedures performed around genitourinary structures vital to reproduction may detrimentally affect fertility. Prior pituitary, retroperitoneal, pelvic, prostatic, inguinal, penile, urethral, scrotal, or testicular surgery should prompt additional investigation. Any of these surgeries can potentially affect the production or delivery of sperm.

A patient's social history should also be discussed. Substances, such as tobacco, excessive alcohol and marijuana,

TABLE 2 Medications with potential detrimental effects on male fertility

• **α-blockers** • **Androgens** – Anabolic steroids – Testosterone • **Anti-androgens** – Biclutaminde – Ketoconazole • **Antibiotics** – Chloraquine – Co-Trimazole – Erythromycin – Minocycline – Nitrofurantoin – Tetracycline • **Anti-depressants** – Fluoxetine – Imiprimine – Paroxetine • **Anti-hypertensives** – Metoprolol – Nifedipine – Spironolactone • **Anti-inflammatory** – Colchicine – Sulfasalazine	• **Anti-psychotics** – Chlorpromazine – Lithium • **Chemotherapeutic agents** – Chlorambucil – Cisplatin – Cyclophosphamide – Melphalen – Methotrexate – Procarbazine • **5α-reductase inhibitors** – Dutasteride – Finasteride • **Gonadotropic releasing Hormone analogs** – Goserelin – Leuprolide • **H_2 blocker** – Cimetidine • **Opiates** – Hydrocodone – Methadone – Morphine – Oxycodone

can affect sperm production and function as well as overall health. Prior anabolic steroid or testosterone use for muscle building or history and treatment of hypogonadism should also be determined. An occupation that exposes a patient to radiation, excessive heat, or chemicals/fumes/toxins/pesticides can also play a role in male infertility.

A family history of infertility should prompt additional history into which family members are affected, the etiology (if available), as well as previous testing (including genetic testing) and therapies used to achieve pregnancy. Cystic fibrosis history is also pertinent to the discussion, as well as any other familial genetic disorders.

A thorough review of systems should include assessment of general well-being (energy, mood, concentration), weight gain or loss, chronic headaches, visual changes, hearing loss, sense of smell, history of recurrent upper respiratory infections, cardiac issues, gastrointestinal problems (constipation or diarrhea), psychiatric abnormalities and neurologic derangements.

Physical

A focused physical examination is performed. The general appearance of the male is noted to assess virilization and body habitus. Special attention is given to those who are obese, tall, or eunuchoid in appearance. The chest is examined for the presence of gynecomastia and nipple discharge, which could be manifestations of a prolactinoma. The abdomen is examined for the presence of prior surgical incisions, hepatic enlargement and masses. The groin is examined for the presence of lymphadenopathy, hernias and surgical incisions indicating prior hernia repairs or surgery for undescended testicles, since these may have occurred at a very young age.

A thorough genital examination is performed noting Tanner stage and genital development. The foreskin of an uncircumcised penis is carefully retracted and the glans penis and location and size of the urethral meatus are noted. The presence of hypospadias, meatal stenosis, or significant penile angulation (Peyronie's disease) may prevent normal deposition of semen within the vagina.

A complete testicular assessment includes assessment of volume, location and lie of each within the scrotum. Abnormally high testicles may be a sign of maldescent, retractile testes, or prior surgical attempts to treat an undescended testicle. The size, shape and consistency of the testicles are noted and compared to each other. Normal testicular size is approximately 18 to 20 cubic centimeters, with a majority of the testicular volume consisting of seminiferous tubules.[3] The epididymis on each side is palpated to assess for fullness or masses. The cord structures are palpated to confirm the presence of a vas deferens bilaterally and to assess for the presence of spermatic cord varicocities called varicoceles. Abnormal or suspicious findings necessitate evaluation with a testicular ultrasound.

A digital rectal examination (DRE) is indicated for patients suspected to have obstructive etiology for their infertility or who are at least 40-years-old. Reduced anal sphincter tone may suggest possible neurologic abnormalities. Attention is given to overall prostate size, consistency, nodules, tenderness or pain with palpation and the presence of abnormal midline structures. Abnormal DREs require additional investigation as to their etiology, which may include serum prostate specific antigen (PSA) levels, a transrectal ultrasound (TRUS) and prostate biopsy.

Diagnostic Studies

The cornerstone of male infertility testing is the semen analysis. At least two specimens separated by 2 to 3 weeks provided after 2 to 3 days of abstinence should be analyzed to ensure consistency in the results. In 2010, the World Health Organization (WHO) released semen analysis criteria updated from their previous publication in 1999. Important normal variables (**Table 3**) include volume of at least 1.5 milliliters (mL), pH of at least 7.2, concentration of at least 15 million sperm per mL, total motility of at least 40% and strict normal morphology of > 4%.[4] Patients with low volume ejaculate and an acidic seminal pH may have ductal obstruction. A positive seminal fructose suggests ejaculatory duct patency, although further evaluation with a transrectal ultrasound is warranted to confirm such a suggestion. Although additional imaging with computed tomography (CT) or magnetic resonance imaging (MRI) could be performed, it is not necessary to achieve the diagnosis.

Abnormalities on or difficulties in performing an adequate scrotal examination due to body habitus or an undescended testicle necessitates evaluation with testicular ultrasonography (US). US can be used to verify the presence of a varicocele or abnormal masses palpated on examination. In patients, who may be surgical candidates, testicular imaging prior to surgery ensures that there is no additional pathology that also requires attention at the time of surgery (i.e. testicular tumors).

TABLE 3: Comparison of WHO semen analysis

	WHO 1999	*WHO 2010*
Volume (mL)	≥2	≥1.5
pH	≥7.2	≥7.2
Concentration (Million/mL)	≥20	≥15
Total count (Million)	≥40	≥22.5
Motility (%)	≥50%	≥40%
Morphology	WHO > 50% Strict > 14%	Strict > 4%
WBC (Million/mL)	< 1	< 1

Adapted from WHO 1999 & WHO 2000[4,67]

Patients with signs and symptoms of an endocrinopathy, warrant additional evaluation to identify underlying pathology contributing to sub-infertility and provide prognostic information that may aid in management. Signs include morbid obesity, gynecomastia, atrophic testicles, underdeveloped genitalia and significant oligospermia. Symptoms include low libido, erectile dysfunction, low energy levels and loss of concentration. Risk factors include use of marijuana, testosterone, or anabolic steroid abuse.

A basic endocrine evaluation includes early morning serum total testosterone and follicle stimulating hormone (FSH) levels. A complete endocrine evaluation additionally includes serum luteinizing hormone (LH), prolactin and estradiol levels. Elevated prolactin levels may be the result of a prolactinoma and requires additional evaluation, including a MRI scan of the head, with special emphasis on the pituitary gland to assess for a possible pituitary adenoma. Patients exhibiting symptoms concerning for hypothyroidism should also have a serum thyroid stimulating hormone (TSH) level evaluated. Patients with the presence of glucose on screening urinalysis should be referred to their primary care physicians for evaluation and treatment of diabetes mellitus.

Genetic testing is reserved for males with severe oligospermia of < 5 million sperm per milliliter without any identifiable cause and those with non-obstructive azoospermia.[5] Couples with recurrent unexplained miscarriages may also benefit from testing. Genetic testing includes serum karyotype as well as a Y chromosome-linked microdeletion assay. Men with congenital bilateral absence of the vas deferens (CBAVD) require testing for mutations of the cystic fibrosis transmembrane conductance regulator (CFTR) located on chromosome 7 (7q31.2) 6. In addition to identification of genetic abnormalities in the patient, these tests provide crucial information regarding transmissible conditions.

Transrectal ultrasonography is reserved for patients with obstructive azoospermia with suspicion of ejaculatory duct obstruction (EDO), based on findings on semen analysis (low volume ejaculate, acidic pH) and physical examination. Imaging signs of ductal obstruction include the presence of ejaculatory duct stones, a midline obstructing cyst, or dilation of the seminal vesicles greater than 15 mm in width.[7] Needle aspiration of the seminal vesicles during TRUS can also be performed to evaluate for the presence of sperm that may be present with ejaculatory duct obstruction.

Flexible cystourethroscopy may be undertaken to evaluate the ejaculatory ducts and veru montanum if the TRUS is non-diagnostic. The presence of a cystic mass confirms the presence of EDO.

Male infertility patients are also screened with a routine urinalysis. The presence of microscopic hematuria, proteinuria, or glucosuria requires further investigative testing and referrals for evaluation. Men with risk factors for retrograde ejaculation (diabetes mellitus, spinal cord injury, etc.) and low volume ejaculate on semen analysis should have a postejaculatory urinalysis examined for the presence of sperm.

PATHOLOGY

Genitourinary (GU) Anomalies

Cryptorchidism

The incidence of cryptorchidism, or undescended testicle (UDT), is approximately 3–5% in full-term newborn boys.[8] Up to 33% of premature boys have cryptorchidism. The incidence decreases to less than 1% by one year of age.[9] Up to 25% of males with cryptorchidism will have bilateral undescended testes.

Unilateral cryptorchidism does not appear to effect spermatogenesis as severely as bilateral cryptorchidism.[10,11] Thirty percent of men with unilateral UDT will have decreased sperm density and 85% will have normal fertility despite early orchiopexy. In comparison, 50% of men with bilateral UDT will have decreased sperm density and up to 65% will have normal fertility after bilateral orchiopexy. Post-pubertal men with persistent bilateral UDTs usually have azoospermia, although 28% of them will have normal sperm counts if they have undergone bilateral orchidopexy.[12]

Early surgical correction of unilateral UDT has not been demonstrated to improve fertility rates in the pre-pubertal male, although a significant difference was seen in males with bilateral UDT.[13] Males with surgical correction of UDT are likely to have antisperm antibodies affecting sperm function.[12] Males with a history of UDT should be instructed to perform regular self-examinations given the higher lifetime risk of testicular cancer.[14] Early orchiopexy does not negate the risk of cancer, but improves the ability to monitor the testicles with regular examinations. Testicular US should be obtained on initial evaluation to identify any non-palpable masses, prior to any surgical intervention for infertility treatment.

Varicocele

Varicoceles are the most commonly diagnosed reversible cause of male infertility. Varicoceles are abnormally dilated internal spermatic veins due to incompetent valves and usually appear around the time of puberty. Testicular function appears to be detrimentally affected by elevated scrotal temperature secondary to retrograde pooling of blood in the testicle.[15] This can result in sperm abnormalities, sub-fertility, as well as lower testosterone levels.[16] Exposure to known gonadotoxins (tobacco, chemotherapy, etc.), with the presence of a varicocele, may result in increased testicular insult than the varicocele or gonadotoxin alone.[17]

Varicoceles are diagnosed in approximately 15 to 20% of the general male population, 40% of males with primary infertility, and up to 80% of males with secondary infertility.[18] Pediatric patients with varicoceles should be considered for therapy if there is reduced testicular volume of the ipsilateral testicle.[19] Up to 75% of men with varicoceles are fertile.[20]

Varicoceles are diagnosed by physical examination or scrotal US. They are graded on physical examination in the standing position by the Dubin grading system on a scale from 1 to 3:[18]

Grade 1: Only palpable during valsalva

Grade 2: Palpable without valsalva

Grade 3: Visible through scrotal skin

Palpable varicoceles are known as clinical varicoceles. A non-palpable varicocele diagnosed solely on US is a sub-clinical varicocele. US criteria for a varicocele includes vein diameter $\geq$3.0 mm and reversal of blood flow with valsalva.[21]

According to the American Society for Reproductive Medicine (ASRM), varicocele treatment should be considered if the following four criteria are met: (a) the varicocele is palpable on physical examination; (b) the couple has infertility; (c) the female partner has normal fertility or treatable cause of infertility; and (d) there are abnormalities in semen analysis results or sperm function tests.[19] Males with normal semen analysis or subclinical varicoceles should not undergo varicocele repair.[15,19]

Varicoceles can be treated with surgical or interventional radiology (IR) approaches. There are many different surgical approaches, but the core principle involves ligating the internal spermatic vein(s) to prevent reflux back to the testicles. Different approaches include open subinguinal, inguinal, retroperitoneal, and laparoscopic. IR guided percutaneous embolization can also be employed to stop reflux primarily or as a salvage technique for a failed surgical repair.

Approximately 66% (range 51–78%) and 43% (range of 24–53%) of patients undergoing varicocele treatment will demonstrate improvements in semen parameters and overall pregnancy rate, respectively.[22] Other studies also demonstrate improvements in hormone parameters and pregnancy rates with intrauterine insemination and in vitro fertilization (IVF).[16,23] Many clinicians believe that untreated varicoceles will have a progressive negative effect on testicular function, although the available data is not conclusive.[15]

Ductal Obstruction

Ductal obstruction can occur anywhere along the genital tract starting in the testicle and proceeding distally to the ejaculatory duct in the prostatic urethra and can result in azoospermia. Forty percent of azoospermia can be attributed to ductal obstruction.[24] Etiologies include congenital, traumatic or iatrogenic, inflammatory and idiopathic causes. Treatment approaches range from surgical sperm retrieval with testicular biopsy and sperm extraction (TESE) or percutaneous sperm aspiration (PESA), as well as microsurgical reconstruction with vasovasostomy or vasoepididymostomy.

The most common congenital cause of ductal obstruction is congenital bilateral absence of the vas deferens (CBAVD). It is found in approximately 1% of males presenting for infertility evaluation and in 1 to 2% of men with azoospermia.[6] This is often associated with cystic fibrosis and can result in non-development of the mesonephric (Wolffian) structures, including the vas deferens, seminal vesicles and epididymis. CBAVD is associated with mutations of the CFTR gene located on chromosome 7 (7q31.2).[6] Greater than 65% of males with cystic fibrosis have CBAVD. Conversely, over 75% of males with CBAVD will be found have mutations on the CFTR gene.[25]

Patients usually present with low volume azoospermia with acidic pH because of atretic seminal vesicles and secretion of acidic prostatic fluid. These patients and their partners should undergo genetic evaluation for CFTR mutations prior to attempting any ART. Surgical reconstruction is not appropriate for these patients and they must rely on surgical sperm retrieval and IVF to achieve pregnancy.

Obstruction can also occur due to trauma, iatrogenic causes, and infection. The vas deferens can be inadvertently injured during hernia surgeries or obstructed secondary to scarring from mesh placement.[26] One of the most common iatrogenic causes of vasal obstruction is vasectomy, performed for permanent sterilization. The site of obstruction is primarily located at the surgical site, but high intraluminal pressures can be transmitted to the delicate epididymal tubules proximally resulting in secondary obstruction.[27] Infections with Chlamydia can cause infectious epididymitis. Tuberculosis and sarcoidosis can also result in a granulomatous infection and subsequent epididymal obstruction. Oftentimes, these obstructions can be bypassed with microsurgical correction with primary vasovasostomy or vasoepididymostomy. Empty epididymis syndrome can also result from prolonged distal obstruction resulting in obstruction at the level of the rete testis. These patients are best treated with TESE and IVF.

Patients can also have ejaculatory duct obstruction, occurring at the most distal portion of the excurrent ductal system. EDO occurs in approximately 1–5% of patients with infertility.[28] Patients may present with infertility, hematospermia, or pain with ejaculation. Physical examination may reveal dilated epididymides bilaterally. In some patients, there may be palpable seminal vesicles and a midline mass on rectal examination. Patients with partial obstruction may have a completely normal examination on one or both sides.

Semen analysis may demonstrate low volume (<1.0 mL) azoospermia, an acidic pH of <7.2, and the absence of fructose in the seminal fluid. Evaluation with TRUS will reveal dilated seminal vesicles >1.5 cm in diameter in the anterior-posterior orientation, as well as a dilated ejaculatory duct >2.3 mm, confirming EDO.[28] Calcifications or a midline cyst may also be seen on a transverse image of the prostate. Seminal vesicle aspiration at the time of TRUS demonstrating >3 sperm per high powered field is also suggestive of EDO. Cystoscopy does not usually provide additional information. Non-conclusive evaluations may necessitate pelvic MRI.[28]

Patients diagnosed with EDO can be treated with a transurethral resection of the ejaculatory duct (TURED) to unroof the obstruction, allowing ejaculate to enter the urethra.

Ejaculatory Disorders

Ejaculation is an important physiologic delivery mechanism for sperm to enter the female reproductive tract during intercourse. The involved organs include the epididymis, vas deferens, prostate, seminal vesicles, bladder neck, and bulbourethral glands.[29] Prior to ejaculation, sperm is stored in the epididymis. During arousal and sexual stimulation, sperm slowly flows into the vas deferens. During ejaculation, the sperm is rapidly transmitted to the urethra through vasal peristalsis and mixes with the seminal and prostatic fluid to form semen. Normal ejaculation requires bladder neck contraction to prevent retrograde ejaculation, as well as rhythmic contractions of the periurethral muscles to propel the bolus of semen through the urethra. Natural ejaculation requires the presence of an intact coordinated interaction of the parasympathetic and sympathetic autonomic nervous systems. Failures in any of these areas result in ejaculatory dysfunction.

Premature ejaculation (PE) is described with three common characteristics, as outlined by the International Society for Sexual Medicine (ISSM): (1) short ejaculatory latency, (2) lack of perceived self-efficacy or control of the timing of ejaculation, and (3) distress and interpersonal difficulties relating to the short ejaculatory latency.[30] The definition for PE according to the latest ISSM guidelines is "male sexual dysfunction characterized by ejaculation which always or nearly always occurs prior to or within about one minute of vaginal penetration and the inability to delay ejaculation on all or nearly all vaginal penetrations, and negative personal consequences, such as distress, bother, frustration and/or the avoidance of sexual intimacy."[30] PE may prevent the ability to deposit semen within the female reproductive tract. It is a common sexual complaint and affects up to one-third of men with sexual dysfunction.[31] Treatment options include the squeeze technique, stop-start technique, behavioral/sexual therapy and counseling. Pharmacologic therapy includes topical anesthetics and oral medications (antidepressants) to extend ejaculatory latency time.[30]

Retrograde ejaculation (RE) describes a process in which part or all of the semen is propelled backward into the bladder rather than forward into the vagina during intercourse. Infertility may arise due to the decrease in or completely absent ejaculate. Etiologies include chronic diabetes mellitus and diseases causing peripheral neuropathy, spinal cord injury, previous bladder neck or prostate surgery, prior pelvic/retroperitoneal surgery and alpha-antagonist medications often used for benign prostatic hypertrophy.

Evaluation for RE includes a semen analysis and a post ejaculatory urinalysis in order to evaluate the urine for the presence of sperm. Treatments include alpha agonists and tricyclic antidepressants to stimulate bladder neck closure. If these measures are unsuccessful, sperm can be retrieved from the urine after ejaculation. Since urinary acidity is toxic to sperm, patients are instructed to empty their bladder prior to ejaculation. The patient is pretreated with urinary alkalinization using oral sodium bicarbonate to improve sperm viability. The post-ejaculatory urine is collected and can be used for intrauterine insemination or IVF.

Delayed ejaculation is characterized by a spectrum of disorders including retarded ejaculation, anejaculation, or anorgasmia. Delayed ejaculation occurs in approximately 8% of men between 18–59 years of age.[31] Etiologies include psychogenic, neurogenic, endocrinologic, surgical, medications (antidepressants) or idiopathic. Treatments include penile vibratory stimulation, electroejaculation, or surgical sperm retrieval with PESA or TESE.

Endocrinopathies

Hyperprolactinemia

Hyperprolactinemia can be a result of many causes, including pituitary adenoma, physiological or pathological changes, medications (i.e. antipsychotic agents, antidepressants, antiemetics, antihistamines, hormones, antihypertensives, opiates, etc.) or illicit drugs (i.e. marijuana).[32] Prolactinomas are the most common functional pituitary tumors, accounting for 40% of all pituitary tumors, although their incidence is quite low.[32] Physiologic and pathological causes include psychological and physical stress, renal failure, hepatic failure, hypothyroidism, adrenal insufficiency, sarcoidosis, spinal cord lesions, meningiomas, craniopharyngiomas and chest wall injury.[33]

Elevated prolactin levels disturb the delicate hormonal balance within the hypothalamic-pituitary-gonadal axis by decreasing GnRH secretion and inhibiting the action of LH on Leydig cells, thereby suppressing testosterone production.[32] Presenting symptoms include impotence, loss of libido, infertility, gynecomastia and galactorrhea.[34] Headaches and visual impairment due to optic nerve impingement may be the present symptoms if there is a large space occupying pituitary adenoma.

Because of the marked physiologic variation in prolactin levels, patients with a single elevated serum prolactin level should have their levels repeated. Continued elevation requires additional evaluation. Once medical, medicinal and illicit drug etiologies have been ruled out, a MRI of the head with a pituitary gland protocol should be performed.

Patients with medical problems as the etiology for hyperprolactinemia should have their underlying pathology treated first. Any medications or drugs causing the problem should be stopped, if possible, with assistance from the prescribing physician. The indications for therapy in patients with a prolactinoma include macroadenoma, enlarging microadenoma, infertility, galactorrhea, gynecomastia and hypogonadism.[34]

Treatment options include surveillance, medical therapy, surgery, or radiation therapy. Microadenomas do not generally enlarge in 90% of patients over a 5-year observation period.[33] Asymptomatic patients with no treatment indications can be observed with careful follow-up and serum prolactin levels and imaging as needed.

Medical therapy is the primary modality utilized in patients with pituitary adenomas. Medications include bromocriptine, pergolide and cabergoline.[32] These medications stimulate dopamine receptors and decrease prolactin production with resultant tumor shrinkage. Optimal duration of therapy is unknown.[34]

Patients who are refractory to medical therapy may benefit from trans-sphenoidal surgery to remove the pituitary tumor. Absolute indications for surgery include rapidly increasing tumor size, continued size-related neurological symptoms despite maximal medical therapy, pituitary infarction, hemorrhage, loss of consciousness, sudden loss of vision with headache and cerebrospinal fluid leak.[32] Morbidity and mortality are low at 0.4% and 0.3%, respectively.[33] Surgery requiring craniotomy, however, have higher complication rates. Radiation therapy is generally not considered a main treatment modality due to the excellent success rates with medical and surgical therapy.[33]

Diabetes Mellitus

Diabetes mellitus (DM) can affect male fertility potential in multiple ways.[35] Up to one-third of males with DM are found to have fertility issues.[36,37] Because of its widespread prevalence, it is important to screen at-risk males for DM in order to initiate an aggressive treatment regimen to prevent progression of sexual dysfunction and other medical problems.

The data regarding the effect of DM on spermatogenesis has been conflicting. Animal studies have suggested a decline in semen parameters with chronically uncontrolled or poorly controlled blood glucose levels, although this has not been found to be consistent in human studies.[35,38] Men with DM are at risk for developing hypogonadism due to low testosterone and increased sex hormone binding globulin levels.[36] DM can result in neurogenic and vasculogenic changes, resulting in sexual dysfunction.[38] Manifestations include erectile dysfunction and ejaculatory dysfunction (retrograde ejaculation, anorgasmia, etc.). Patients may also complain of decreased vibratory sensation to the penis, resulting in decreased arousal from physical stimulation. These disorders may prevent normal deposition of sperm within the female reproductive tract, resulting in infertility.

Treatment of males with DM includes strict glucose control to prevent continuing decline in sexual function. Specific treatments for retrograde ejaculation include α-agonists and tricyclic antidepressants to stimulate bladder neck closure. If these are unsuccessful, urinary alkalinization with oral sodium bicarbonate can decrease the caustic effects of urine on sperm function and viability. The postejaculatory urine can be processed and the collected sperm used for insemination or IVF. Erectile dysfunction can be treated with various medications including phosphodiesterase inhibitors (i.e. sildenafil, vardenafil, tadalafil), prostaglandin E1 intraurethral suppository, or intracavernosal injection. Surgical therapy includes placement of a penile prosthesis. Unfortunately, decreased penile sensation and anorgasmia are untreatable, although surgical sperm retrieval can be performed in this setting for IVF.

Thyroid Abnormalities

Normal thyroid function is imperative to maintain normal male fertility. Hyper- and hypothyroidism can result in alterations in sex hormone binding globulin (SHBG) and sex steroids and can result in gonadal dysfunction. Alterations in thyroid function appear to affect female fertility more severely compared to male fertility.[39] Thyroid hormones have also been found to play a role in Sertoli and Leydig cell proliferation, testicular maturation and steroidogenesis.[40]

Hyperthyroidism can result in decreased sperm concentration and motility, as well as increased SHBG levels, thereby decreasing bioavailable testosterone levels.[39] Although total testosterone concentration can increase, free testosterone levels were found to remain stable.[41] Total and free estradiol levels are also often elevated and may contribute to the development of gynecomastia.[42] Despite normal to increased total testosterone and normal free testosterone levels, males with hyperthyroidism can also exhibit symptoms of sexual dysfunction, including hypoactive sexual disorder, erectile dysfunction, premature ejaculation, or delayed ejaculation.[43] Treatment for thyrotoxicosis results in hormonal normalization and improvements in semen parameters and symptoms of sexual dysfunction.

Hypothyroidism can cause abnormalities in morphology.[39] Hypothyroidism results in decreased SHBG levels, leading to reduced total testosterone concentration. Free testosterone levels are also reduced in 60% of men with hypothyroidism. Sexual dysfunction is also prevalent with hypothyroidism and can include similar symptoms as described for hyperthyroidism.[43] Like hyperthyroidism, hormonal and seminal aberrations along with sexual dysfunction symptoms have been noted to normalize after initiating thyroid replacement therapy.[44]

Genetic Anomalies

Kallmann Syndrome

Kallmann syndrome is defined by anosmia or hyposmia associated with hypogonadotrophic hypogonadism. The underlying etiology is a result of faulty migration of gonadotropin releasing hormone (GnRH) and olfactory neurons to the hypothalamus during fetal neuronal development.[45] Patients may also present with eunuchoidism, midline facial defects like cleft lip and/or palate, color blindness, deafness, microphallus, cryptorchidism and infertility.

The estimated incidence is 1 in 8000–10,000 males.[45] Most patients are diagnosed at evaluation for delayed puberty. This disorder can be inherited as an X-linked, autosomal dominant or recessive, or a sporadic mutation on the GnRH receptor. The X-linked form is related to the *KAL1* gene that guides LH secreting neurons to the basal hypothalamus.[46] The GnRH and LH abnormalities result in the lack of LH production from the pituitary gland, leading to hypogonadism and infertility.

Men diagnosed with Kallmann syndrome desiring fertility require medications to stimulate androgen production and spermatogenesis. Treatment commonly includes combination human chorionic gonadotropin (hCG) and human menopausal gonadotropin (hMG) injection therapy.

Klinefelter Syndrome

Klinefelter syndrome (KS) is the most common chromosomal abnormality in humans occurring in 1 in 500–1000 males.[47] The reported prevalence is 0.1–0.2% in the general population, 4% in infertile men, and upto 12% in azoospermic men.[48,49] It is the most common genetic cause of hypogonadism and male infertility.[50] Approximately 80–90% of cases are due to X chromosomal aneuploidy resulting in a 47, XXY karyotype.[51] The remaining 10–20% are made up of other aneuploidies (48,XXXY; 48,XXYY; 49,XXXXY), mosaicism (46,XY/47,XXY), or abnormalities on the X chromosome.[48]

Only one-third of cases are diagnosed because of the variable presentation, with < 10% diagnosed prior to puberty.[48] Diagnosis is usually made during evaluation for gynecomastia, hypogonadism, or infertility with peripheral karyotype testing. Most KS males maintain a low normal testosterone level and undergo normal secondary sexual development.[50] After puberty, these men are often found to have hypergonadotropic hypogonadism, with increased gonadotropin levels in >90% and decreased testosterone levels in >65% of patients.[47]

Pathognomonic physical characteristics include a tall male, eunuchoid body proportions, gynecomastia and small, firm testes.[52] Additional KS findings include azoospermia and elevated FSH.[49] The testicles are small and firm due to progressive hyalinization and fibrosis of the seminiferous tubules and absence of spermatogenesis, resulting in azoospermia. There is also Leydig cell and interstitial hyperplasia.[50] Some tubules may retain small foci of spermatogenesis, resulting in positive sperm in a testicular biopsy or severe oligospermia on semen analysis, although fewer than 10% will have sperm in their ejaculate.[48]

Men with KS were considered sterile in the past, due to azoospermia, with donor insemination and adoption as the only options available for fatherhood. However, a small percentage of KS men have been found to have severe oligospermia or cryptospermia and have been able achieve spontaneous pregnancy.[48] The clinical approach to the KS male has changed with the introduction of intracytoplasmic sperm injection (ICSI). Sperm obtained through TESE or microscopic TESE can now be used for ICSI to achieve pregnancy. The sperm retrieval rate of TESE is approximately 44% and the rate is higher at 55% when utilizing microscopic TESE.[49] Some institutions have published TESE retrieval success rates up to 72%.[53] Pregnancy rates with ICSI have been reported to be greater than 50%.[54]

There is a higher risk of offspring also having genetic aberrations. The incidence of sex chromosomal hyperploidy ranges from 0.9–2.5% in the mosaic form and 2.5–21.6% in the non-mosaic form.[48] KS patients desiring fertility need to be counseled on the genetic risks of having children by a genetics counselor prior to proceeding with any treatment. If available, preimplantation genetic diagnosis by embryo biopsy can also be considered for embryo selection.[48]

Medical management of KS men with low testosterone levels desiring fertility presents a challenge to the clinician. Testosterone supplementation should be started as early as possible to prevent the consequences of chronic hypogonadism and to improve quality of life.[50] However, exogenous testosterone supplementation will suppress any existing spermatogenesis via negative feedback on pituitary hormonal production and should be avoided in men desiring fertility.[48] During the fertility treatment period, treatment with testolactone, anastrazole, clomiphene citrate, recombinant FSH, or hCG can be used to raise testosterone levels and maintain spermatogenesis.[53] Once fertility is achieved men are transitioned to exogenous testosterone replacement therapy.

KS patients also require long term follow up due to a significantly higher frequency of developing other medically morbid conditions compared to the general population. These include breast cancer, mediastinal tumors, osteoporosis, metabolic syndrome (reduced glucose tolerance, elevated triglycerides, low high-density lipoproteins, increased waist adipose tissue, and hypertension) resulting in obesity and diabetes, psychiatric disorders, cardiovascular problems, anemia, pulmonary disease, hypothyroidism, skin, gastrointestinal disease, rheumatic disease, and vascular disease.[49]

Other Genetic Abnormalities

Other sex chromosome abnormalities include Y-linked chromosome microdeletions; 47,XYY; XX male syndrome, mixed gonadal dysgenesis and translocations.[51] XYY syndrome occurs in approximately in 1 in 1000 live births and can result in infertility. Men with 47,XYY can exhibit increased height, decreased intelligence, aggressive or antisocial behavior and a higher risk of developing leukemia. Infertility may result from severe oligospermia or azoospermia.

Malignancy

Testicular Cancer

Testicular cancer is the most common malignancy occurring in young men in industrialized countries. According to the most recent data from the Surveillance Epidemiology and End Results (SEER), the age-adjusted incidence is 5.4 per 100,000 men per year for all races.[55] The lifetime risk of developing testicular cancer is 0.37%, with the median age at diagnosis of approximately 34 years.

Risk factors for testicular cancer include history of cryptorchidism, contralateral testicular cancer, familial history of testicular cancer, as well as a history of subfertility.[56] Most testicular tumors are diagnosed on physical examination, revealing a painless scrotal mass. Non-palpable masses are often detected on screening US for infertility evaluation for other findings on physical examination or based on past medical history. Patients diagnosed with testicular tumors should have serum tumor markers obtained, which include: alpha fetoprotein (αFP), beta human chorionic gonadotropin (βhCG) and lactate dehydrogenase (LDH).

The gold standard treatment for testicular tumors is a radical inguinal orchiectomy. However, not all testicular masses are malignant. Therefore, partial orchiectomy has been gaining support in an attempt to spare benign testicular tissue and to preserve fertility and testosterone production.[57] Those who are found to have testicular cancer should undergo chest, abdominal and pelvic imaging to evaluate for metastasis.

Over the past several decades, there has been a steady increase in the incidence of testicular cancer.[58] There has also been evidence of declining fertility and sperm quality during this same time period.[59] There is increasing evidence suggesting that men with infertility have higher risks of developing testicular cancer.[60]

A recent retrospective cohort study of 22,562 men seeking infertility evaluation demonstrated that men of infertile couples were 1.3 times (standardized incidence ratio = 1.3; 95% confidence interval (CI) = 0.9 - 1.9) more likely to subsequently develop testicular cancer than the general population, regardless of male fertility status.[61] Those with male factor infertility were 2.8 times (Incidence ratio = 2.8; 95% CI = 1.5–4.8) more likely to develop testicular cancer.

Because men with UDT have a higher risk of developing testicular cancer, cryptorchidism may be a confounding factor when trying to link testicular cancer and male infertility. A recent analysis of 5 studies excluding patients with UDT found a positive correlation between testicular cancer and male infertility (Relative risk = 1.59; 95% CI = 1.28–1.98).[62]

Different mechanisms linking testicular cancer and male infertility have been studied. Carcinoma-in-situ (CIS) of the testicles precedes most testicular cancers. CIS cell proliferation consumes resources normally reserved for normal gonocyte maturation to spermatogonia.[63] Because fewer gonocytes are maturing to spermatocytes, sperm counts are lower, potentially resulting in male infertility. Men with testicular dysgenesis syndrome (TDS) are also at a higher risk for male infertility. This syndrome is associated with multiple genitourinary disorders including UDT, hypospadias, male infertility and testicular cancer.[64] Many genetic etiologies can result in TDS, including defects in DNA repair genes, SRY mutations, 45X/46XY karyotype, and androgen insensitivity.

Other Malignancies

Hematologic malignancies such as lymphomas and leukemias are commonly diagnosed in young male patients. More than 50% of men with cancer have expressed their desire for future fertility, with 77% of them with untested fertility at the time of cancer diagnosis. The presence of malignancy can cause nutritional, metabolic and endocrinologic derangements, resulting in infertility.[65]

Many malignancies are readily treated with chemotherapy with excellent oncologic outcomes. These chemotherapeutic agents (i.e. alkylating agents, platinum analogs, antibiotics, antimetabolites and plant derivatives) (**Table 2**) are gonadotoxic and can result in azoospermia.[65] Approximately 50% of men will recover spermatogenesis within two years and 80% at eight years, after stopping therapy.[66] Although spermatogenesis may recover over time, the gonadotoxic effects may persist with potentially elevated risks of fetal malformations and malignancies, as well as sperm DNA damage resulting in other genetic diseases.[65]

It is therefore important to address fertility preservation prior to definitive malignancy therapy. The treating physician should initiate discussions about sperm cryopreservation. A multi-disciplinary approach, including a male fertility specialist, should be employed to ensure adequate patient education as to the available options to preserve future fertility.

SUMMARY

A systematic evaluation of the male is undertaken to identify the presence of any pathology that may cause infertility. Any reversible conditions are treated. Life-threatening conditions are addressed to minimize morbidity and mortality. A combination of empiric therapy and ART may be utilized to achieve pregnancy.

REFERENCES

1. Sharlip ID, Jarow JP, Belker AM, et al. Best practice policies for male infertility. Fertil Steril. 2002;77:873-82.
2. Male Infertility Best Practice Policy Committee of the American Urological Association; Practice Committee of the American Society of Reproductive Medicine. Report on optimal evaluation of the infertile male. Fertil Steril. 2006;86(5 Suppl 1):S202-09.
3. Spyropoulos E, Borousas D, Mavrikos S, et al. Size of external genital organs and somatometric parameters among physically normal men younger than 40 years old. Urology. 2002;60:485-9.
4. World Health Organization. WHO Laboratory Manual for the Examination and Processing of Human Semen, 5th ed. Geneva: World Health Organization; 2010.
5. Oates RD, Lamb D. Genetic Aspects of Male Infertility. In: LI Lipshultz, SS Howards, CS Niederberger, eds. Infertility in the Male, 4th ed. Cambridge: Cambridge University Press; 2009.
6. Samli H, Samli MM, Yilmaz E, Imirzalioglu N. Clinical andrological and genetic characteristics of patients with congenital bilateral absence of vas deferens (CBAVD). Arch Androl. 2006;52:471-7.
7. Onur MR, Orhan I, Firdolas F, et al. Clinical and radiological evaluation of ejaculatory duct obstruction. Arch Androl. 2007;53:179-86.
8. Murphy F, Paran TS, Puri P. Orchidopexy and its impact on fertility. Pediatr Surg Int. 2007;23:625-32.
9. Barthold JS, Gonzalez R. The epidemiology of congenital cryptorchidism, testicular ascent and orchiopexy. J Urol. 2003;170: 2396-401.
10. Lee PA. Fertility in cryptorchidism: does treatment make a difference? Endocrinol Metab Clin North Am. 1993;22:479-90.
11. Lee PA. Fertility after cryptorchidism: epidemiology and other outcome studies. Urology. 2005;66:427-31.
12. Kurpisz M, Havryluk A, Nakonechnyj A, et al. Cryptorchidism and long-term consequences. Reprod Biol. 2010;10:19-35.
13. Virtanen HE, Bierknes R, Cortes D, et al. Cryptorchidism: classification, prevalence and long-term consequences. Acta Paediatrica 2007;96: 611-6.
14. Swerdlow AJ, Higgins CD, Pike MC. Risk of testicular cancer in cohort of boys with cryptorchidism. BMJ. 1997;314:1507-11.
15. Jarrow JP. Effects of varicocele on male fertility. Hum Reprod Update. 2001;7:59-64.
16. Hsiao W, Rosoff JS, Pale JR, et al. Older age is associated with similar improvements in semen parameters and testosterone after subinguinal microsurgical varicocelectomy. J Urol. 2011;185:620-5.
17. Peng BC, Tomashefsky P, Nagler HM. The cofactor effect: varicocele and infertility. Fertil Steril. 1990;54:143-8.
18. Will MA, Swain J, Fode M, et al. The great debate: varicocele treatment and impact on fertility. Fertil Steril. 2011;95(3):841-52.
19. Practice Committee of American Society for Reproductive Medicine. Report on varicocele and infertility. Fertil Steril. 2008;90:S247-9.
20. Pasqualotto FF, Borges E, Roth F, Lara LV, Pasqualotto EB. Varicocele: To fix or not to fix. In: Sabanegh ES, ed. Current Clinical Urology: Male Infertility: Problems and Solutions. New York: Humana Press; 2011.
21. Lee J, Binsaleh S, Lo K, Jarvi K. Varicoceles: the diagnostic dilemma. J Androl. 2008;29:143-6.
22. Pryor JL, Howards SS. Varicocele. Urol Clin North Am. 1987;14:499-513.
23. Daitch JA, Bedaiwy MA, Pasqualotto EB, et al. Varicocelectomy improves intrauterine insemination success rates in men with varicocele. J Urol. 2001;165:1510-3.
24. Practice Committee of American Society for Reproductive Medicine. The management of infertility due to obstructive azoospermia. Fertil Steril. 2008;90:S121-4.
25. Daudin M, Bieth E, Bujan L, et al. Congenital bilateral absence of the vas deferens: clinical characteristics, biological parameters, cystic fibrosis transmembrane conductance regulator gene mutations, and implications for genetic counseling. Fertil Steril. 2000;74:1164-74.
26. Shin D, Lipshultz LI, Goldstein M, et al. Herniorrhaphy with polypropylene mesh causing inguinal vasal obstruction: a preventable cause of obstructive azoospermia. Ann Surg. 2005;241: 553-8.
27. Kolettis PN, Sabanegh ES, D'amico AM, et al. Outcomes for vasectomy reversal performed after obstructive intervals of at least 10 years. Urology. 2002;60:885-8.
28. Smith JF, Walsh TJ, Turek PJ. Ejaculatory duct obstruction. Urol Clin North Am. 2008;77:873-82.
29. Thomas AJ. Ejaculatory dysfunction. Fertil Steril. 1983;39:445-53.
30. Althof SE, Abdo CH, Dean J, et al. International Society for Sexual edicine's guidelines for the diagnosis and treatment of premature ejaculation. J Sex Med. 2010;7:2947-69.
31. Laumann EO, Paik A, Rosen RC. Sexual dysfunction in the United States: prevalence and predictors. JAMA. 1999;281:537-44.
32. Mann WA. Treatment for prolactinomas and hyperprolactinaemia: a lifetime approach. Eur J Clin Invest. 2011;41:334-42.
33. Molitch ME. Medical management of prolactin-secreting pituitary adenomas. Pituitary. 2002;5:55-65.
34. Klibanski A. Clinical Practice. Prolactinomas. N Engl J Med. 2010;362:1219-26.
35. Agbaje IM, Rogers DA, McVicar CM, et al. Insulin dependant diabetes mellitus: implications for male reproductive function. Hum Reprod. 2007;22:1871-77.
36. Kasturi SS, Tannir J, Brannigan RE. The metabolic syndrome and male infertility. J Androl. 2008;29:251-9.
37. Bener A, Al-Ansari AA, Zirie M, Al-Hamaq AO. Is male fertility associated with type 2 diabetes mellitus? Int Urol Nephrol. 2009;41:777-84.
38. Mulholland J, Mallidis C, Agbaje I, McClure N. Male diabetes mellitus nd assisted reproduction treatment outcome. Reprod Biomed Online. 2011;22:215-9.
39. Krassas GE, Poppe K, Glinoer D. Thyroid function and human reproductive health. Endocr Rev. 2010;31:702-55.
40. Wajner SM, Wagner MS, Maia AL. Clinical implications of altered thyroid status in male testicular function. Arq bras Endocrinol Metabol. 2009;53:976-82.

41. Ruder H, Corvol P, Mahoudeau JA, et al. Effects of induced hyperthyroidism on steroid metabolism in man. J Clin Endocrinol Metab. 1971;33:382-7.
42. Krassas GE, Pontikides N, Deligianni V, Miras K. A prospective controlled study of the impact of hyperthyroidism on reproductive function in males. J Clin Endocrinol Metab. 2002;87:3667-71.
43. Carani C, Isidori AM, Granata A, et al. Multicenter study on the prevalence of sexual symptoms in male hypo- and hyperthyroid patients. J Clin Endocrinol Metab. 2005;90:6472-9.
44. Donnelly P, White C. Testicular dysfunction in men with primary ypothyroidism; reversal of hypogonadotrophic hypogonadism with replacement thyroxine. Clin Endocrinol. 2000;52:197-201.
45. Kaplan JD, Bernstein JA, Kwan A, Hudgins L. Clues to an early diagnosis of Kallmann syndrome. Am J Med Genet A. 2010;152A:2796-801.
46. Cadman SM, Kim SH, Hu Y, et al. Molecular pathogenesis of Kallmann's syndrome. Horm Res. 2007;67:231-42.
47. Giltay JC, Maiburg MC. Klinefelter syndrome: clinical and molecular aspects. Expert Rev Mol Diagn. 2010;10:765-76.
48. Lanfranco F, Kamischke A, Zitzmann M, Nieschlag E. Klinefelter's syndrome. Lancet. 2004;364:273-83.
49. Forti G, Corona G, Vignozzi L, et al. Klinefelter's syndrome: a clinical and therapeutical update. Sex Dev. 2010;4:249-58.
50. Wikstrom AM, Dunkel L. Testicular function in Klinefelter Syndrome. Horm Res. 2008; 69:317-26.
51. Walsh TJ, Pera RR, Turek PJ. The genetics of male infertility. Semin Reprod Med. 2009;27:124-36.
52. Varella J. Effects of X chromosome on size and shape of body: an anthropometric investigation in 47,XXY males. Am J Phys Anthropol. 1984;64:233-42.
53. Schiff JD, Palermo GD, Veeck LL, et al. Success of testicular sperm extraction corrected and intracytoplasmic sperm injection in men with Klinefelter syndrome. J Clin Endocrinol Metab. 2005;90: 6263-7.
54. Paduch DA, Bolyakov, Cohen P, Travis A. Reproduction in men with Klinefelter syndrome: the past, the present, and the future. Semin Reprod Med. 2009;27(2):137-48.
55. Altekruse SF, Kosary CL, Krapcho M, et al. (Eds) SEER Cancer Statistics Review, 1975-2007, National Cancer Institute. Bathesda, MD, http://seer.cancer.gov/csr/1975_2007/, based on November 2009 SEER data submission, posted to the SEER web site, 2010.
56. Dieckmann KP, Pichlmeier U. Clinical epidemiology of testicular germ cell tumors. World J Urol. 2004;22:2-14.
57. Zuniga A, Lawrentschuk N, Jewett MA. Organ-sparing approaches for testicular masses. Nat Rev Urol. 2010;7:454-64.
58. Huyghe E, Matsuda T, Thonneau P. Increasing incidence of testicular cancer worldwide: a review. J Urol. 2003;170:5-11.
59. Carlsen E, Giwercman A, Keiding N, Skakkebæk NE. Evidence for decreasing quality of semen during past 50 years. BMJ. 1992;305:609-13.
60. Doria-Rose VP, Biggs ML, Weiss NS. Subfertility and the risk of testicular germ cell tumors (United States). Cancer Causes Control. 2005;16:651-6.
61. Walsh TJ, Croughan MS, Schembri M, et al. Increased risk of testicular germ cell cancer among infertile men. Arch Intern Med. 2009;169:351-6.
62. Peng X, Zeng X, Peng S, et al. The association risk of male subfertility and testicular cancer: a systematic review. PLoS One. 2009;4:e5591.
63. Rørth M, Rajpert-De Meyts E, Andersson L, et al.: Carcinoma in situ in the testis. Scand J Urol Nephrol Suppl. 2000;205:166-86.
64. Burns WR, Sabanegh E, Dada R, et al. Is male infertility a forerunner to cancer? Int Braz J Urol. 2010;36:527-36.
65. Sabanegh ES Jr, Ragheb AM. Male fertility after cancer. Urology. 2009;73:225-31.
66. Howell SJ, Shalet SM. Spermatogenesis after cancer treatment: Damage and recovery. J Natl Cancer Inst Monogr. 2005;34:12-7.
67. World Health Organization. WHO Laboratory Manual for the Examination of Human Semen and Sperm-Cervical Mucus Interaction, 4th ed. Cambridge: Cambridge University Press. 1999.

16

Cryopreservation of Spermatozoa, Individual Sperm and Testicular Tissue

Faten F Abdelhafez, Rachel Pope, Mohamed A Bedaiwy, Nina Desai

CHAPTER OUTLINE

INTRODUCTION

In the history of cryopreservation of reproductive cells and tissues, sperm cryopreservation is considered to be the oldest and the most widely applied technique in human and animal reproductive medicine.[1-4] In 1949, the accidental discovery of glycerol as a cryopreservation agent (CPA) for bovine spermatozoa revolutionized the field.[5] In 1953, the first human pregnancy from insemination of cryopreserved spermatozoa was reported.[2,6] A yolk medium CPA for human spermatozoa was introduced in 1978.[7] Since then, many other CPAs were introduced, such as ethylene glycol (EG), dimethyl sulphoxide (DMSO) and propylene glycol; yet glycerol is still the most commonly used.[8] Various techniques have been used for sperm cryopreservation, such as vapor freezing, programmable controlled rate cooling and, more recently, vitrification. With each of these techniques there is still a good deal of interlaboratory variation in cooling and warming rates. Variations also include the type of vessel selected for sperm storage.

EFFECT OF CRYOPRESERVATION ON HUMAN SPERMATOZOA

Cryopreservation significantly reduces viability of cryopreserved, thawed sperm.[9-10] This effect may be due to extracellular ice formation[11] or extreme volume excursions resulting from unbalanced osmotic pressure.[12] Human sperm membrane has a characteristic lipid composition. Low temperatures may affect the way the membrane lipids are organized, causing a decreased permeability and loss of fluidity. This effect in turn can cause a low post-thaw sperm survival. Decreased viability can also be due to CPA toxicity.[1,13] Despite acting as protectants to increase cell survival during the cryopreservation process, CPAs can result in potentially lethal volume excursions as an effect of osmotic stress.[13] This danger, however, can be avoided by the gradual addition and removal of CPA.

Cryopreservation also results in a significant decrease in post-thaw motility, which is probably related to CPA concentration and the temperature at which they are added.[14,15] When glycerol was added at a concentration of 5%, post-thaw motility improved over that observed with 7.5%. Also, when glycerol was added at -5ºC, post-thaw sperm motility was better than when it was added at room temperature.[14] A decrease between 25–75% in post-thaw sperm motility was reported, depending on the prefreeze sperm quality and freezing protocol.[16-19] Nonetheless, when viability studies were performed on the post-thaw specimen, 20 to 30% of the immotile sperm were found to be viable.[17-18] It remains, however, important to mention that sperm from different individuals will react differently to cryopreservation/thawing processes.[20]

Additionally, structural changes like changes of acrosomal structure and activity,[21] nuclear swelling or shrinkage, cytoplasmic membrane swelling and loss of plasma membrane integrity[22] were reported. The effect of cryopreservation on sperm DNA and chromatin structure is controversial. While some studies reported a deleterious effect of freezing on sperm DNA,[9,23] other studies found no statistically significant changes related to chromatin structure and morphology.[24,25] Additional studies are needed to resolve this issue.

Unfortunately, the cryopreservation thawing procedure can cause some structural and ultrastructural damage to sperm. This damage can subsequently reduce viability, motility and thus, fertilizing potential of cryopreserved/thawed sperm.[11,18,26]

CLINICAL APPLICATIONS OF SPERM CRYOPRESERVATION

Donor banking: Sperm Cryopreservation to be Offered for Others

Cryopreservation of donor sperm is mandatory because it must be quarantined and screened for infectious diseases, such as HIV and hepatitis, before being used for artificial insemination.[27]

Autoconservation: Sperm Cryopreservation for one's Future use

Convenience Cryobanking

In some cases, the male partner will not be able to give ejaculate on the day of oocyte retrieval or intrauterine insemination (IUI). Thus, in these cases it is helpful to cryopreserve sperm and use it on the day of oocyte retrieval or IUI. Some men also ask for cryopreservation of their sperm so that it can be used by their partners during their absence while working in a foreign country or performing military service.

Freezing of Surgically Retrieved Spermatozoa

Another form of convenience cryobanking is the freezing of surgically retrieved spermatozoa. Surgically retrieved spermatozoa can be used for intracytoplasmic sperm injection (ICSI) while fresh, or can be cryopreserved and stored for later use. Cryopreservation of epididymal and testicular sperm eliminates the need to coordinate the women's treatment cycle with a urologist's availability for sperm extraction. Moreover, spermatogenesis can be assessed before ovarian stimulation[28] and thus, the risk of not finding viable sperm on the day of egg retrieval can be avoided. Cryopreservation of surgically retrieved sperm also avoids the necessity of performing a repeated surgery, with its potential complications any further expenses.[18,29,30]

Fertility Preservation

Sperm cryopreservation is used as a means of fertility preservation before surgical sterilization, varicocele ligation, or reconstructive surgery. Besides, males at risk of losing their future fecundity secondary to a malignant or non-malignant disease, such as autoimmune, inflammatory bowel disease and kidney diseases that require radio and/or chemotherapy, can store their sperm prior to therapy.

SPERM CRYOPRESERVATION FOR CANCER PATIENTS

With the recent advances in the management of different malignancies and cancers, more patients are surviving and having a longer life span. Unfortunately, some of the chemotherapies are gonadotoxic, leaving the patient sterile.[31] In testicular cancer patients, infertility may be caused by the tumor itself.[32]

The most common cancers in childhood and early adulthood include leukemia, Hodgkin's lymphoma and testicular germ cell tumors. Other malignancies can affect gonadal function even prior to the start of cancer treatment. Different mechanisms of action include hormonal and metabolic alterations, and direct invasion in cases of central nervous system tumors.[33] Another mechanism of action may also be malnutrition associated with malignancy, which in turn results in hypovitaminosis and deficiency in minerals and other trace elements needed for spermatogenesis. Besides, some tumors release cytokines and other chemicals that can adversely affect spermatogenesis. Finally, fever may be present with some malignancies and can also impair proper gonadal function.

Thus, about 12% of men with malignancies are found to have poor sperm quality in the form of azoospermia or severe oligospermia with poor motility—even before the start of chemo- or radiotherapy.[34] In about 50% of testicular cancer patients, spermatogenesis will return after the patient is in remission.[35,36] However, it is not possible to predict which patients will recover. Therefore, it is preferable to bank sperm for all patients with testicular cancers, or any other malignant or non-malignant disease that requires chemo and/or radiotherapy.

Available Options for Men and Postpubertal Boys

Currently, sperm banking is the only fertility preservation modality for these patients. However, it is still not widely applied. In a 2006 study, only 67% of cancer patients of reproductive age had their sperm cryopreserved prior to treatment.[37] The remainder of these cancer patients were of younger age and were too anxious to discuss their future fertility options. The success rate of assisted reproductive technology (ART) using cryopreserved sperm from cancer patients ranges from 33% to 56 %.[38]

Another fertility preservation option for these patients is through the creation of a pre-pubertal testicular state via hormonal treatment.[39] Hormones used include testosterone alone,[40] testosterone in conjunction with gonadotropin releasing hormone agonist (GnRH-a)[41] or estradiol[42] and GnRH-a in conjunction with antiandrogen flutamide.[43] However, only a few clinical studies were performed[39,41] and the majority of these were experimental studies using rats. Thus, more clinical trials are needed in this direction before this application of hormonal treatment for fertility preservation in male patients becomes routine.

Options for Prepubertal Boys

To date, all options to preserve future fertility in pre-pubertal patients with cancer remain experimental.[28] Spermatogonial stem cells can be retrieved from testicular tissue before cancer therapy, cryopreserved and then transplanted back after remission. Spermatogonial stem cell transplantation was successfully performed in rodents.[44] Recently, the xenografting of human post-pubertal testicular tissue resulted in high germ cell survival.[45] The major drawback of this procedure is the possibility of re-introduction of malignant cells after remission in the patient.[46] Cell sorting and in vitro maturation (IVM) of spermatogonial stem cells followed by cryopreservation until future use are the other alternatives.[47] However, testicular tissue harvesting in pre-pubertal boys may affect the recovery of the testis after completion of cancer treatment. Knowing that in many cases spermatogenesis may completely or at least partially recover after cancer therapy, this group of pre-pubertal boys is at risk of unrecovered spermatogenesis after puberty.

Effect of Cancer Therapy on Gonadal Function

The gonadotoxic effect will depend on the type of chemotherapy used and cumulative dose administered. The effect of chemotherapy on spermatogenesis is variable. During the pre-pubertal period, the gonads can still be affected by the toxic effect of cancer therapies, which contradicts the previous hypothesis that the gonads are quiescent at that young age.[48]

Sertoli cells are very sensitive to irradiation. A >4 Gy dose can cause permanent sterility. Meanwhile, Leydig cells are less radiosensitive and a >20 Gy dose will cause hypogonadism. Testes are exposed to radiotherapy in cases of total body irradiation, and testicular carcinoma.[49]

Offspring of Cancer Survivors

Cancer treatment can cause germ cell mutations and thus, may result in congenital malformations in offspring. Luckily, the data in the literature shows no difference between offspring of cancer patients and the normal population regarding rates of congenital diseases and juvenile malignancies.[50] However, these children were conceived spontaneously and not after ART procedures. The chance of passing the defective genes to offspring may increase with the use of ICSI because the natural selection mechanism is no longer in effect.[51]

LABORATORY TECHNIQUES FOR SPERM CRYOPRESERVATION

Theoretically, human sperm is an ideal cell for cryopreservation as it is small in volume and has a large surface area. It has a small amount of cytoplasm and consequently minimal intracellular water. Common cryopreservation protocols use a cooling rate between –10 and –100ºC/min.[8] Great inter- and even intra-individual variations exist regarding sperm cryosurvival using various CPAs and cryopreservation methods.[52] The addition and removal of CPAs need to be performed in a gradual manner in order to avoid extreme volume excursions in sperm that can result in cell lysis[53].

To Wash or Not to Wash

Sperm cryopreservation can be performed for unwashed sperm, i.e. within seminal plasma, or after washing. Whether this choice contributes to the post-thaw results is still controversial. Proponents of freezing native semen claim that it allows the antioxidant protective effect of seminal plasma to guard against reactive oxygen species.[10,54,55] Others report better results with washed sperm.[56,57] Yet, some researchers found no significant differences between freezing native and washed sperm samples.[58]

Cytoprotective Agents

In general, CPAs can be divided into permeating and non-permeating CPAs. Permeating CPAs include glycerol, EG, DMSO and propandiol. They act by replacing the intracellular water and thus, prevent intracellular ice formation. However, since the discovery of glycerol's cryoprotectant properties in 1948, it remains the most commonly used CPA for sperm cryopreservation. EG, however, is an alternate CPA which has provided promising results. Higher rates of motile sperm recovery after cryopreservation with 1.0M EG as compared to 1.0M glycerol have been reported.[13] Although it has been proposed as a viable substitute for glycerol, it has received little attention.[59]

Non-permeating CPAs like sucrose and raffinose exert their cryoprotectant effect by dehydrating the cell via osmosis. Hen`s egg yolk is a non-permeating CPA that is commonly used in sperm cryopreservation. It maintains the fluidity of sperm membrane and has been shown to have a cryoprotective effect even in the absence of glycerol.

Different Sperm Cryopreservation Techniques

Vapor Freezing

Vapor freezing is the classic method of sperm cryopreservation. The CPA (usually glycerol at a concentration of 5–10%) is added to the sperm sample in a 1:1 ratio at room temperature for 5–10 minutes. Vials or straws are then suspended in liquid nitrogen (LN_2) vapor for 15 minutes before being immerged in LN_2 for storage. It is quick and simple because there is no need for any expensive machines.

Slow Programmable Freezing

This method uses a chamber controlled by a programmable computer to lower the temperature in a controlled step-wise fashion. Optimal results were obtained with a cooling rate of -8°C to -10°C per minute from 4°C to -80°C.[53] Slow programmable sperm freezing has been reported to yield better results for sub- or infertile males, when compared to the classic vapor freezing method.[60,61]

Sperm Vitrification

With vitrification, the cell is cryopreserved without a phase change. Vitrification can be achieved using either relatively slow or moderate cooling rates, but with the addition of a very high concentration of CPA. Alternatively, the rate of cooling/thawing can be high enough to prevent formation of intra- and/or extracellular ice. This process usually involves the use of a CPA, but at a lower concentration. Alternatively, it can be applied using no CPAs. To date, vitrification was only achieved for human spermatozoa. Human spermatozoa were vitrified using only non-permeable CPAs[62,63] or without any CPA, which is known as "Cryoprotectant free vitrification." This methodology was first proposed by Luyet and his colleagues in 1930's.[64] However, because achieving very rapid cooling and warming rates at that time was very difficult, it was abandoned until recently. Due to the development of new vessels which allow vitrification of very small sample sizes, the idea was revisited and applied on human spermatozoa.[29,65-67] While numerous studies indicate better survival and outcomes with oocyte/embryo vitrification as compared to conventional slow cooling, this has not been the case with sperm vitrification.

Special Concerns of Sperm Cryopreservation

Cryopreservation of Surgically Retrieved Spermatozoa

With the new advances in cryotechnology, the cryopreservation of surgically retrieved spermatozoa has become a very appealing and occasionally indispensable approach for managing infertility due to severe male factor. There are some notable advantages in the efficient cryopreservation of a small amount of sperm. Specifically, it decreases the amount of surgical interventions needed so that expenses and risks are also reduced. Moreover, the use of cryopreserved sperm removes the issue of planning egg retrieval to coincide with a urologist's schedule for the surgical retrieval of sperm. Moreover, performing the sperm retrieval prior to initiation of the in vitro fertilization (IVF) stimulation cycle eliminates the risk of no sperm being found on the day of egg retrieval.

Sperm extraction procedures are usually performed by a urologist. Subsequently, the retrieved sperm are transferred to the laboratory for assessment and freezing. For cryopreservation, epididymal and testicular sperm samples are diluted 1:1 with test yolk buffer-glycerol cryoprotectant and aliquotted into cryovials. Vials are vapor frozen for 30 minutes prior to immersion in LN_2. It is also helpful to freeze a separate 25 μL "test" aliquot for post-thaw evaluation. Before IVF cycle initiation, the "test aliquot" is thawed and assessed. This process allows patients to be adequately counseled before cycle initiation. Plans could be made for back-up donor specimens, fresh sperm harvest and oocyte freezing, in the event that the laboratory cannot locate motile sperm after extensive searching.

Single Sperm Freezing

Because epididymal and testicular spermatozoa have distinctive qualities, traditional techniques of sperm cryopreservation may not be the most appropriate. In specimens that have been surgically retrieved, often large amounts of red blood cells, cellular debris, testicular cells and dead or immotile sperm are present. For the small amount of observed motile sperm in such a sample, the process of concentrating the sample for cryopreservation can in fact harm the existing viable sperm in the sample.[68,69] It is clear that conventional methodology cannot effectively address these problems. Thus, for these exceedingly compromised sperm specimens, innovative cryopreservation approaches need to be devised in order to enhance the recovery and post-thaw parameters. The lack of easily implemented technology to handle single sperm freezing remains a major deterrent to maximizing outcomes in such cycles.

Freezing individually selected sperm or small numbers of sperm is a challenge. Many different types of vessels or carriers have been tried for sequestering and freezing small numbers of sperm.[70-72] These include biological carriers like zona pellucida from evacuated hamster[73-77] or human oocytes,[73,74,78-84] as well as non-biological carriers like straws,[29,85,86] media microdroplets,[87-89] ENREF 58,[90,91] ENREF 78, ICSI pipettes,[92,93] alginate beads,[94] cryoloop,[29,66,67,95-98] agarose microspheres[99] and the sleeper cell.

Additional research into cryopreservation technology particularly focused on small numbers and quantities of sperm is essential. Over a decade ago, human and hamster zonae that were used to store small samples of spermatozoa resulted in pregnancies. Despite the passage of time, hardly any studies have been published on the cryopreservation of small amounts of testicular or epididymal sperm in very impaired surgical specimens. Moreover, very few of these studies have reported on the use of these individually selected and cryopreserved sperm for a subsequent ICSI cycle and the resulting pregnancy outcomes.[70] Currently there is insufficient evidence to establish one technology as better than another. Thus, in order to appropriately consider the viability and efficacy of the available methodologies for single sperm cryopreservation, well-designed clinical trials are needed.

In the majority of IVF programs currently, urologists and gynecologists only limitedly use single sperm cryotechnology. Such failure to take advantage of the available technology is a missed opportunity, because it can improve the care options for an important subset of patients. This technology likely has failed to become mainstream because of the labor intensive nature of single sperm isolation and cryopreservation, the lack of an ideal vessel for such freezing and the scarcity of clinical data on its efficacy.

STORAGE AND TRANSPORTATION OF CRYOPRESERVED SPERM

The storage duration of cryopreserved sperm in LN_2 has no impact on post-thaw progressive motility rates and concentrations (100). Live births from ICSI and IUI using cryopreserved sperm stored for 21 years[101] and 28 years[102] have been reported.

In 1996, a case reported on LN_2 contamination of blood bags, resulting in Hepatitis B virus infection in 6 cases. Since then, theoretical concerns regarding contamination during direct exposure and storage of cryopreserved samples in LN_2 have been raised.[103] The source of microbial and/or viral contamination could be from the LN_2 source itself or cross-contamination from an infected sample in the storage dewar. Although, to-date there is no report of sample cross-contamination or infection in a LN_2 storage dewar in either commercial sperm banks or in an IVF setting, proper precautions need to be taken.

The use of sealed cryopreservation containers can minimize this risk. Unscreened and infected semen samples should be stored separately in quarantine tanks. Another method that has been proposed is vapor storage of samples, rather than storage directly in LN_2.[104-105] The investigators concluded that vapor phase storage was as efficient as liquid phase storage. However, a recent study suggests that storage in the vapor phase still presents an inherent risk for pathogen transmission and cross-contamination.[106]

Cryopreserved specimens are transported using "dry shippers." These are storage dewars with an absorbent inner layer that retains LN_2, keeping the chamber cooled without the danger of LN_2 spilling during transport. Under certain regulations, cryopreserved samples that are stored in dry shippers are considered "non-hazardous" and can be safely transported by air. The dry shipper can keep the temperature of nitrogen vapor around 150°C for up to 1 week, depending on the manufacturer's specifications.[23]

CONCLUSION

Sperm cryopreservation is useful in several settings. Specifically, preservation is useful in the following circumstances: (a) when male partners are unable to give a fresh sperm sample on the day of oocyte retrieval, (b) in cases where spermatozoa are surgically retrieved, and (c) as a fertility preservation method for males with malignant diseases requiring chemo- and/or radiotherapy. Several techniques exist for preparation and storage of the spermatogonia. Freezing, vitrification, vapor freezing and the use of cryoprotectants each have advantages and disadvantages. Despite the long-standing history of cryopreservation, no single protocol has been identified as superior. Several investigators are leading the field in designing techniques with successful outcomes; however, evidence by means of research is lagging behind.

REFERENCES

1. Buhr MM, Fiser P, Bailey JL, Curtis EF. Cryopreservation in different concentrations of glycerol alters boar sperm and their membranes. J Androl. 2001;22:961-9.
2. Aboulghar MA, Mansour RT, Serour GI, et al. Fertilization and pregnancy rates after intracytoplasmic sperm injection using ejaculate semen and surgically retrieved sperm. Fertil Steril. 1997;68:108-11.
3. Critser JK, Mobraaten LE. Cryopreservation of murine spermatozoa. ILAR J. 2000;41:197-206.
4. Woelders H. Fundamentals and recent development in cryopreservation of bull and boar semen. Vet Q. 1997;19:135-8.
5. Polge C, Smith A, Parkes A. Revival of spermatozoa after vitrification and dehydration at low temperature. Nature. 1949;164:666-76.
6. Bunge RG, Sherman JK. Fertilizing capacity of frozen human spermatozoa. Nature. 1953;172:767-8.
7. Graham E, Crabo B. Some methods of evaluating human spermatozoa. In: Integrity of Frozen Spermatozoa. Natl Acad Sci. 1978:274-304.
8. Agca Y, Critser JK. Cryopreservation of spermatozoa in assisted reproduction. Semin Reprod Med. 2002;20:15-23.
9. Hammadeh ME, Askari AS, Georg T. Effect of freeze-thawing procedure on chromatin stability, morphological alteration and membrane integrity of human spermatozoa in fertile and subfertile men. Int J Androl. 1999;22:155-62.
10. Ozkavukcu S, Erdemli E, Isik A, et al. Effects of cryopreservation on sperm parameters and ultrastructural morphology of human spermatozoa. J Assist Reprod Genet. 2008;25:403-11.
11. Morris GJ. Rapidly cooled human sperm: no evidence of intracellular ice formation. Hum Reprod. 2006;21:2075-83.
12. Medeiros CM, Forell F, Oliveira AT, Rodrigues JL. Current status of sperm cryopreservation: why isn't it better? Theriogenology. 2002;57:327-44.
13. Gilmore JA, Liu J, Gao DY, Critser JK. Determination of optimal cryoprotectants and procedures for their addition and removal from human spermatozoa. Hum Reprod. 1997;12:112-8.
14. Critser JK, Huse-Benda AR, Aaker DV, et al. Cryopreservation of human spermatozoa. III. The effect of cryoprotectants on motility. Fertil Steril. 1988;50:314-20.
15. Watson PF. Recent developments and concepts in the cryopreservation of spermatozoa and the assessment of their post-thawing function. Reprod Fertil Dev. 1995;7:871-91.
16. Esteves SC, Sharma RK, Thomas AJ Jr., Agarwal A. Improvement in motion characteristics and acrosome status in cryopreserved human spermatozoa by swim-up processing before freezing. Hum Reprod. 2000;15:2173-9.
17. Nijs M, Ombelet W. Cryopreservation of human sperm. Hum Fertil. (Camb) 2001;4:158-63.

18. Yildiz C, Ottaviani P, Law N, et al. Effects of cryopreservation on sperm quality, nuclear DNA integrity, in vitro fertilization, and in vitro embryo development in the mouse. Reprod. 2007;133:585-95.
19. Nijs M, Creemers E, Cox A, et al. Influence of freeze-thawing on hyaluronic acid binding of human spermatozoa. Reprod Biomed Online. 2009;19:202-6.
20. Holt WV. Fundamental aspects of sperm cryobiology: the importance of species and individual differences. Theriogenology. 2000;53:47-58.
21. Meijer D, Hermans A, von Lindern M, et al. Molecular characterization of the testis specific c-abl mRNA in mouse. EMBO. J. 1987;6:4041-8.
22. Barthelemy C, Royere D, Hammahah S, et al. Ultrastructural changes in membranes and acrosome of human sperm during cryopreservation. Arch Androl. 1990;25:29-40.
23. Bielanski A. Experimental microbial contamination and disinfection of dry (vapour) shipper dewars designed for short-term storage and transportation of cryopreserved germplasm and other biological specimens. Theriogenology. 2005;63:1946-57.
24. Donnelly ET, Steele EK, McClure N, Lewis SE. Assessment of DNA integrity and morphology of ejaculated spermatozoa from fertile and infertile men before and after cryopreservation. Hum Reprod. 2001;16:1191-9.
25. Atabekoglu C, Sonmezer M, Ozkavukcu S, Isbacar S. Unexpected pregnancy despite extremely decreased estradiol levels during ovarian stimulation. Fertil Steril. 2008;90:2003 e5-9.
26. Morris GJ, Acton E, Avery S. A novel approach to sperm cryopreservation. Hum Reprod. 1999;14:1013-21.
27. Mascola L, Guinan ME. Screening to reduce transmission of sexually transmitted diseases in semen used for artificial insemination. N Engl J Med. 1986;314:1354-9.
28. Kupker W, Schlegel PN, Al-Hasani S, et al. Use of frozen-thawed testicular sperm for intracytoplasmic sperm injection. Fertil Steril. 2000;73:453-8.
29. Isachenko V, Isachenko E, Montag M, et al. Clean technique for cryoprotectant-free vitrification of human spermatozoa. Reprod Biomed Online. 2005;10:350-4.
30. Nudell DM, Conaghan J, Pedersen RA, et al. The mini-micro-epididymal sperm aspiration for sperm retrieval: a study of urological outcomes. Hum Reprod. 1998;13:1260-5.
31. Shrader WD, Young WB, Sprengeler PA, et al. Neutral inhibitors of the serine protease factor Xa. Bioorg Med Chem Lett. 2001;11:1801-4.
32. Kuczyk M, Machtens S, Bokemeyer C, et al. Sexual function and fertility after treatment of testicular cancer. Curr Opin Urol. 2000;10:473-7.
33. AbdelHafez F, Bedaiwy M, El-Nashar SA, et al. Techniques for cryopreservation of individual or small numbers of human spermatozoa: a systematic review. Hum Reprod Update. 2009;15:153-64.
34. van Casteren NJ, Boellaard WP, Romijn JC, Dohle GR. Gonadal dysfunction in male cancer patients before cytotoxic treatment. Int J Androl. 2010;33:73-9.
35. Aass N, Fossa SD, Theodorsen L, Norman N. Prediction of long-term gonadal toxicity after standard treatment for testicular cancer. Eur J Cancer. 1991;27:1087-91.
36. Lampe H, Horwich A, Norman A, et al. Fertility after chemotherapy for testicular germ cell cancers. J Clin Oncol. 1997;15:239-45.
37. Edge B, Holmes D, Makin G. Sperm banking in adolescent cancer patients. Arch Dis Child. 2006;91:149-52.
38. Medeiros CM, Parrish JJ. Changes in lectin binding to bovine sperm during heparin-induced capacitation. Mol Reprod Dev. 1996;44:525-32.
39. Masala A, Faedda R, Alagna S, et al. Use of testosterone to prevent cyclophosphamide-induced azoospermia. Ann Intern Med. 1997;126:292-5.
40. Delic JI, Bush C, Steel GG. Influence of timing of cytotoxic drug treatment on the response of murine clonogenic spermatogonia to X-irradiation. Radiother Oncol. 1986;7:341-8.
41. Cigni A, Faedda R, Atzeni MM, et al. Hormonal strategies for fertility preservation in patients receiving cyclophosphamide to treat glomerulonephritis: a nonrandomized trial and review of the literature. Am J Kidney Dis. 2008;52:887-96.
42. Kurdoglu B, Wilson G, Parchuri N, et al. Protection from radiation-induced damage to spermatogenesis by hormone treatment. Radiat Res. 1994;139:97-102.
43. Meistrich ML, Parchuri N, Wilson G, et al. Hormonal protection from cyclophosphamide-induced inactivation of rat stem spermatogonia. J Androl. 1995;16:334-41.
44. Brinster RL, Zimmermann JW. Spermatogenesis following male germ-cell transplantation. Proc Natl Acad Sci U S A. 1994;91:11298-302.
45. Van Saen D, Goossens E, Bourgain C, et al. Meiotic activity in orthotopic xenografts derived from human postpubertal testicular tissue. Hum Reprod. 2011;26:282-93.
46. Jahnukainen K, Hou M, Petersen C, et al. Intratesticular transplantation of testicular cells from leukemic rats causes transmission of leukemia. Cancer Res. 2001;61:706-10.
47. Geens M, Goossens E, De Block G, et al. Autologous spermatogonial stem cell transplantation in man: current obstacles for a future clinical application. Hum Reprod Update. 2008;14:121-30.
48. Chemes HE. Infancy is not a quiescent period of testicular development. Int J Androl. 2001;24:2-7.
49. Wallace WH, Anderson RA, Irvine DS. Fertility preservation for young patients with cancer: who is at risk and what can be offered? Lancet Oncol. 2005;6:209-18.
50. Madanat-Harjuoja LM, Malila N, Lahteenmaki P, et al. Risk of cancer among children of cancer patients - a nationwide study in Finland. Int J Cancer. 2010;126:1196-205.
51. Dohle GR. Male infertility in cancer patients: Review of the literature. Int J Urol. 2010;17:327-31.
52. Friberg J, Gemzell C. Sperm-freezing and donor insemination. Int J Fertil. 1977;22:148-54.
53. Mortimer D. Current and future concepts and practices in human sperm cryobanking. Reprod Biomed Online. 2004;9:134-51.
54. Zini A, Fischer MA, Sharir S, et al. Prevalence of abnormal sperm DNA denaturation in fertile and infertile men. Urology. 2002;60:1069-72.
55. Koca Y, Ozdal OL, Celik M, et al. Antioxidant activity of seminal plasma in fertile and infertile men. Arch Androl. 2003;49:355-9.
56. Donnelly ET, McClure N, Lewis SE. Cryopreservation of human semen and prepared sperm: effects on motility parameters and DNA integrity. Fertil Steril. 2001;76:892-900.
57. Saritha KR, Bongso A. Comparative evaluation of fresh and washed human sperm cryopreserved in vapor and liquid phases of liquid nitrogen. J Androl. 2001;22:857-62.
58. Fraczek M, Sanocka D, Kamieniczna M, Kurpisz M. Proinflammatory cytokines as an intermediate factor enhancing lipid sperm membrane peroxidation in in vitro conditions. J Androl. 2008;29:85-92.
59. Gao D, Mazur P, Critser J. Fundamental cryobiology of mammalian spermatozoa. In: Karow A, Critser J, Eds. Reproductive tissue banking. London: Academic Press, 1997:263-328.
60. Verheyen G, Pletincx I, Van Steirteghem A. Effect of freezing method, thawing temperature and post-thaw dilution/washing on motility (CASA) and morphology characteristics of high-quality human sperm. Hum Reprod. 1993;8:1678-84.
61. Hammadeh ME, Greiner S, Rosenbaum P, Schmidt W. Comparison between human sperm preservation medium and TEST-yolk buffer on protecting chromatin and morphology integrity of human spermatozoa in fertile and subfertile men after freeze-thawing procedure. J Androl. 2001;22:1012-8.
62. Hossain AM, Osuamkpe CO. Sole use of sucrose in human sperm cryopreservation. Arch Androl. 2007;53:99-103.
63. Isachenko E, Isachenko V, Weiss JM, et al. Acrosomal status and mitochondrial activity of human spermatozoa vitrified with sucrose. Reprod. 2008;136:167-73.
64. Fahy GM, Lilley TH, Linsdell H, et al. Cryoprotectant toxicity and cryoprotectant toxicity reduction: in search of molecular mechanisms. Cryobiology. 1990;27:247-68.

65. Isachenko E, Isachenko V, Katkov II, et al. Vitrification of mammalian spermatozoa in the absence of cryoprotectants: from past practical difficulties to present success. Reprod Biomed Online. 2003;6:191-200.
66. Isachenko E, Isachenko V, Katkov II, et al. DNA integrity and motility of human spermatozoa after standard slow freezing versus cryoprotectant-free vitrification. Hum Reprod. 2004;19:932-9.
67. Isachenko V, Isachenko E, Katkov II, et al. Cryoprotectant-free cryopreservation of human spermatozoa by vitrification and freezing in vapor: effect on motility, DNA integrity, and fertilization ability. Biol Reprod. 2004;71:1167-73.
68. Aitken RJ, Clarkson JS. Significance of reactive oxygen species and antioxidants in defining the efficacy of sperm preparation techniques. J Androl. 1988;9:367-76.
69. Mortimer D, Mortimer ST. Methods of sperm preparation for assisted reproduction. Ann Acad Med Singapore. 1992;21:517-24.
70. Desai N, Goldberg J, Austin C, et al. Cryopreservation of individually selected sperm: methodology and case report of a clinical pregnancy. J Assist Reprod Genet. 2012;29:375-9.
71. Endo Y, Fujii Y, Kurotsuchi S, et al. Successful delivery derived from vitrified-warmed spermatozoa from a patient with nonobstructive azoospermia. Fertil Steril. 2012;98:1423-7.
72. Endo Y, Fujii Y, Shintani K, et al. Simple vitrification for small numbers of human spermatozoa. Reprod Biomed Online. 2012;24:301-7.
73. Cohen J, Garrisi GJ, Congedo-Ferrara TA, et al. Cryopreservation of single human spermatozoa. Hum Reprod. 1997;12:994-1001.
74. Walmsley R, Cohen J, Ferrara-Congedo T, et al. The first births and ongoing pregnancies associated with sperm cryopreservation within evacuated egg zonae. Hum Reprod. 1998;13 Suppl 4:61-70.
75. Suzuki T, Sumantri C, Khan NH, et al. Development of a simple, portable carbon dioxide incubator for in vitro production of bovine embryos. Anim Reprod Sci. 1999;54:149-57.
76. Hsieh YY, Tsai HD, Chang CC, Lo HY. Sperm cryopreservation with empty human or mouse zona pellucidae. A comparison. J Reprod Med. 2000;45:383-6.
77. Liu J, Zheng XZ, Baramki TA, et al. Cryopreservation of a small number of fresh human testicular spermatozoa and testicular spermatozoa cultured in vitro for 3 days in an empty zona pellucida. J Androl. 2000;21:409-13.
78. Montag M, Rink K, Dieckmann U, et al. Laser-assisted cryopreservation of single human spermatozoa in cell-free zona pellucida. Andrologia. 1999;31:49-53.
79. Hsieh Y, Tsai H, Chang C, Lo H. Cryopreservation of human spermatozoa within human or mouse empty zona pellucidae. Fertil Steril. 2000;73:694-8.
80. Borini A, Sereni E, Bonu E, Flamigni C. Freezing a few testicular spermatozoa retrieved by TESA. Mol Cell Endocrinol. 2000;169:27-32.
81. Fusi F, Saponara S, Gagov H, Sgaragli G. 2,5-Di-t-butyl-1,4-benzohydroquinone (BHQ) inhibits vascular L-type Ca(2+) channel via superoxide anion generation. Br J Pharmacol. 2001;133:988-96.
82. Cesana C, Miqueleiz S, Bernuzzi P, et al. Smouldering Waldenstrom's macroglobulinemia: factors predicting evolution to symptomatic disease. Semin Oncol. 2003;30:231-5.
83. Levi-Setti PE, Albani E, Negri L, et al. Cryopreservation of a small number of spermatozoa in yolk-filled human zonae pellucidae. Arch Ital Urol Androl. 2003;75:195-8.
84. Hassa H, Gurer F, Yildirm A, et al. A new protection solution for freezing small numbers of sperm inside empty zona pellucida: Osmangazi-Turk solution. Cell Preservation Tech. 2006;4:199-208.
85. Desai N, J G, J G. A Convenient Technique for Cryopreservation of Micro Quantities of Sperm. Fertil Steril. 1998; Annual meeting program supplement:S197-8.
86. Koscinski I, Wittemer C, Lefebvre-Khalil V, et al. Optimal management of extreme oligozoospermia by an appropriate cryopreservation programme. Hum Reprod. 2007;22:2679-84.
87. Gil-Salom M, Romero J, Rubio C, et al. Intracytoplasmic sperm injection with cryopreserved testicular spermatozoa. Mol Cell Endocrinol. 2000;169:15-9.
88. Quintans LN, Castro GD, Castro JA. Oxidation of ethanol to acetaldehyde and free radicals by rat testicular microsomes. Arch Toxicol. 2005;79:25-30.
89. Bouamama N, Briot P, Testart J. Comparison of two methods of cryoconservation of sperm when in very small numbers. Gynecol Obstet Fertil. 2003;31:132-5.
90. Chmura SJ, Nodzenski E, Kharbanda S, et al. Down-regulation of ceramide production abrogates ionizing radiation-induced cytochrome c release and apoptosis. Mol Pharmacol. 2000;57:792-6.
91. Sereni E, Bonu MA, Fava L, et al. Freezing spermatozoa obtained by testicular fine needle aspiration: a new technique. Reprod Biomed Online. 2008;16:89-95.
92. Gvakharia M, Adamson GD. A method of successful cryopreservation of small numbers of human spermatozoa. Fertil Steril. 2001;76:S101.
93. Sohn JO, Jun SH, Park LS, et al. Comparison of recovery and viability of sperm in ICSI pipette after ultra rapid freezing or slow freezing. Fertil Steril. 2003; 80(3): 128.
94. Herrler A, Eisner S, Bach V, et al. Cryopreservation of spermatozoa in alginic acid capsules. Fertil Steril. 2006;85:208-13.
95. Nawroth F, Isachenko V, Dessole S, et al. Vitrification of human spermatozoa without cryoprotectants. Cryo Letters. 2002;23:93-102.
96. Schuster TG, Keller LM, Dunn RL, et al. Ultra-rapid freezing of very low numbers of sperm using cryoloops. Hum Reprod. 2003;18:788-95.
97. Lane M, Bavister BD, Lyons EA, Forest KT. Containerless vitrification of mammalian oocytes and embryos. Nat Biotechnol. 1999;17:1234-6.
98. Desai NN, Blackmon H, Goldfarb J. Single sperm cryopreservation on cryoloops: an alternative to hamster zona for freezing individual spermatozoa. Reprod Biomed Online. 2004;9:47-53.
99. Isaev DA, Zaletov SY, Zaeva VV, et al. Artificial microcontainers for cryopreservation of solitary spermatozoa. Hum Reprod. 2007;22:i154.
100. Yogev L, Kleiman SE, Shabtai E, et al. Long-term cryostorage of sperm in a human sperm bank does not damage progressive motility concentration. Hum Reprod. 2010;25:1097-103.
101. Horne G, Atkinson AD, Pease EH, et al. Live birth with sperm cryopreserved for 21 years prior to cancer treatment: case report. Hum Reprod. 2004;19:1448-9.
102. Feldschuh J, Brassel J, Durso N, Levine A. Successful sperm storage for 28 years. Fertil Steril. 2005;84:1017.
103. Bielanski A, Lalonde A. Effect of cryopreservation by slow cooling and vitrification on viral contamination of IVF embryos experimentally exposed to bovine viral diarrhea virus and bovine herpesvirus-1. Theriogenology. 2009;72:919-25.
104. Lim JJ, Shin TE, Song SH, et al. Effect of liquid nitrogen vapor storage on the motility, viability, morphology, deoxyribonucleic acid integrity, and mitochondrial potential of frozen-thawed human spermatozoa. Fertil Steril. 2010;94:2736-41.
105. Punyatanasakchai P, Sophonsritsuk A, Weerakiet S, et al. Comparison of cryopreserved human sperm in vapor and liquid phases of liquid nitrogen: effect on motility parameters, morphology, and sperm function. Fertil Steril. 2008;90:1978-82.
106. Grout BW, Morris GJ. Contaminated liquid nitrogen vapour as a risk factor in pathogen transfer. Theriogenology. 2009;71:1079-82.

17

Strategies for Fertility Preservation in the Male Cancer Patient

Wayland Hsiao, Peter N Schlegel

CHAPTER OUTLINE

INTRODUCTION

As advances in cancer treatment have led to significantly better cancer survival, there is an increasing recognition that quality of life issues such as paternity are increasingly more important to cancer survivors. While advances in assisted reproductive techniques have greatly increased options for men rendered azoospermic after systemic treatment for cancer, it is our opinion that sperm cryopreservation prior to treatment is the preferred management for preservation of fertility in men planning treatment that may affect future fertility. While cryopreservation of an ejaculated specimen is the most straight-forward way to preserve fertility in a cancer patient, in this chapter we will go on to discuss treatment options available to cancer patients who are found to be azoospermic at the time of cancer diagnosis as well treatment options for those patients who are found to be persistently azoospermic after systemic therapy.

With advances in in vitro fertilization (IVF) and specifically intracytoplasmic sperm injection (ICSI), paternity is now possible for men using exceedingly small numbers of testicular sperm. Post-treatment azoospermic men who previously only faced the options of donor sperm, cryopreserved sperm, or adoption now have the option of surgical sperm retrieval coupled with IVF-ICSI. This chapter will deal with the treatment options available to the cancer patient who remains persistently azoospermic after systemic therapy (whether due to chemotherapy, radiation or surgery).

The challenges for the azoospermic cancer patient are unique, however, because the urgency of getting the necessary chemotherapy must be balanced with the need to undergo procedures to successfully preserve sperm. Any fertility treatment offered must be of minimal morbidity, while not significantly delaying the needed chemotherapeutic treatment.

CRYOPRESERVATION OF EJACULATED SPERM

Men with normal or even low sperm counts in their ejaculate can relatively easily present an ejaculated sample for cryopreservation; and cryopreservation of ejaculated sperm remains the cornerstone of fertility preservation in a man with cancer.

Previously cryopreserved sperm greatly simplifies the algorithm for the post-chemotherapeutic azoospermic man, such that the couple can go directly to IVF. While in the past, there were rather strict criterion for cryopreservation of spermatozoa for subsequent use in assisted reproduction, the widespread application of ICSI has made it possible to cryopreserve even severely oligospermic samples that still result in pregnancy and live birth. In 1992, Sanger et al. reviewed the literature and a survey of nine semen banks and identified 115 live births from the use of cryopreserved sperm from cancer survivors.[1] In addition, Agarwal reported his success with the use of cryopreserved sperm in 29 men wi th a variety of malignancies.[2] Underlying the importance of cryopreservation prior to therapy is a study by Schmidt et al.[3] While examining a population of patients reporting to a Danish fertility clinic for testis cancer, lymphoma and leukemia, Schmidt et al. noted that 57% of their population was azoospermic after systemic treatment. Of the 35 live births in their series, 22 of them were due to the use of cryopreserved sperm. Thus, the use of cryopreserved sperm is both viable and successful and cryopreservation should be offered to all patients prior to systemic chemotherapy or radiation treatment.

The use of ICSI with cryopreserved sperm in cancer survivors has also significantly increased the fertilization and delivery rates. Hurvitz reported on 118 couples undergoing 169 IVF-ICSI cycles at Weill Cornell. From 1994 to 2005, using cryopreserved sperm and ICSI, there was a fertilization rate (per injected egg) of 77.6%, a clinical pregnancy rate (defined as heartbeat seen on transvaginal ultrasound 32 days after embryo transfer) of 57% (96/169) and a 50% delivery rate (85/169).[4] As a historical control, a similar population was evaluated from 1992 to 1994 at the same institution prior to the routine use of ICSI. Using conventional IVF, the fertilization rate was 32% and the delivery rate was 24% (13/54).[4]

While cryopreservation at present is the only proven method to preserve fertility in the pre-treatment setting, it should be noted that cryopreservation is not without its limitations. Cryopreservation can result in significant loss of sperm viability and motility,[5] though the advent of ICSI has made the number of sperm needed for treatment much lower. In addition, it is controversial as to how long sperm are able to be effectively cryopreserved. In a large study by Yogev et al., cryopreservation of spermatozoa in liquid nitrogen did not seem to affect the concentration of post-thaw motile sperm for storage periods of up to 14 years[6] Tel Aviv Sourasky Medical Center, 6 Weizman Street, However, the success of these long-term stored spermatozoa in assisted reproduction remains to be seen.

Another limitation of cryopreservation is the low percentage of patients who cryopreserved spermatozoa who actually use the sample. In a large study of 629 cancer patients who were referred for semen cryopreservation, 557 men eventually cryopreserved sperm. Of these men, only 7.5% used their banked semen with a mean follow up of seven years.[7] This statistic agrees with other reports from sperm banking facilities that less than 20% of men who store sperm before cancer treatment end up using it to try to conceive.[2,8-10] Of course, this number could be artificially low because of death due to cancer, a long delay between medical therapy for cancer and attempts at childbearing, recovery of sperm production in some men, or limited access to assisted reproductive treatments.

AZOOSPERMIA AT PRESENTATION

However, cancer patients may be azoospermic at the time of their diagnosis for a number of reasons. One possibility is that malignancy itself may disrupt fertility even prior to the initiation of anti-neoplastic treatment. Suboptimal semen analysis parameters have been seen even before systemic treatment in patients with leukemia, lymphoma and testicular cancer.[11-16] In fact, up to 13.8% of all patients who attempt to bank sperm prior to cancer treatment are azoospermic.[10,17] It remains controversial, however, whether the type of malignancy predicts lower sperm quality or affects assisted reproduction outcomes.[15,17-19] Even if the cancer does not involve the reproductive tract itself (testis, seminal vesicles, prostate, or urethra), cancer may affect the reproductive tract, though the mechanism of this remains unknown.

In the pre-ICSI era, successful IVF required millions of motile sperm capable of the acrosome reaction. In that era, the use of surgically retrieved sperm was limited. With the advent of ICSI,[20] exceedingly low numbers of surgically retrieved sperm (even non-motile testicular sperm) could be used for successful assisted reproduction. Therefore, in the modern era of widespread application of ICSI, the ability to preserve fertility has been expanded even to those men who lack sperm in their ejaculate. With surgically retrieved sperm, we are able to preserve fertility potential as long as we are able to find sperm in the reproductive tract. For azoospermic patients, fertility preservation options include: cryopreservation of testicular spermatozoa from normal testis, cryopreservation of spermatozoa from the diseased testis (in cases of testicular cancer), or cryopreservation of epididymal or vasal sperm. We will now discuss the various methods available to retrieve sperm for cryopreservation as well as the available data.

PERCUTANEOUS TESTICULAR AND EPIDIDYMAL ASPIRATION

Patients who have normal levels of sperm production and who are either azoospermic (obstructive azoospermia) or anejaculate are potential candidates for percutaneous testicular or epididymal aspiration under local anesthesia. Percutaneous techniques for sperm retrieval include fine needle aspiration of the testis, percutaneous epididymal aspiration of sperm and percutaneous biopsy of the testis. A local skin block combined with a spermatic cord nerve block usually provides adequate anesthesia. We believe, these procedures should not be performed on patients with non-obstructive azoospermia, because of the potentially low yield of sperm due to poor sperm production. Cancer patients with a history of vasectomy, those with inguinopelvic surgery and those with congenital absence of the vas deferens would be good candidates for percutaneous procedures. Also, any patients who have malignancies which would preclude masturbation or electroejaculation may be good candidates for these procedures, assuming adequate levels of sperm production.

Fine needle aspiration of the testis is the easiest of these procedures to perform, but yields much lower numbers of sperm when compared to open surgical retrieval.[21] After local anesthesia is given, the testis is stabilized and a needle is inserted into the testis along the long axis of the testis. The needle is withdrawn slightly and redirected in order to disrupt the testicular architecture while aspiration is performed. This procedure can be repeated to increase the yield of testicular tissue.

Percutaneous aspiration of the epididymis can also be performed under local anesthesia. For this procedure, we use a 21 gauge butterfly needle attached to a 20 mL syringe. The needle is inserted into the caput epididymis and then slowly withdrawn until fluid can be seen in the tubing. The tubing is then clamped and the fluid flushed with medium. Difficulties in the procedure include being able to palpate and stabilize the epididymis effectively, failure to retrieve sperm and the admixture of degenerating sperm with better quality sperm samples.

The final percutaneous procedure is biopsy of the testicle using a 15-gauge biopsy gun with a short (1 cm) excursion. We usually start by making a small nick in the scrotal skin overlying the trapped testis or use a larger bore needle to make a small hole in the scrotal skin. The biopsy gun is then advanced along that same tract right up to the tunica albugina of the testis and the biopsy gun is fired. Multiple biopsies can be obtained through a single entry site. It is best to avoid performing the biopsy along the midline longitudinal plane and we angle our biopsies, because of the large longitudinal vessel that is commonly on the midline of the anterior testis. This procedure can provide higher sperm yield than needle aspiration, but it provides fewer sperm with lower motility than microsurgical epididymal sperm aspiration.[22]

SURGICAL RETRIEVAL OF VASAL OR EPIDIDYMAL SPERM

Patients with epididymal obstruction, but with normal sperm production, are candidates for surgical retrieval of epididymal sperm. Our preferred approach is the microscopic technique by which the epididymis is exposed and punctured with a pulled glass pipet and epididymal fluid is aspirated. Using the microscopic approach, millions of sperm can be retrieved and cryopreserved. While theoretically sperm can also be aspirated and preserved from the vas deferens by performing a hemivasotomy, aspiration of the epididymis is our preferred approach because any vasal obstruction would also cause epididymal dilation and sperm quality (motility) is generally better closer to the testis in obstructed patients. Baniel reported on three testicular cancer patients in whom vasal and epididymal sperm were successfully aspirated from the cancer bearing testis and cryopreserved at the time of orchiectomy.[23] In this small series, two pregnancies were achieved using cryopreserved sperm.

SURGICAL RETRIEVAL OF TESTICULAR SPERM

In those patients who have primary testicular failure (non-obstructive azoospermia), surgical retrieval of testicular sperm coupled with IVF-ICSI may represent the only hope of fertility preservation. The traditional approach to testicular sperm extraction involved a random testicular biopsy followed by evaluation for sperm in the andrology lab. The risk of testicular injury along with low spermatozoa yields in conventional testicular sperm extraction (TESE) led to the development of microsurgical TESE (mTESE). The technique involves placing a wide incision in the tunica albuginea in an avascular region and eversion of the testicular parenchyma allowing for microscopic inspection of the testicular parenchyma and identification of sperm producing tubules (**Figure 1**). Under high power (25X) magnification, tubules with spermatozoa appear larger and more opaque than the fibrotic Sertoli cell-only tubules (**Figure 2**). Subtunical vessels as well as intratesticular vessels can also be identified and better preserved using the operating microscope. Overall, mTESE has been shown to result in an increased chance of retrieving sperm, a higher number of sperm harvested and a decrease in testicular tissue removed.[24,25]

SPECIAL CONSIDERATIONS IN TESTICULAR CANCER PATIENTS

Testicular cancer patients face unique challenges in fertility preservation because at least one testis will typically be removed during cancer treatment. There remains, however, a variety of options available to these patients. Sperm retrieval is possible at the time of orchiectomy from either the contralateral normal testis or the normal parenchyma of the affected testis (such retrieval is done on a sterile "backtable" after extirpation of the testis from the patient to avoid spillage and contamination). Vasal or epididymal sperm can also be retrieved from the orchiectomy specimen. In cases of partial orchiectomy, the surrounding normal testicular parenchyma can be examined and specimens collected for cryopreservation as well.

A number of case reports have shown that testicular sperm from the testicle harboring testis cancer can result in successful live birth,[26-28] but more research with larger numbers of patients is needed before this becomes routine practice. Sperm can also be retrieved from the epididymis or vas deferens in testicular orchiectomy specimens. In a fascinating study, Delouya et al. reviewed pathologic specimens of 39 radical orchiectomy specimens with an emphasis on the extent of spermatogenesis present in the normal surrounding parenchyma. In this study, 50% of evaluable epididymal sections contained sperm. When the testicular parenchyma was examined, 40% of the specimens had full spermatogenesis as the dominant histological pattern, and nearly 80% of the testes revealed evidence of focally complete spermatogenesis.[29] This study suggests that in up to 50% of orchiectomy specimens, epididymal or vasal sperm can be successfully retrieved and cryopreserved.

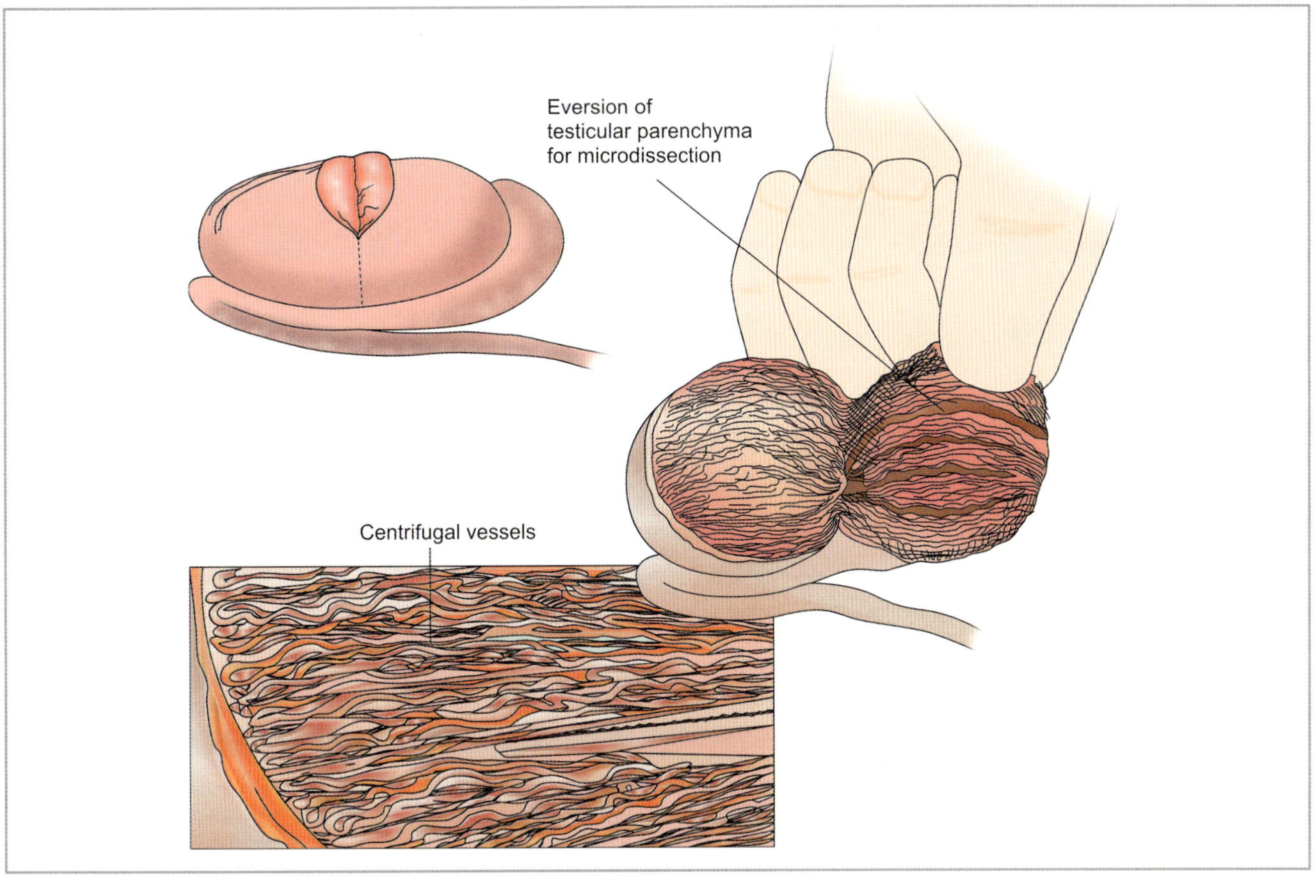

FIGURE 1 mTESE involves a incision along the equator of the testis. The parenchyma is everted for inspection under the operating microscope.

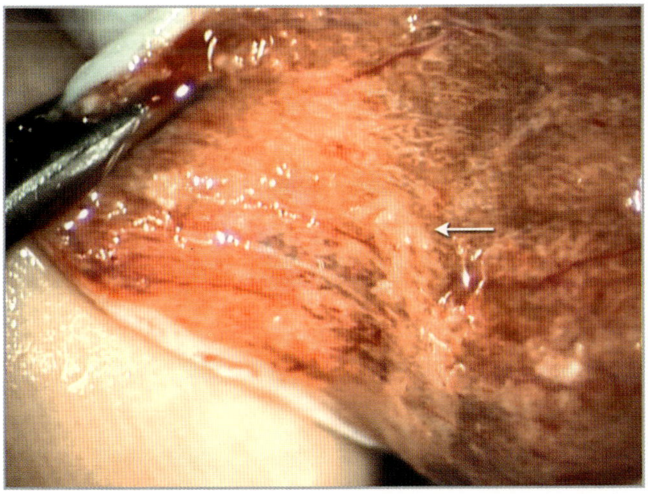

FIGURE 2 Picture of intraoperative view. The arrow points to a tubule that is larger in diameter and more likely to harbor spermatogenesis.

For those patients whose production is so low that there is no sperm in the epididymis, sperm should be found in about 40% of patients with random biopsy. Theoretically, however, sperm can be found in up to 80% of specimens with a testicular microdissection approach in a sterile field after removal of the radical orchiectomy specimen from the patient. Interestingly, these numbers agree with data generated by Schrader et al. in one of the largest studies of preoperative sperm retrieval outcomes. Schrader reported on 31 azoospermic men with either testicular cancer or lymphoma prior to chemotherapy. In testicular cancer patients, standard testicular sperm extraction was performed on the contralateral testicle. Lymphoma patients underwent bilateral standard testicular sperm extraction prior to chemotherapy. The sperm retrieval rate was 43% (6/14) in testicular cancer and 47% (8/17) in patients with Hodgkin's or non-Hodgkin's lymphoma.[30]

Routine testicular sperm extraction after orchiectomy, though, is not without its disadvantages. As Delouya et al. wisely noted, the violation of the tunica albuginea for testis dissection for sperm retrieval may affect pathologic staging. Therefore, cryopreservation of vasal or epididymal sperm on a backtable may be the preferred first-line approach in this setting because of higher sperm yields, the provision of sperm which are more likely to survive cryopreservation and better preservation of pathologic staging.

PERSISTENT AZOOSPERMIA AFTER SYSTEMIC TREATMENT

For the persistently azoospermic man after chemotherapy, there needs to be an evaluation of both the ejaculatory status as well as levels of spermatogenesis. Patients with good sperm production who have ejaculatory dysfunction may benefit from electroejaculation, while those men with spermatogenic compromise will most likely benefit from testicular sperm extraction. If a patient is unable or unwilling to successfully pursue any of the previous options, the use of donor sperm remains an alternative approach to fatherhood.

RETRIEVAL OF SPERM IN ANEJACULATE PATIENT

Any retroperitoneal surgery, such as retroperitoneal lymphadenectomy, could affect the sympathetic chain or structurally compromise the bladder neck and thus, affecting antegrade ejaculation. Partial ejaculatory function may be preserved depending on the degree of nerve sparing. The preservation of ejaculatory function obviously has a tremendous impact on fertility rates. In Norwegian testicular cancer survivors who had chemotherapy, those with intact antegrade ejaculation had an 83% paternity rate, while rates for paternity were only 10% in the anejaculate group.[31] Patients who present with "anejaculation" (defined as a failure of ejaculation of semen from the urinary meatus during orgasm) may have retrograde ejaculation (in which all of the seminal fluid flows retrograde into the bladder) or failure of emission (in which there is lack of any seminal fluid during orgasm).

For patients with retrograde ejaculation, the first line treatment is largely medical with the use of sympathomimetic drugs. Ephedrine sulfate, imipramine hydrochloride, midodin hydrochloride and pseudoephedrine hydrochloride have been successfully used in the treatment of retrograde ejaculation. If attempts at medical conversion to antegrade ejaculation are unsuccessful, sperm may be obtained by bladder sperm harvesting. The night before and the morning of scheduled harvest, patients should alkalinize their urine with 5–10 cc of poly-citra since acidity is toxic to sperm. The patient should also stay well hydrated the day before and the day of harvest. On the day of harvest, the patient is instructed to void and then masturbate. After orgasm, the patient should void into a collection cup and this sample will contain sperm.

For patients with failure of emission, one treatment option is to undergo electroejaculation. This is a procedure generally performed under general anesthesia in the sensate patient. We do not routinely catheterize the patient prior to electroejaculation. The patient is placed in the lateral decubitus position. Anoscopy is performed to confirm that the rectum is empty and no rectal mucosal abnormalities are present. The rectal probe is inserted completely into the rectum with the electrodes oriented anteriorly over the prostate and seminal vesicles. Stimulation is carried out with a standard electrical stimulation system.

The pattern of electrical stimulation tends to work best by gradually increasing voltage "peaked" sine wave stimulation that is abruptly ceased, with at least 5–7 second delays between stimulations. Maximum stimulation at the peak of the sine wave is increased by one volt for each stimulation, with a baseline of 0 volts (no electrical stimulation). Penile tumescence and rectal temperature are observed. Typically, penile tumescence is noted first, followed by seminal emission. When seminal emission ceases, rectal temperature of 38°C is observed, or a maximum of 30 volts is attained, electrostimulation is stopped. Anoscopy is performed again to ensure that there is no rectal mucosal injury, which is a potential complication of this procedure. The patient is turned supine and urethral catheterization is performed. An initial retrograde specimen is diluted in human tubal fluid (HTF) buffered with HEPES and plasmanate, pH 7.4 and sent for immediate processing, as is the antegrade ejaculate. The bladder is then irrigated with HTF and this second retrograde specimen is sent for immediate processing as well.

Ohl et al. performed electroejaculation in 24 testicular cancer patients (23 of whom had undergone retroperitoneal lymphadenectomy) and observed seminal emission in all 24 patients. Greater than 10 million motile and progressive sperm were obtained in 88% (21/24) of patients. Seventeen couples underwent intrauterine insemination and the overall cycle fecundity rate was 9% per IUI attempt.[32] Seven clinical pregnancies were established and there were 5 live births. Electroejaculation has also been successfully combined with IVF (and obtained a 53% fertilization rate per inseminated oocyte[33]) as well as IVF/ICSI (with a 75.5% fertilization rate per injected oocyte[34]). Rosenlund (1998) looked at 17 couples treated for testicular cancer where most patients (14/17) received chemotherapy and acquired sperm through electroejaculation. Rosenlund employed both IVF and ICSI and had a fertilization rate of 55–57% in both groups. The ongoing pregnancy rate for the whole cohort was 57% per cycle.[35] Finally, at Weill Cornell, we reported a clinical pregnancy rate of 56% per retrieval and an implantation rate of 33% per embryo transferred.[34] Taken together, these studies demonstrate that treated testicular cancer patients can successfully undergo assisted reproductive technology (ART) with electroejaculated spermatozoa.

SPERM RETRIEVAL IN THE AZOOSPERMIC PATIENT AFTER CHEMOTHERAPY

For men who are azoospermic after chemotherapy, spontaneous recovery may occur in at least a subset of patients within 2–8 years. For men treated with alkylating agents, the duration of azoospermia may be longer, so a period of observation prior to attempted testicular sperm extraction is recommended. For men treated with platinum-based regimens, most men who will have sperm return to the ejaculate will have sperm detected within two years. However, the persistently azoospermic patient with good ejaculatory function most likely has impaired spermatogenesis due to the patient's chemotherapeutic regimen, the use of radiation, the extent of surgery, the disease itself, the baseline function of the patient, or any combination of the aforementioned factors.

Percutaneous aspirations or biopsies, while possible, are more likely to yield low numbers of sperm and require multiple treatments for patients with non-obstructive azoospermia. In our view, the low yield, uncertainty of sperm retrieval and intratesticular bleeding and scarring make these procedures less favorable, especially in this patient population with multiple insults to spermatogenesis. The risk of testicular injury along with low spermatozoa yields led to the development of mTESE.[24] Our data and that of others suggest that mTESE yields the highest sperm retrieval rate in this population.[36-38]

Evaluation prior to mTESE includes a thorough history (including sexual history), chemotherapy history, physical exam and hormonal profile. On physical exam, attention is paid to the fullness of the epididymis as well as testicular volumes. In our practice, we prefer to perform mTESE in conjunction with a programmed IVF cycle to optimize the use of freshly retrieved viable sperm. The mTESE procedure involves placing a wide incision in the tunica albuginea in an avascular region to allow subsequent eversion of the testicular parenchyma for microdissection. Using high power magnification through an operating microscope (25X), subtunical vessels as well as intratesticular vessels can be identified and preserved. Microscopic dissection and direct examination of seminiferous tubules allow identification of the rare regions that contain sperm in men with non obstructive azospermia (NOA). The tubules harboring spermatozoa are usually wider and more opaque than the fibrotic Sertoli cell-only tubules. Overall, mTESE has been shown to result in an increased chance of retrieving sperm, higher number of sperm harvested and decreased testicular tissue removed.[24,25]

The only predictor of successful treatment is the most advanced stage seen on biopsy.[39] Testicular volume, serum FSH levels and etiology of NOA appear to have little to no effect on the chance of sperm retrieval.[39-41] Postoperative ultrasound has demonstrated fewer acute and chronic changes after microdissection as compared to conventional TESE.[42] The clinically significant risk of damage to testicular androgen production is 5-10%, depending on the number of prior interventions and the baseline level of serum testosterone.

At Weill Cornell Medical College, we have performed 84 mTESE in 73 post-chemotherapy patients. These patients presented with a history of prior treatment for malignancies with the most common being Hodgkin's lymphoma, leukemia, testicular cancer and non-Hodgkin's lymphoma. The mean number of years since chemotherapy was 18.6 years. Sperm were found in 37% of patients and in 42.9% of mTESE attempts. Fertilization rate per injected oocyte during IVF was 57%. Clinical pregnancy rate was 50%. The live birth rate was 42% with ten singleton deliveries and five twin deliveries. The sperm retrieval rate was highest in patients with a history of testicular cancer at 85%, while patients with lymphoma had a sperm retrieval rate of 33%.Patients with sarcoma had the lowest sperm retrieval rate at 14%.[43]

Other groups have had similar results using testicular sperm. Damani et al. reported on 23 patients who underwent chemotherapy, mostly for testicular cancer. The patients underwent either conventional testicular sperm extraction or fine needle aspiration mapping and subsequent TESE. Sperm was successfully extracted in 65% (15/23) and a total of 26 cycles of ICSI were performed. The mean fertilization rate was 65%, with a delivery/ongoing pregnancy rate of 20.8% in 11 couples.[44] In another study, a multibiopsy approach TESE was undertaken in 12 post-chemotherapy men and sperm was successfully retrieved in 29.4% (5/17) of attempts. Eight ICSI cycles were performed with a fertilization rate per injected oocyte of 68%. There was one live birth from seven embryo transfers.[45] All this would seem to indicate that testicular sperm extraction is an effective form of fertility "salvage" after chemotherapy for men with non-obstructive azoospermia due to oncologic or treatment related causes.

SPERM RETRIEVAL IN THE AZOOSPERMIC PATIENT AFTER RADIATION THERAPY

Radiation therapy is widely used for a number of malignancies, including but not limited to, hematologic cancer, testis cancers (with retroperitoneal exposure fields), prostate cancer, bladder cancer and rectal cancer. Both treatment fields and scatter radiation can reach the testis, though levels are lower with scatter radiation. The testes are exquisitely radiosensitive and changes in sperm production can be affected by even very low doses of radiation, with permanent damage to spermatogenesis caused by doses over 2 gray.[46] In testis cancer patients, there seems to be a higher risk of infertility in those patients who received radiation therapy to the retroperitoneum (for seminoma) when compared to those who were treated with only chemotherapy (for non-seminomatous tumors).[47]

There is scant literature regarding outcomes of infertility treatments specifically due to radiation induced azoospermia. Most studies combine patients with chemotherapy with patients with radiation therapy and do not give specific success rates for radiation patients.[3] In our practice, radiation to any other site, including the abdomen and mediastinum, does not preclude attempts at sperm retrieval with mTESE and we have been able to successfully retrieve sperm in these patients. However, in the cases where the testis itself has been irradiated or in patients receiving whole body radiation for bone marrow transplants, to date we have been unable to find sperm, even with mTESE.

USE OF SPERMATOZOA FROM MEN WHO HAVE RECEIVED CHEMOTHERAPY OR RADIATION

Men who have received chemotherapy and even men who had non-gonadal radiation therapy, will have increased rates of sperm aneuploidy for six months or longer after treatment.[48] An increase in sperm DNA fragmentation has also been observed after chemotherapy and sperm DNA may remain abnormal up to 24 months after chemotherapy.[49] In addition, studies have shown that when adult male rats are administered chemotherapy typical for either testicular cancer (bleomycin, etoposide and cisplatinum) or non-Hodgkin's lymphoma (cyclophosphamide, doxorubicin, vincristine and prednisone), they have lower weight, decreased spermatogenesis and smaller litter sizes.[50,51] Although, limited in number and quality, observational studies in humans have not demonstrated an increased risk of congenital or genetic anomalies in offspring of men who have received chemotherapy or non-gonadal radiation.[52-54] Taken together, the data on sperm aneuploidy after chemotherapy and radiation may suggest a cautious approach for patients who desire to have children soon after completion of gonadotoxic therapy. However, there is a need for more research on the long-term effects of chemotherapy on the quality of sperm produced, and the specific time course of chemotherapy-mediated damage caused by different chemotherapeutic regimens.

CONCLUSION

The challenges of sperm retrieval are unique in the cancer population. This cancer subpopulation faces the challenge of balancing the temporal rush to get essential chemotherapy with the need to undergo sperm preservation procedures. A number of treatment options are open for the post-treatment male seeking fertility treatment. A summary of selected studies is presented in **Table 1**. For those anejaculatory males, electroejaculation represents a viable and effective treatment, especially when coupled with IVF-ICSI. For the post-chemotherapeutic man who remains persistently azoospermic, mTESE, coupled with ICSI, is also an effective treatment option.

TABLE 1 Selected articles reporting reproductive outcomes for anejculatory and azoospermic men after cancer treatment

	Sperm retrieval technique	*Patient population*	*Patient number*	*Sperm retrieval*	*ART and birth outcomes*
Hsiao et al.[43]	Microdissection TESE	Testicular cancer, Lymphomas, Leukemia, others	73	37% per patient 43% overall	Fertilization 57% Clinical pregnancy 50%; Live birth 42%
Damani et al.[44]	TESE	Testicular cancer, Lymphoma others	23	65% per patient	Fertilization rate 65% Ongoing/Delivered Pregnancies 31%
Chan et al.[55]	TESE, microdissection TESE	Testicular cancer, Lymphoma, Leukemia, others	17	45% sperm retrieval	Biochemical Pregnancy 45%, Live birth 33%
Rosenlund et al.[35]	EEJ, 1 TESE	Testicular cancer	15		Fertilization 57%, Pregnancy 57%, per cycle Live birth 11/15
Chung et al.[34]	EEJ	Testicular cancer, spinal cord injury, psychogenic anejaculation	13		ICSI Fertilization 76%, Clinical pregnancy 55.6%, Implantation rate 33%
Hultling et al.[33]	EEJ	Testicular cancer	10	90%	Fertilization rate 54% Pregnancy 5/6 Live birth 4/6
Ohl et al.[32]	EEJ	Testis cancer	24	21/24 patients	Using IUI Pregnancy in 36.9% of couples

REFERENCES

1. Sanger WG, Olson JH, Sherman JK. Semen cryobanking for men with cancer--criteria change. Fertil Steril. 1992 Nov;58(5):1024-7.
2. Agarwal A, Ranganathan P, Kattal N, et al. Fertility after cancer: a prospective review of assisted reproductive outcome with banked semen specimens. Fertil Steril. 2004 Feb;81(2):342-8.
3. Schmidt KL, Larsen E, Bangsboll S, et al. Assisted reproduction in male cancer survivors: fertility treatment and outcome in 67 couples. Hum Reprod. 2004 Dec;19(12):2806-10.
4. Hourvitz A, Goldschlag DE, Davis OK, et al. Intracytoplasmic sperm injection (ICSI) using cryopreserved sperm from men with malignant neoplasm yields high pregnancy rates. Fertil Steril. 2008 Sep;90(3):557-63.
5. McLaughlin EA, Ford WC, Hull MG. Motility characteristics and membrane integrity of cryopreserved human spermatozoa. J Reprod Fertil. 1992 Jul;95(2):527-34.
6. Yogev L, Kleiman SE, Shabtai E, et al. Long-term cryostorage of sperm in a human sperm bank does not damage progressive motility concentration. Hum Reprod. May; 25(5):1097-103.
7. van Casteren NJ, van Santbrink EJ, van Inzen W, et al. Use rate and assisted reproduction technologies outcome of cryopreserved semen from 629 cancer patients. Fertil Steril. 2008 Dec;90(6):2245-50.
8. Kelleher S, Wishart SM, Liu PY, et al. Long-term outcomes of elective human sperm cryostorage. Hum Reprod. 2001 Dec;16(12):2632-9.
9. Blackhall FH, Atkinson AD, Maaya MB, et al. Semen cryopreservation, utilisation and reproductive outcome in men treated for Hodgkin's disease. Br J Cancer. 2002 Aug 12;87(4):381-4.
10. Ragni G, Somigliana E, Restelli L, et al. Sperm banking and rate of assisted reproduction treatment: insights from a 15-year cryopreservation program for male cancer patients. Cancer. 2003 Apr 1;97(7):1624-9.

11. Spermon JR, Ramos L, Wetzels AM, et al. Sperm integrity pre- and post-chemotherapy in men with testicular germ cell cancer. Hum Reprod. 2006 Jul;21(7):1781-6.
12. Berthelsen JG, Skakkebaek NE. Gonadal function in men with testis cancer. Fertil Steril. 1983 Jan;39(1):68-75.
13. Sanger WG, Armitage JO, Schmidt MA. Feasibility of semen cryopreservation in patients with malignant disease. JAMA. 1980 Aug 22-29;244(8):789-90.
14. Viviani S, Ragni G, Santoro A, et al. Testicular dysfunction in Hodgkin's disease before and after treatment. Eur J Cancer. 1991;27(11):1389-92.
15. Williams DH, Karpman E, Sander JC, et al. Pretreatment semen parameters in men with cancer. J Urol. 2009 Feb;181(2):736-40.
16. van Casteren NJ, Boellaard WP, Romijn JC, Dohle GR. Gonadal dysfunction in male cancer patients before cytotoxic treatment. Int J Androl. Feb;33(1):73-9.
17. Lass A, Akagbosu F, Abusheikha N, et al. A programme of semen cryopreservation for patients with malignant disease in a tertiary infertility centre: lessons from 8 years' experience. Hum Reprod. 1998 Nov;13(11):3256-61.
18. Khalifa E, Oehninger S, Acosta AA, et al. Successful fertilization and pregnancy outcome in in-vitro fertilization using cryopreserved/ thawed spermatozoa from patients with malignant diseases. Hum Reprod. 1992 Jan;7(1):105-8.
19. Padron OF, Sharma RK, Thomas AJ Jr, Agarwal A. Effects of cancer on spermatozoa quality after cryopreservation: a 12-year experience. Fertil Steril. 1997 Feb;67(2):326-31.
20. Palermo G, Joris H, Devroey P, Van Steirteghem AC. Pregnancies after intracytoplasmic injection of single spermatozoon into an oocyte. Lancet. 1992 Jul 4;340(8810):17-8.
21. Friedler S, Raziel A, Strassburger D, et al. Testicular sperm retrieval by percutaneous fine needle sperm aspiration compared with testicular sperm extraction by open biopsy in men with non-obstructive azoospermia. Human Reprod. 1997 Jul;12(7):1488-93.
22. Sheynkin YR, Ye Z, Menendez S, et al. Controlled comparison of percutaneous and microsurgical sperm retrieval in men with obstructive azoospermia. Human Reprod. 1998 Nov;13(11):3086-9.
23. Baniel J, Sella A. Sperm extraction at orchiectomy for testis cancer. Fertil Steril. 2001 Feb;75(2):260-2.
24. Schlegel PN. Testicular sperm extraction: microdissection improves sperm yield with minimal tissue excision. Human Reprod. 1999 Jan;14(1):131-5.
25. Tsujimura A, Matsumiya K, Miyagawa Y, et al. Conventional multiple or microdissection testicular sperm extraction: a comparative study. Human Reprod. 2002 Nov;17(11):2924-9.
26. Carmignani L, Gadda F, Gazzano G, et al. Testicular sperm extraction in cancerous testicle in patients with azoospermia: a case report. Hum Reprod. 2007 Apr;22(4):1068-72.
27. Descombe L, Chauleur C, Gentil-Perret A, et al. Testicular sperm extraction in a single cancerous testicle in patients with azoospermia: a case report. Fertil Steril. 2008 Aug;90(2):443 e1-4.
28. Kohn FM, Schroeder-Printzen I, Weidner W, et al. Testicular sperm extraction in a patient with metachronous bilateral testicular cancer. Hum Reprod. 2001 Nov;16(11):2343-6.
29. Delouya G, Baazeem A, Boman JM, et al. Identification of spermatozoa in archived testicular cancer specimens: implications for bench side sperm retrieval at orchiectomy. Urology. Jun;75(6):1436-40.
30. Schrader M, Muller M, Sofikitis N, et al. "Onco-tese": testicular sperm extraction in azoospermic cancer patients before chemotherapy-new guidelines? Urology. 2003 Feb;61(2):421-5.
31. Brydoy M, Fossa SD, Klepp O, et al. Paternity following treatment for testicular cancer. J Natl Cancer Inst. 2005 Nov 2;97(21):1580-8.
32. Ohl DA, Denil J, Bennett CJ, et al. Electroejaculation following retroperitoneal lymphadenectomy. J Urol. 1991 May;145(5):980-3.
33. Hultling C, Rosenlund B, Tornblom M, et al. Transrectal electroejaculation in combination with in-vitro fertilization: an effective treatment of anejaculatory infertility after testicular cancer. Hum Reprod. 1995 Apr;10(4):847-50.
34. Chung PH, Palermo G, Schlegel PN, et al. The use of intracytoplasmic sperm injection with electroejaculates from anejaculatory men. Hum Reprod. 1998 Jul;13(7):1854-8.
35. Rosenlund B, Sjoblom P, Tornblom M, et al. In-vitro fertilization and intracytoplasmic sperm injection in the treatment of infertility after testicular cancer. Hum Reprod. 1998 Feb;13(2):414-8.
36. Ghalayini IF, Al-Ghazo MA, Hani OB, et al. Clinical comparison of conventional testicular sperm extraction and microdissection techniques for non-obstructive azoospermia. J Clin Med Res. 2011 May 19;3(3):124-31.
37. Okada H, Dobashi M, Yamazaki T, et al. Conventional versus microdissection testicular sperm extraction for nonobstructive azoospermia. J Urol [Comparative Study]. 2002 Sep;168(3):1063-7.
38. Schlegel PN. Testicular sperm extraction: microdissection improves sperm yield with minimal tissue excision. Human Reprod. 1999 Jan;14(1):131-5.
39. Su LM, Palermo GD, Goldstein M, et al. Testicular sperm extraction with intracytoplasmic sperm injection for nonobstructive azoospermia: testicular histology can predict success of sperm retrieval. J Urol. 1999 Jan;161(1):112-6.
40. Ramasamy R, Lin K, Gosden LV, et al. High serum FSH levels in men with nonobstructive azoospermia does not affect success of microdissection testicular sperm extraction. Fertil Steril. 2009 Aug;92(2):590-3.
41. Ramasamy R, Schlegel PN. Microdissection testicular sperm extraction: effect of prior biopsy on success of sperm retrieval. J Urol. 2007 Apr;177(4):1447-9.
42. Ramasamy R, Yagan N, Schlegel PN. Structural and functional changes to the testis after conventional versus microdissection testicular sperm extraction. Urol [Comparative Study]. 2005 Jun;65(6):1190-4.
43. Hsiao W, Stahl PJ, Osterberg EC, et al. Successful treatment of postchemotherapy azoospermia with microsurgical testicular sperm extraction: the weill cornell experience. J Clin Oncol Apr. 20;29(12):1607-11.
44. Damani MN, Master V, Meng MV, et al. Postchemotherapy ejaculatory azoospermia: fatherhood with sperm from testis tissue with intracytoplasmic sperm injection. J Clin Oncol. 2002 Feb 15;20(4):930-6.
45. Meseguer M, Garrido N, Remohi J, et al. Testicular sperm extraction (TESE) and ICSI in patients with permanent azoospermia after chemotherapy. Hum Reprod. 2003 Jun;18(6):1281-5.
46. Shalet SM. Effect of irradiation treatment on gonadal function in men treated for germ cell cancer. Eur Urol. 1993;23(1):148-51; discussion 52.
47. Huyghe E, Matsuda T, Daudin M, et al. Fertility after testicular cancer treatments: results of a large multicenter study. Cancer. 2004 Feb 15;100(4):732-7.
48. Burrello N, Vicari E, La Vignera S, et al. Effects of anti-neoplastic treatment on sperm aneuploidy rate in patients with testicular tumor: a longitudinal study. J Endocrinol Invest. 2011 Jun;34(6):e121-5.
49. O'Flaherty C, Hales BF, Chan P, Robaire B. Impact of chemotherapeutics and advanced testicular cancer or Hodgkin lymphoma on sperm deoxyribonucleic acid integrity. Fertil Steril. Sep;94(4):1374-9.
50. Bieber AM, Marcon L, Hales BF, Robaire B. Effects of chemotherapeutic agents for testicular cancer on the male rat reproductive system, spermatozoa, and fertility. J Androl. 2006 Mar-Apr;27(2):189-200.

51. Vaisheva F, Delbes G, Hales BF, Robaire B. Effects of the chemotherapeutic agents for non-Hodgkin lymphoma, cyclophosphamide, doxorubicin, vincristine, and prednisone (CHOP), on the male rat reproductive system and progeny outcome. J Androl. 2007 Jul-Aug;28(4):578-87.
52. Byrne J, Rasmussen SA, Steinhorn SC, et al. Genetic disease in offspring of long-term survivors of childhood and adolescent cancer. Am J Hum Genet. 1998 Jan;62(1):45-52.
53. Boice JD, Jr., Tawn EJ, Winther JF, et al. Genetic effects of radiotherapy for childhood cancer. Health Phys. 2003 Jul;85(1):65-80.
54. Winther JF, Boice JD, Jr., Mulvihill JJ, et al. Chromosomal abnormalities among offspring of childhood-cancer survivors in Denmark: a population-based study. Am J Hum Genet. 2004 Jun;74(6):1282-5.
55. Chan PT, Palermo GD, Veeck LL, et al. Testicular sperm extraction combined with intracytoplasmic sperm injection in the treatment of men with persistent azoospermia postchemotherapy. Cancer. 2001 Sep 15;92(6):1632-7.

INDEX

Page numbers followed by **f** refer to figure and *t* refer to table, respectively.